The Science of Homeopathy

by
GEORGE VITHOULKAS

With a Foreword by
WILLIAM A. TILLER

GROVE PRESS, INC. · NEW YORK

First Edition 1980
First Evergreen Edition 1980
Second Printing 1985

Library of Congress Cataloging in Publication Data

Vithoulkas, George.
  The Science of homeopathy.
  1. Homeopathy. I. Title.
RX71.V53   615'.532   79-52056
ISBN 0-394-50866-1
ISBN 0-394-17560-3 pbk.

Manufactured in the United States of America

GROVE PRESS, INC., 196 West Houston Street, New York, N.Y. 10014

Dedicated to my Teacher, C.H.

Contents

vii

Foreword

A COUPLE OF centuries ago, before science began to single-mindedly focus its attention on the purely physical aspect of Nature, homeopathy and allopathy walked hand in hand to serve the health needs of humankind. As the physical sciences became more successful, its tolerance for ideas that could not be tested by the same criteria diminished and homeopathy began to feel the pressures of second-class citizenship. Physical science became more and more quantitative and predictably powerful, and homeopathy began to fall out of favor with practicing physicians. Only a small enclave of physicians faithfully persisted in the practice of homeopathy into this century, but now the number is growing because the serious flaws of allopathic medicine are becoming apparent to us all.

One might say that it was the emphasis on disease rather than on health that split apart allopathic and homeopathic practice. The physical body reveals the obvious materialization of disease while the relationship to the more subtle aspects of man are not so easily discriminated. Conventional allopathic medicine deals directly with the chemical and structural components of the physical body. It can be classed as an objective medicine because it deals with Nature on a purely four-dimensional, space–time level and thus has had much direct laboratory evidence to support its physicochemical hypotheses. This has occurred because reliable sensing ability for both humans and instrumentation presently operates on this level.

Homeopathic medicine, on the other hand, deals indirectly with the chemistry and structure of the physical body by dealing directly with substance and energies at the next, and more subtle, level. It must be classed as a subjective medicine at this time, in part because it deals with energy that can be strongly perturbed by the mental and emotional activity of individuals and in part because there has not been any diagnostic equipment to support the homeopathic physician. That situation is expected to change in the near future.

The present transition toward an emphasis upon *health* and *wholeness* rather than upon disease has enhanced the growing awareness, perspective, and importance of a hierarchy of subtle energies and influences that determine human well-being. Along this line, I have devised a reaction equation connecting the various levels of energy in Nature that influence humankind:

$$\begin{array}{c} \text{Function} \rightleftarrows \text{Structure} \rightleftarrows \text{Chemistry} \rightleftarrows \\ \hline \text{Positive Space/Time} \rightleftarrows \text{Negative Space/Time} \rightleftarrows \text{Mind} \rightleftarrows \\ \text{Energies} \qquad\qquad \text{Energies} \\ \hline \text{Spirit} \rightleftarrows \text{Divine} \end{array}$$

This equation expresses that humankind comprise multidimensional beings living in a multidimensional universe and that a disturbance of the energy chain at any level causes ripples of effect to flow both ways along the chain. Complete homeostasis at the physical level requires homeostasis at all the underlying levels as well. If they are out of balance, then complete homeostasis cannot exist at the physical level and disease *must* eventually materialize in one form or another.

If we start at the lower right, with the Divine, this equation illustrates that we are essentially elements of Spirit, multiplexed in the Divine. That Spirit, in order to have a mechanism for experiencing, has mind imbedded within it. Mind is the builder, and, in order to have a learning experience, Mind has imbedded within two interpenetrating frames of reference in the universe which I call the "positive space/time frame" and the "negative space/time frame." Springing from these is substance. Substance, which we associate with chemical components, takes on various structural forms, forms that have function. Physical substance manifests itself in the positive space/time frame—it is electrical in nature, has positive mass, travels slower than the velocity of electromagnetic light, gives rise to the gravitational force, and is the substance prescribed and utilized in allopathic medicine. Etheric substance is postulated to manifest itself in the negative space/time frame—it is magnetic in nature, has negative mass, travels faster than the velocity of electromagnetic light, gives rise to the levitational force, and is the substance prescribed and utilized in homeopathic medicine.

The human being communicates with his environment via a variety of built-in sensing and response networks functioning over a wide spectrum of relative integrity. The greater the degree of integrity of the networks and the lower the firing threshold for internal signal generation, the more sensitive is the individual to disturbances in the environment. The more organized and coherent we become at the physical level, the more apparent is our disorganization, incoherence and imbalance at more subtle levels. As we evolve and become more integrated, the coherence extends to the more subtle levels, which become more energized, and the individual functions in the physical world under conditions of increased energy flux. Thus, smaller and smaller imbalances in the system scatter the energy flow significantly so that they are detected and diagnosed as disease.

This perspective is remarkably similar to the situation one observes during the development and maturation of many technologies. For example, the semiconductor industry, which evolved from the transistor to integrated circuits, is now working toward large-scale integration, where a million circuits will be placed on a single silicon chip. In the early days, the quality of the silicon material that performed well in circuit applications of that time would fail miserably if tested today. Today's integrated circuits are orders of magnitude more demanding than those of a decade ago, our understanding of materials is more sophisticated, and our ability to sense departures from perfection is correspondingly greater. Thus, the greater degree of coherence of the system means that departures from perfection are more catastrophic to the function of the system and show up more readily.

In the past, we have not had adequate instrumentation to detect these subtle levels of energy that are so relevant to homeopathy. In the present, we are just beginning to develop instrumentation of an electrical nature to monitor physiological responses to a network of skin points. These points correlate well with imbalances in the body at the physical and at the next, more subtle level. In the laboratory and on the drawing board, devices are being developed that will directly reveal the interaction of mental intention and healing. Thus, our future medicine will proceed toward the development of techniques and treatments that can utilize successively finer and finer energies. A wider range of devices will develop which monitor or perturb at all the key levels.

A rigorous science of these subtle energies is developing. Many new techniques and new procedures will join the present equipment and methods of practicing homeopathic physicians. We must make room for many changes in both understanding and technique. It is to be hoped that adequate testing of these new procedures will be allowed and encouraged by the present homeopathic establishment and that they will not be prejudiced against the "new" in the same way that they, in turn, have been discriminated against in the past by the powerful allopathic medical establishment.

As the tide shifts in favor of homeopathy, I can think of no better leader and teacher of the subject than George Vithoulkas to guide it toward its predestined role of leadership in the health care field. The arrival of this great textbook, which I have thoroughly enjoyed reading, is timely; it provides us with a set of scientific concepts and experimental observations to form a strong foundation upon which to build the science of homeopathy. It is a new beginning—and has an exciting future!

—William A. Tiller
Department of Materials Science and Engineering
Stanford University

Preface

THIS BOOK HAS been born out of twenty years of experience in the application of homeopathy—twenty years of real dedication, study, close observation, and constant meditation on the many challenging problems that the young and emerging science of homeopathy presented to my inquiring mind. I could perceive from the very beginning that there existed in its theory and application many missing points and many confusing issues, many unknown links about which I was in vain seeking illumination from the masters of the time. Yet, in spite of existing blanks in its theory, the therapeutic results that its application could give were more than miraculous.

Eventually, after all these years of intensive study, application, and observation, many important factors, many missing links, started one by one to be illuminated. With time, the whole theory and practice of homeopathy emerged as I present it in this textbook. Important issues like a complete definition of health, the understanding of the human being in its three levels of existence, the hierarchical importance of the symptoms or syndromes and their interrelation, the understanding of the defense mechanism, the comprehension of the theory of the miasms in its true perspective—and many other problems were clarified.

It did not take me long to understand that homeopathy, in comparison to orthodox medicine, has—on therapeutic grounds—the same differences that quantum mechanics bear to Newtonian physics. It was obvious that after the entrance of homeopathy into the therapeutic field, the physician was able to affect in a curative way, through the energized homeopathic remedy, the electromagnetic field of the patient. I realized that through the concepts that homeopathy has been introducing to medicine, the grounds on which therapeutics has so far been operating were transferred from the physical body to its electromagnetic level. Sure enough, with the introduction of homeopathy into the field of therapeutics, a new era in medicine is dawning. The truth of this bold statement is difficult to be realized by everybody at this time, yet its meaning will be totally understood by the coming generations.

There is only one handicap to homeopathy, and this is that it is extremely difficult to master. Recalling my own experience, I can say with certainty that I can hardly remember a day in my life all these years when this really Divine Science has not occupied the best part of my thoughts. It was soon that I realized that I was living only for homeopathy. I knew that this was the secret for therapeutic effectiveness and even personal gratification. Homeopathy is a living dynamic science and can be effective only if it becomes a living pulsating knowledge within the mind and heart of the practicing homeopath.

This present exposition of homeopathy is my small contribution toward an easier and more complete learning for prospective students. In preparing this English edition, I was helped by the American doctor Bill Gray (a graduate of Stanford University) whose real dedication to the cause of homeopathy and whose scientific thoroughness have tremendously impressed me. Dr. Gray remained for over a year in our school working very hard indeed. My contact with him left me with the strong belief that, after all, this chaotic world of ours is not devoid of men of dignity and high caliber who are ready to sacrifice personal comfort for a good cause. I am aware that along with him other pioneering scientists are working today to prepare the medical establishment for a major change, a great revolution in therapeutics.

It is absolutely certain, and every visionary man or woman is sensing it, that medicine today stands on the threshold of a deep and radical change and that soon it will embrace the new and unique possibilities that homeopathy is offering to it. It is also certain that people of today more than anything else want to gain back their lost health. They are not concerned about empty speculations. One can say that contemporary people are demanding a way to regain their lost psychosomatic equilibrium in order to face the challenges that technological civilization has imposed on them. It is my strong belief and my experience that homeopathy can effectively help ailing humanity in this endeavor and be an invaluable asset for a speedy spiritual evolution of mankind.

—George Vithoulkas
March 1979

Section I:

The Laws and Principles of Cure

Introduction

AT FIRST GLANCE, the basic content of this book will appear to be somewhat ambitious. Health and disease, especially in rela-ion to fundamental questions of the nature of Man, are indeed deep and ponderous issues upon which innumerable volumes have been written throughout the ages. Nevertheless, there have been discoveries made in modern times which shed new light on the basic principles and methods involved in such issues. This book is an endeavor to elucidate the relatively simple principles and methods involved in healing, not only for the professional but also for the general reader who wishes to enter the subject in depth.

An effort has been made in this book to:

A. Outline the basic laws of healing that, while they have always operated and are valid for all ages, have only in modern times been discovered and formulated in systematic fashion.

B. Show the underlying and verifiable connection between hu-manity's spiritual evolution and its state of health, without the understanding of which the physician will not be able to effect a radical and lasting cure.

C. Show in some detail the method through which Man can be helped to attain permanently a better state of health.

Until only recently, it would appear that the human race has done very little to effectively insure good health. Despite modern advances in dealing with acute illness, the virtually crisis proportions of chronic disease have aroused fears that the human race may be in danger of losing its health for good. As throughout history, modern therapy is helpless when faced with crippling chronic diseases, and it is consequently reduced to providing merely palliative, rather than curative, treatment. Great interest has been aroused in all quarters concerning the fundamental assumptions underlying medical care, a result, I believe, of the enormous amount of suffering people are undergoing today in the face of a disproportionately small amount of relief available through the various accepted therapies.

Because of the arousal of such doubts, alternative therapies have once again become popular, and people are in desperation trying them indiscriminately. Once disenchantment with orthodox approaches occurs, one is then at a loss to evaluate accurately and dependably the efficacy and safety of the alternatives. Thus, by contrast it becomes clear that the prevailing medical system has not explained the laws and principles governing health and disease. Such an explanation has not been forthcoming because it has in fact not been formulated, even within the medical profession itself. If we search back into medical history, we shall find volumes of empirical data and experimental results, but no general laws or principles to support them, or arising from them. It is not unfair to conclude that medicine is the only branch of science that has based its structure on opinions and suppositions rather than on laws and principles.

Due to such a weakness in its conception, the prevailing medical system fails either to persuade the populace as to its efficacy or to provide satisfactory and continuous therapeutic results, especially in the face of one of the most frustrating and rapidly increasing crises facing medicine today: chronic disease.

The purpose of this book is to attempt to restate the universal principles of health and disease into a comprehensive rational system, readily verifiable by actual clinical results, that understands and can effect radical cure whenever that is possible. These principles must be known and respected by any practitioner, no matter which therapeutic modality is used. By understanding clearly these simple principles, people will be able to judge any therapeutic method as to its curative action, and thus will be able to find their way to better health by choosing to take advantage of a system that offers the most efficacious possibilities.

During the course of this exposition, readers will doubtless

4

come across fragments of ideas they remember having discovered in one or another healing system proposed in the past. However, it is only in relatively recent times that such a comprehensive description of the natural laws governing health and disease has been formulated into one methodology.

At this point, let us touch on the highlights of medical thought throughout history. It is not within the scope of this book to present an exhaustive description of the different phases through which medicine has passed in its development, but we can at least review some well-known generalities. One would have thought that as Western man progressed from his primitive state toward higher and higher civilizations, medicine would naturally have kept pace in its own evolution. Yet the facts do not verify this assumption. Despite the strides made by humanity in many fields over many epochs in Western history, medicine has never kept pace with the general progress in thought.

For example, when Greece, having progressed beyond all other Western primitive civilizations during the sixth, fifth, and fourth centuries before Christ, reached a state of inner evolution unsurpassed perhaps even today, humanity nevertheless was forced to continue the most primitive and unreliable methods to recover its health. The great insights and deductions that permitted those giants of thought to plunge into unparalleled philosophical and spiritual speculation did not help them to unravel the secrets governing health and disease.

Again, during the Christian era, when a massive and profound spiritual evolution took place, medicine remained in the dark. As humanity proceeded further to reach new heights of religious and artistic expression during the eras of the Byzantine and Renaissance, medicine was busy developing and applying bloodletting and cathartics.

In the eighteenth and nineteenth centuries, the scientific spirit made tremendous leaps in discovery, yet that spirit sanctioned the use of healing methods that were more than primitive, and on a massive scale. It is during this time, significantly, that a German doctor, Samuel Hahnemann, formulated for the first time in the history of medicine the complete laws and principles governing health and disease, and proved them in actual clinical experience. Yet nobody listened to him. Apparently his ideas were too advanced for the primitive state of mind in which his colleagues lived. They seemed unable to make the leap necessary to grasp an idea centuries in advance of their thinking.

5

Instead, the more materialistic concepts put forward by Louis Pasteur were widely accepted. His concepts fit more adequately the need for a concrete Newtonian conceptualization. Pasteur's theories and research into the nature of microbes led everyone to believe that the cause of illness had been explained. As the modern science of bacteriology has advanced, however, it has come to the conclusion that both the microbe and constitutional susceptibility are necessary to initiate the disease process. Yet modern physicians seem to have closed their eyes to this fact. They continue to hunt down new microbes, bacteria, viruses, etc., and then develop powerful drugs with which to kill them. Witness the massive effort to explain the "cause" of the recent Legionnaire's Disease; the entire effort has been focused on the microbial cause, and has largely ignored the constitutional susceptibility of the victims. Another perfectly valid approach, which might even produce better results, would be to study the relative resistance of the survivors to the supposedly virulent organism.

Unfortunately, the obsession of medical researchers with their determination to pursue this erroneous idea of microbes and concrete causative factors in illness, despite increasingly disappointing results especially in chronic disease, is leading progressively to the development of increasingly toxic drugs, which themselves are becoming a significant public health menace.

It is evident to all thoughtful patients of today, furthermore, that the obsessive search for a concrete cause of illness is, in fact, not really the basis of modern therapeutics anyway. The vast majority of drugs prescribed for illnesses such as arthritis, asthma, colitis, ulcers, heart disease, epilepsy, anxiety, and depression are not designed to be curative, even in their original conception. They do not strike at the cause at all but merely offer a rather pallid hope for palliation, even if we disregard the danger of side effects. This in itself is a sign of the helplessness of modern medicine to deal effectively with disease.

Thus we see that orthodox medicine (referred to throughout this book as allopathy, derived from the Greek roots signifying "other" and "suffering") has built for itself a structure strong in finances, institutional inertia, and political connections but simultaneously weak in basic laws and principles. In general, medicine has found itself in the midst of a scientific society experiencing the greatest technological advances ever witnessed in history, yet ironically with almost no laws or principles to justify its methods. Any science is a system based on laws and principles verified by continuous experimental and experiential data. Orthodox medicine calls itself a "science," but does it really deserve that name? Where are its laws and principles, which are the foundation of any science?

Consider, for a moment, what the ideal therapeutic system should be. Of course, it must be effective, but it must be effective with minimal or, ideally, no risk to the patient. Its effectiveness must be based upon not merely the alleviation or the absence of symptoms but on the enhanced constitutional strength and well-being of the individual—on the increased ability of the individual to live to the fullest. It should not be prohibitively expensive, of course, and it should be readily accessible and understandable to all members of the population.

Most importantly, though, the ideal therapeutic system must have a clear conception of the following questions:

What exactly, and in the fullest sense, is a human being?
What does it truly mean to be healthy?
What precisely is a diseased state?

Unless these questions are completely understood, any therapy will be unlikely to produce solid, reliable, and verifiable results, or even to recognize real progress if it were to occur.

This book is divided into four major sections. In the first, we set out in the early chapters to understand the three most basic concepts as developed by the science of homeopathy, but which apply equally to all other healing disciplines: Man, Health, and Disease. Next, we attempt to understand the laws and principles of their interrelationship in health and disease. The second section will study in considerable detail the precise, systematic method and technique by which these concepts are applied. The third section will present the *materia medica* "essences" of the major homeopathic medicines, and the final section, the appendices, will give actual clinical cases with detailed analysis for study.

Before proceeding further, we must discuss another vital question which cannot be separated from the others: *What is the objective of human life?* We cannot talk cogently of health and disease in an individual without first knowing clearly the fundamental purpose of life. So, for what are we searching in our lives?

The answer to such a question will naturally be a bit superficial at first, such as: *Man wants money, power, fame, land, sex, absence of suffering, and release from anxiety and tension.* If we meditate on these desires further, however, we come readily to the answer that everyone, through these desires, seeks an inner state of being which is *happiness*, a happiness that is unconditional and continuous—a happiness that will depend very little upon external conditions and persist despite the transient changes which kaleidoscopically march past us in life.

Upon further reflection, it is clear that if a person experiences a limitation of the sense of well-being on either physical, emotional, or mental levels of existence, the possibility for this state of inner happiness to manifest itself is prevented. In serious illness, awareness is mobilized to deal with the disease process and its manifestations and is therefore unavailable to help the person grow and transform itself into a state of true happiness. In this sense, we can see that the attainment of health is an essential prerequisite to Man's attainment of the fundamental objective in life: unconditional happiness, which can then help the individual to attain the highest evolutionary states.

Thus the human spirit is intimately connected with the physical organism in a single integrated totality. This concept is a fundamental tenet which will be expressed again and again throughout this book. Despite modern trends to the contrary, this holistic perspective has been understood very clearly throughout history, as illustrated by the following quotation from a very ancient Sumari text, *The Sacred Script of the Covenant*:

> *Honor your body, which is your representative in this universe. Its magnificence is no accident. It is the framework through which your works must come; through which the spirit and the spirit within the spirit speaks. The flesh and the spirit are two phases of your actuality in space and time. Who ignores one, falls apart in shambles. So it is written . . .*

Summary of Introduction

1. There are laws and principles according to which a disease or a series of diseases arise in a person.

2. There are also laws and principles governing a cure, and every therapist, no matter which therapeutic method is being used, should know and apply these laws and principles.

3. A human being's main and final objective is continuous and unconditional happiness. Any therapeutic system should lead a person toward this objective.

Annotated Bibliography to Introduction

1. Janssens, Paul A., *Paleopathology* (London: John Baker, 1970), p. 150. Documents the presence of many chronic diseases into prehistoric times. Studies of bone repair, metastasis in skeletons, remains of mummies, etc., show that basic defense and repair mechanisms have changed little throughout history. It might have been expected that evolution would have made protective mechanisms more efficient, but the evidence suggests that modern man possesses *less* efficient defense and repair mechanisms than primitive beings. Whatever protection we have occurs because of external means rather than because of internal immunity.

2. Henschen, Folke, *The History of Diseases* (London: Longmans, Green, 1966). Extensive and well-documented review of evidence for various diseases in ancient history; for example, tuberculosis found in bones dated from 5000 B.C. and infectious diseases such as gonorrhea, malaria, and leprosy found many thousands of years ago. Syphilis began in North America about 13,000 B.C. and spread to Europe via Columbus. Cancer has been found all over the world since earliest times. Also includes a chart of mortality from major diseases in Scandinavia, comparing rates from 1911 to 1961—a dramatic decrease in infectious diseases, and a dramatic increase in cardiovascular disease and cancer (p. 31).

3. Gordon, Benjamin L., *Medicine Throughout Antiquity* (Philadelphia: F.A. Davis, 1949). Evidence for epilepsy, mental disorders, arthritis since earliest Man.

4. Raven, Ronald W., ed., *Cancer*, Vol. I (London: Butterworth, 1957). Cancer documented since 3000 B.C. in Edwin Smith Surgical Papyrus.

5. Himwich, *Biochemistry, Schizophrenias, and Affective Illness* (Baltimore: Williams & Wilkins, 1970), p. 153. Schizophrenia is one of oldest diseases in human race. Well-described and differentiated from other mental disorders as early as 3300 B.C. First described in Indian Ayura Veda.

6. Lilienfeld and Gifford, eds., *Chronic Disease and Public Health* (Baltimore: Johns Hopkins Press, 1966). Excellent documentation of changing rates of incidence and mortality of major chronic diseases, especially in relation to infectious disease rates. It is commonly stated that chronic disease rates are only apparently increased because of the success of antibiotics in reducing infectious disease rates. Rates of ten leading causes of death in the U.S. in 1900 and 1960 clearly demonstrate an *absolute* increase in the mortality rate of chronic diseases, not merely a relative increase (p. 8). This increase is not due to a relative increase in age of the population, contrary to popular opinion. For example, mortality rates for heart disease and cancer increased by about 25% in absolute rate from 1900 to

9

1960; the effect of age changes in the population would have accounted for an increase of only 12%.

7. International Agency for Research on Cancer and John E. Fogarty International Center of the National Institutes of Health, USA, *Host Environment Interactions in the Etiology of Cancer in Man* (Lyons: International Agency for Research on Cancer, 1973), p. 17. One of the best studies available on the specific changes in rate of individual cancers, with specific reference to age, sex, and geographic differences. Compares cancer rates from 1937 to 1969.

8. Curriel et al., *Trends in the Study of Morbidity and Mortality*, Public Health Papers No. 27 (Geneva: WHO, 1965). An extensive summary of morbidity and mortality rate changes for a wide variety of diseases. Corroborates studies quoted above.

9. Health Information Foundation Research Series No. 11, *Measuring Health Levels in the United States, 1900–1956* (New York: Foundation, 1960). A technical book on vital statistics, elucidating the strengths and weaknesses in morbidity and mortality rate studies.

10. Combined Staff of Clinic, "Recent Advances in Hypertension," *American Journal of Medicine* 39: 634-638 (Oct. 1965). An excellent review of the effectiveness of drug therapy in treating hypertension. Demonstrates improved survival among malignant hypertensives, but no benefit (while increased morbidity from drug side effects) in ordinary hypertensive patients. Treatment may actually accelerate angina or cerebral ischemic attacks in some patients. Even among the severe malignant hypertension patients, untreated patients with no end-organ damage have a good prognosis—again demonstrating the variability in susceptibility from patient to patient.

11. Dubos, René, *Mirage of Health: Utopian Progress and Biological Change* (New York: Anchor Books, 1959). Probably the major work contradicting the myth that allopathic medicine has affected therapeutically the health of populations.

12. Dubos, René and Jean, *The White Plague: Tuberculosis, Man, and Society* (Boston: Little, Brown, 1953), pp. 186, 231. Well-documented account of the rise and fall of tuberculosis. Demonstrates clearly that the tuberculosis mortality rates had already declined 50% on their own by the time the tubercle bacillus was isolated, 75% by the time the first sanatorium was established in the U.S., and 90% by the time antibiotics were developed to combat it. Therefore, medical science cannot claim to have conquered tuberculosis by its methods.

13. Porter, R.R., "The Contribution of the Biological and Medical Sciences to Human Welfare," Presidential Address to the British Association for the Advancement of Science, Swansea Meeting, 1971 (London:

The Association, 1972), p. 95. Comments on the decline in death rate of children under 15 from scarlet fever, diphtheria, whooping cough, and measles. Between 1860 and 1965, 90% of the decline occurred before antibiotics and immunization.

14. LaLonde, M., *A New Perspective on the Health of Canadians* (Ottawa: Government of Canada, April 1974). Demonstrates that public health measures are far more effective in improving health of a population than medical therapy.

15. McKinnon, R.R., "The Effects of Control Programs on Cancer Mortality," *Canadian Medical Association Journal* 82: 1308–1312 (1960). Extensive study in Canada considering age- and sex-specific cancer rate comparisons between 1931 and 1957. It is shown that cancer control programs have no effect whatsoever on cancer mortality rates.

16. Lewison, Edwin F., "An Appraisal of Long-Term Results in Surgical Treatment of Breast Cancer," *Journal of the American Medical Association* 186: 975-978 (1963). Compares cancer survival rates at Johns Hopkins between 1935 and 1950 in relation to several modes of therapy. No difference in survival rates by different modes, or even in comparison with therapies prior to 1935.

17. Illich, Ivan, *Medical Nemesis* (New York: Bantam, 1976). A landmark work challenging the monopolistic role and effectiveness claims of the medical profession. Very well-documented and thoughtful. Presents considerable evidence that improvements in sanitation and public health measures have had the primary effect on the health of populations, while allopathic therapy has had little effect—actually a damaging effect.

18. Frobisher and Fuerst, *Microbiology in Health and Disease* (Philadelphia: W.B. Saunders, 1973), p. 276. Describes the susceptibility factor. A person in robust health may easily resist exposure to even the most virulent microorganisms. The degree of resistance can change from hour to hour and day to day depending upon exhaustion, starvation, cold, overwork, etc. This is a standard textbook on microbiology used in virtually all universities and medical schools in the U.S., and it states clearly that the susceptibility factor is so significant that it is virtually impossible to decide the infective dose of a specific microorganism.

19. Dubos, *Mirage of Health*, pp. 66-67. *"Similarly, almost all human beings, Americans included, become infected with a host of microbial parasites of one sort or another. Bacteria such as tubercle bacilli, streptococcus, or staphylococcus, many types of viruses potentially capable of producing influenza, intestinal disorders, or various forms of paralysis, all kinds of protozoa and worms, are commonly present in the tissues of individuals who consider themselves hale and hearty. A generation ago each and every person lived in almost constant daily contact with tubercle bacilli, became a little tuberculous, yet had a fair chance of enjoying a normal, creative life. In brief, the presence of pathogens in the body can bring about disease,*

but usually does not. The world is obsessed—naturally so—by the fact that pol-iomyelitis can kill and maim several thousand unfortunate victims every year. But more extraordinary, even though less dramatic, is the fact that millions upon millions of young people become infected with polio viruses all over the world, yet suffer no harm from the infection."

20. Smith, J.W., et al., "Studies on the Epidemiology of Adverse Drug Reactions. V. Clinical Factors Influencing Susceptibility," *Annals of Internal Medicine* 65: 629-640 (Oct. 1966). *"Nine hundred hospitalized medical patients were surveyed over one year for adverse drug reactions. Reactions were detected in 10.8%. Reactions were most common in patients with serious illness who received many drugs. Patients with abnormal renal function, infections, or with previous drug reactions appeared predisposed to drug reactions."*

21. Ferguson, M., *Brain Revolution* (New York: Taplinger, 1973). Eighty-four percent of patients with asthma who died had used aerosols: a study in England, p. 133.

22. Shader and Di Mascio, *Psychotropic Drug Side Effects* (Baltimore: Williams & Wilkins, 1970). A large work enumerating the voluminous actions of all types of drugs and drug combinations on the mental and emotional state.

23. Martin, E.W., *Hazards of Medication* (Philadelphia: Lippincott, 1971). The standard reference work on drug side effects.

Chapter 1

The Human Being in the Environment

THE FIRST and fundamental task of a professional who has decided to devote himself or herself to the study and practice of a true therapeutic science is above all else to reestablish health in a diseased individual. It is therefore crucial for such a professional to first ask the following questions:

What is a human being?
How is the human being constructed?
How does the human being function in the context of his universe?
What are the laws and principles governing the function of the human being in both health and disease?

It is only through understanding the answers to these questions that the practitioner can bring about cure in the individual, thereby restoring the patient to harmony with himself and the universe surrounding him. Moreover, understanding his answers is necessary in order to be able to recognize and appreciate a true cure as it is emerging in the patient.

To begin with, we must recognize that the human organism is not an isolated entity, sufficient unto itself. Every individual is born, lives, and dies inseparably from the larger contexts of physical, social, political, and spiritual influences. The laws governing the physical universe are not separate from those governing the functions of living organisms. So, we must begin by comprehending clearly the setting in which the human being is found, how it influences him, and in turn how he affects it.

As with all things, the human organism was originally designed to function harmoniously and compatibly in the environment. The intention of this design obviously was to establish a dynamic balance in which both the individual and the environment are mutually benefited. Any imbalance inevitably leads to destruction, which diminishes both the human being and the universe in which he or she lives. Since human beings are endowed with consciousness and awareness, they carry a great responsibility, both for their own benefit and for that of the Cosmos, to live according to the laws of Nature. Ideally, the human race should have enough consciousness and awareness to live within and contribute to the order of the universe, and thereby be freed to achieve the highest possibilities of evolution.

Instead, we find ourselves in the midst of disorder and disease. In the midst of an age of unprecedented technological advancement, we also see unprecedented damage being done to the atmosphere, the water, and the land. Socially, it is easy to pessimistically conjecture that the modern epidemics of competition, violence, and war may well lead to the actual destruction of the human race. And individually—instead of rejoicing in an increasing degree of vibrant health from generation to generation—we witness a continuous decline in health.[1]

Why is this so? In the most basic analysis, we can ascribe this state of degeneration to two dynamics:

1) Human violations of laws of nature, resulting in contamination of the environment, which in turn places increased stress on the ability of the individual to function.
2) Mankind has gradually lost the inner awareness which would have enabled correct perception of the laws of nature, which must be respected.

Thus we see that both collectively and individually human beings are simultaneously affecting and are affected by the environment; as we deviate increasingly from the laws of nature, a vicious cycle is established which requires great insight and energy to correct.

---

1. See Bibliography following the Introduction to this book.

For each individual in this situation, there may be a wide variety of possible responses to external stresses. Some people seem to be relatively unaffected by external or internal disturbances; their organisms are in a state of relative balance which is maintained with minimal effort. Most people, on the other hand, experience degrees of imbalance ranging from slight to very severe; these are the individuals we consider dis-eased, in the broadest use of the term. In such people, the disturbance manifests itself in a highly individualistic and varied manner, but always the disturbance can be viewed as an imbalance in the organism's ability to cope with internal and external influences. If we consider the individual as a *totality*, it is clear that the disturbances do not manifest themselves solely on the physical level of existence, as assumed in modern allopathic medical practice. The entire person is disturbed on all levels of existence, to varying degrees.

It is a common observation made by everyone that people vary in their sensitivity to environmental influences. Some people throughout life are blessed with the capacity to maintain a high level of creative living despite minimal hours of sleep, erratic diet, heavy work responsibilities, family pressures, and perhaps even major griefs in life. Other people, on the other hand, feel overwhelmed by minimal stresses, must get many hours of sleep and rest every day, and suffer a variety of symptoms after even a slight deviation from their usual diet. Some people barely notice heat and cold, while others are so sensitive that they can predict weather changes a day in advance.

Why is it that some people can cope with stresses effortlessly, and others become disturbed very easily? This is a very basic question which has separated two major traditions of medical thinking througout Western history. On the one hand, the Rationalist tradition which led to modern orthodox medical thinking focuses on what concrete factors lead to sickness in a person, in the hope that somehow understanding the "exciting cause" of illness will enable curative intervention; this approach has been tested and applied quite adequately through history, yet we still see a steady and alarming increase of crippling degenerative diseases.

On the other hand, the Empiric tradition of thought focuses on the question, What enables a person to remain healthy despite many noxious influences?

Consideration of this question leads quickly to recognition of the fact that every organism possesses a defense mechanism which is constantly coping with stimuli from both internal and external sources. This defense mechanism is responsible for maintaining a state of *homeostasis,* which is a state of equilibrium between processes tending to disorder the organism and processes which tend to maintain order. Understanding precisely how this defense mechanism works is vital, for any significant impairment of its function rapidly leads to imbalance and finally death. It is the action of the defense mechanism with which we will be dealing throughout this book, so in this chapter we will content ourselves with just a brief overview.

All environmental influences produce stimuli of a particular type. These stimuli are perceived by the organism by *receptors* on the mental, emotional, and physical levels of existence.

The core of human existence depends on the ability of the organism to keep its dynamic equilibrium with a minimum of disturbance and in maximum constancy. The defense mechanism is constantly trying to create and maintain this balance, but it is not always completely successful. If the defense mechanism were always functioning perfectly, there would never be any suffering, symptoms, or disease.

This mechanism in most people, however, does not function perfectly, for reasons which will be discussed extensively in later chapters. If the stimuli are stronger than the organism's natural resistance, a state of imbalance is created which then manifests itself as signs and symptoms. Although the *effects* are experienced by the entire person on all levels, the *manifestations* are expressed with relatively greater force on either mental, emotional, or physical levels, depending upon the individual predisposition of the person. These symptoms, or groups of symptoms, are erroneously called "diseases," when in reality they represent the result of the struggle of the defense mechanism to counteract the morbific stimulus.

Before proceeding to more extensive descriptions of precisely how the defense mechanism works, let us first consider briefly the nature of the environmental influences with which the defense mechanism must cope, and some examples of the varied types of responses which can be observed in a given individual. Each of the levels of environmental influences has a unique contribution which needs to be understood by the practitioner:

1. The universe as a whole and its laws
2. The solar system
3. The nation

4. The immediate society
5. The geographical location
6. The family

The influence of the universe beyond the solar system is thus far little understood, but considering recent research being conducted on X-rays, cosmic rays, and electromagnetic fields,[2] on not only solar but also galactic levels, we can be confident that their effects will one day be considered important. Increasingly, it is becoming clear both to physicists and metaphysicists that the universe is one interesting whole, each component of which affects the others.

The effects of the solar system are profound and well known. Of greatest importance is the sun itself. Sunspots affect weather, the electromagnetic field of the earth, and the ionization of the atmosphere—all of which, in turn, influence the health of people. The moon, of course, has long been known to have major influences on health; the synchronicity between the menstrual cycle and moon phases has been repeatedly verified; in addition, history has long recorded the effect of moon phases on epileptics and psychotics. It is also an interesting fact that police and emergency crews of many major cities are now strengthened around the time of full moon because of the well-documented increase of violence and accidents during that phase.

The nation also can affect people in a morbific way. Every nation has a kind of "mood" within which the individual is caught. Americans, for instance, are in general too materialistically ambitious, desiring to accomplish and acquire far more than is needed in order to be happy. This constant pressure will eventually undermine their nervous systems, so that by the age of fifty-five or sixty they may require institutionalization in a rest home. Other countries, as well, have national characters which are topics of conversation the world over. The mood of the nation can play a significant role in shaping the expression of illness of the individual.

One's work environment and pressures produce obvious influences which are being studied by the medical profession in great detail. Exposures to noxious substances such as asbestos, lead, silica dust, and radioactive products, are well known. Noise levels, the pressures of deadlines, the effects of repetitive tasks, and even executive responsibilities, are known occupational haz-

2. See Chapter 4 of this book.

17

ards which can produce crippling illnesses. Even inadequacies in education, as we shall see in more detail in a later chapter, have profound influence on the emotional strength or weakness of people.

By geographical conditions, I refer not only to climatic conditions, but also to the ecology of the area (particularly the degree of contamination of the atmosphere, water, and food supply), sanitary conditions, and altitude. These influences give us a good opportunity to consider in some detail precisely how an individual may be affected by external stimuli in a unique manner, depending upon the degree of weakness existing in his or her defense mechanism. Let us examine, for example, what effects a very humid climate can have on people with different levels of health:

1. A quite healthy person's system will resist humidity with minimal disturbance of the existing equilibrium and will recover without any significant sequelae.

2. A person with a lesser degree of health may develop stiffness of muscles, pains in the joints, sinusitis, rhinitis, or asthma. The focus of disturbance in such a case is primarily on the physical body.

3. Another person with an even worse state of health may develop an anxiety state or even depression in such a climate. The focus of disturbance here is on the emotional plane.

4. Someone with very poor health may develop dullness of mind and an inability to concentrate. The focus in this instance is on the mental level.

In each of these examples, the morbific stimulus (humidity) is *received* by receptors on the physical level of the organism. The *effect* is felt by the entire organism on all levels, but the resulting *manifestation* of imbalance or disturbance is expressed on one level or another depending on the predisposing weakness of the individual.

The influence of the family can also be an extremely powerful factor in the health of the individual. Again, let us demonstrate in some detail how the individuality of the person is combined with external circumstances to produce a variety of possible conditions. We will take as an example a stressful relationship between a mother and a daughter due to a subconscious competition or jealousy, considering only the effect on the daughter. In such a situation, the emotional tension can reach an incredible degree. Even unintentional words or actions of the mother can produce extreme pain to the daughter. If such a situation remains unresolved over a long time, the daughter's reaction may take one of the following forms:

1. If the daughter is quite healthy, she may eventually disregard and ignore the mother's influence. She "understands" the whole situation, and the initial stress is easily released. The stimulus in this instance has not overcome the organism's natural resistance, and thus has not created a state of imbalance.

2. If the daughter's organism is constitutionally not quite so healthy, there may well develop a disturbance manifesting as severe acne on the face, or eczema, or duodenal ulcer, etc. Here, the stimulus is stronger than the defense mechanism and is received through the emotional receptors, but manifests solely in the physical body.

3. If the daughter's health has been further undermined, a more serious ailment may develop. In the beginning, it may be an excessive lack of confidence in social situations, later perhaps apathy, and finally a depression. In this instance, the stimulus is received through the emotional receptors, and results in a disturbance manifesting primarily on the same level.

4. If the daughter's health were even further deteriorated due to hereditary predisposition, the same degree of stress overwhelms the resistance even more severely, and a mental disorder is produced. The child is unable to concentrate in school, eventually may lose marks in class, and may complain that she does not comprehend material which previously was understood perfectly well. Such a progression, if continued, may well end in psychosis. This instance demonstrates a stress received by emotional receptors and transmitted to the center of being, the mental level.

A crucial and profound conclusion that can be drawn from such examples is that the human being is a whole, integrated entity, not fragmented into independent parts. Medicine in general has amassed a great deal of information concerning human beings from anatomy, physiology, pathology, psychology, psychiatry, biochemistry, molecular biology, biophysics, and so on. Unfortunately, each of these branches of study has examined the individual from its particular angle. No one denies that what was revealed through these laborious studies has been illuminating and often useful. But such studies have not so far given us a clear, integrated idea of what a human being is, functioning in its *total-*

ity—not merely on its molecular level, nor on the organ level, nor even on the psychological level alone. Consequently, modern therapeutics takes a fragmented view of the human being. If the liver is affected, give something for the liver; if the nose is running, give some medicine for the nose. The knowledge is haphazard, rather than being based on systematically verified laws and principles derived from observation of human beings.

The above examples consider the effects of environmental stimuli on people of varying degrees of ill health; the structure and function of the human being can similarly be described in the healthy state. If we observe a healthy man, we can easily discern that he is an integrated organism *acting* all the time either consciously or unconsciously. Action is the characteristic of a living organism. Action can be either passive or active, and the exact nature of the action is an expression of the individuality of the person. The activity of an individual is manifested primarily on three levels:

1. Mental level
2. Emotional level
3. Physical level

At any moment, the activity of a person is *centered* mainly on one of these three levels. The center of activity may change frequently, even rapidly, depending on the intention or the circumstances of the person, but always there is a dynamic interaction among these three levels.

When a person functions on one of these levels, the whole integrated system cooperates to fulfill its objective in the best possible way. A long distance runner during the activity of running has mobilized fully all functions onto the physical level. The same is true when someone does manual labor. A man who tries to solve a difficult problem has his mental faculties mobilized, while his emotions and physical functions are kept quiet. A man who meets his beloved after a long separation allows full play to his emotions while reducing the mental and physical activities.

Of course, it is always the whole of the person that is acting, but his attention, his awareness, is centered upon the particular plane on which he has elected to function. This concept may seem simplistic and of little practical value, but we shall later see that it has the most profound significance in the process of producing and evaluating a cure of disease.

Summary of Chapter 1

1. The human being is an integrated whole *acting* all the time through three distinct levels: the mental, the emotional, the physical, the mental level being the most important, and the physical the least.

2. The activity of the organism may be passive or active. In disease, the "reactions" of the defense mechanism to various stimuli are of most concern to the practitioner.

3. The human being, from the moment of birth, lives in a dynamic environment which is affecting his organism at all times in many ways, and is, therefore, obliged to adjust continuously in order to maintain a dynamic equilibrium.

4. If the stimuli are stronger than the organism's natural resistance, a state of imbalance will occur with signs and symptoms erroneously labeled "disease."

5. The results of this struggle can be seen primarily upon the mental, emotional, or physical level, depending upon the overall state of health at the moment of the stress.

Annotated Bibliography for Chapter 1

1. Goffman, J.W., and Tamplin, A.R., "Epidemiological Studies of Carcinogenesis by Ionizing Radiation," *Proceedings of the Sixth Berkeley Symposium on Mathematical Statistics and Probability* (Univ. of California, July 1970), pp. 35-77. Definite correlation between ionizing radiation and cancer. Recommends not waiting for epidemiological data to be conclusive before establishing public policy.

2. Duhamel, A.M.F., *Health Physics, Vol. 2, Progress in Nuclear Energy, Series XII* (Oxford: Pergamon Press, 1969). A complete textbook on environmental effects of radiation. Cosmic rays discussed on pp. 126 and 292. Leukemia rate increased in Hiroshima and Nagasaki after atomic bomb, p. 117. Thresholds established for various radiations because of known relationships for cancer production, pp. 2-3.

3. Dubos, René, *Mirage of Health: Utopian Progress and Biological Change* (New York: Anchor Books, 1959). Premature senility occurs in vicinity of atomic explosions, p. 95. Entire section on effects of environment on health, p. 93 ff.

4. Bentov, Itzhak, *Stalking the Wild Pendulum* (New York: Dutton, 1977).

5. Capra, Fritjof, *The Tao of Physics* (New York: Bantam, 1977). An excellent exposition of the correlations between discoveries of modern physics and the ancient knowledge of Eastern and Western mysticism.

6. Dubos, *Mirage of Health*, p. 86. Effect of weather on potato blight, which in turn affects tuberculosis rate in Ireland.

7. Ostrander and Schroeder, *Psychic Discoveries Behind the Iron Curtain* (Englewood Cliffs, N.J.: Prentice-Hall, 1970). An entire chapter describes the remarkable discoveries by the Russians and Czechoslovakians leading to astrological methods of birth control, now proven effective in over 30,000 women at a rate of 98%. This method is based on the moon-sun angle cycles in relation to the same angle at the moment of birth of the woman.

8. "Report of the Advisory Committee on Asbestos Cancers to the Director of the International Agency on Research on Cancer," *British Journal of Industrial Medicine* 30: 180-186 (1973).

9. Selikoff et al., "Carcinogenicity of Amosite Asbestos," *Archives of Environmental Health* 25: 183-186 (1972). Two hundred thirty men studied between 1960–1971; 105 deaths, compared to normal population death-rate of 46.4. Lung cancer and mesothelioma found in "considerable excess." In normal population, would have expected 2 or 3 deaths; actually observed 25.

10. Glensson et al., *Clinical Toxicology of Commercial Products; Acute Poisoning* (Baltimore: Williams & Wilkins, 1969). Standard reference book on effects of toxic exposures from the environment.

11. Vitums et al., "Pulmonary Fibrosis from Amorphous Silica Dust, A Product of Silica Vapor," *Archives of Environmental Health* 32: 62-68 (1977). Definite causative correlation between silica dust and pulmonary fibrosis.

12. Dubos, *Mirage of Health*, p. 95.

13. Goffman and Tamplin, "Epidemiological Studies."

14. Wolf et al., "Hypertension as Reaction Pattern to Stress: Summary of Experimental Data on Variations in Blood Pressure and Renal Blood Flow," *Annals of Internal Medicine* 29: 1056-1076 (1948). A good study demonstrating the effect of executive stress on physical parameters.

15. Hill et al., "Studies on Adrenocortical and Psychological Response in Man," *Archives of Internal Medicine* 97: 269-298 (1956). Thorough study done on a college rowing crew before a major race. Effect existed whether measured on physically stressful days or rest days prior to race. Thus the adrenocortical effect can be surmised to be a result of emotional stress as well as physical stress.

Chapter 2

The Three Levels of
the Human Being

THERE is a readily identifiable hierarchy in the construction of the human being. Most basically, this hierarchy is characterized by three levels:

1. Mental/Spiritual
2. Emotional/Psychic
3. Physical (including sex, sleep, food, and five senses)

These levels are not in reality separate and distinct, but rather there is a complete interaction between them. Nevertheless, the degree of health or disease of the individual can be evaluated from a survey of all three levels. This is a crucial determination for any health practitioner to be able to make, because it is essential for evaluating the progress of the patient.

Of course, there are also hierarchies within these three basic planes. The hierarchies are illustrated in Figure 1. In a simplified one- or two-dimensional representation, the mental plane is seen to be the most central, the highest in the hierarchy, because on this level are the functions most crucial to the expression of the individual as a human being; the physical level, although important, is nevertheless listed as most peripheral (as least significant) in the hierarchy.

Figure 2 is a breakdown of Figure 1 into individual functions. Within each plane, there is a further hierarchy of individual functions. As the practitioner is concerned primarily with disease, the hierarchies listed in Figure 2 show a listing of the symptoms which are the negative aspects of the corresponding functions.

The precise listing is as yet preliminary; much work needs to be done to refine our understanding of the various levels. Nevertheless, this approximation is useful clinically, and it can be verified and refined by detailed chronological history-taking always focused on the whole being. In this chapter, an attempt will be made to describe the three levels in moderate detail, while further illustrations will be elaborated much more exhaustively as we progress through the book.

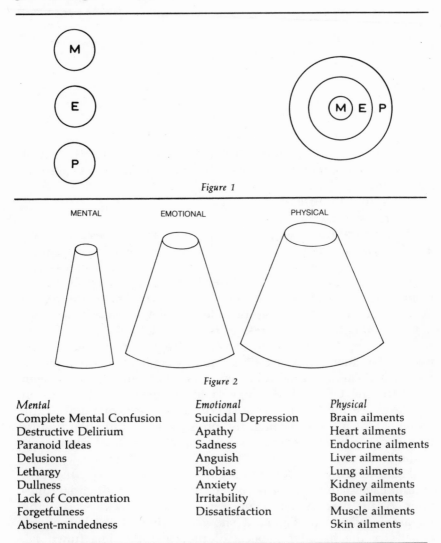

Figure 1

Figure 2

Mental	*Emotional*	*Physical*
Complete Mental Confusion	Suicidal Depression	Brain ailments
Destructive Delirium	Apathy	Heart ailments
Paranoid Ideas	Sadness	Endocrine ailments
Delusions	Anguish	Liver ailments
Lethargy	Phobias	Lung ailments
Dullness	Anxiety	Kidney ailments
Lack of Concentration	Irritability	Bone ailments
Forgetfulness	Dissatisfaction	Muscle ailments
Absent-mindedness		Skin ailments

Each description in the illustration should be considered to be composed of a particular *symptom* and its degree of *intensity*. In the diagram, the sequence of symptoms is listed with the supposition that they are of the same severity. In a given individual, of course, this is not the case. For example, irritability of degree (a) is of less severity to the patient's life than depression also of degree (a). A great irritability of degree (x) is of course worse than a depression of degree (a). On the other hand, if a patient progresses from this state into one in which there is depression of intensity (x) while irritability falls back to intensity (a), an adverse direction has occurred in the patient's health.

By combining both the hierarchical level on which the main disturbance rests and the intensity of symptoms, it is possible to construct a rough idea of the *center of gravity* of a patient's illness. To the extent that both the level and intensity of symptoms progress upward in the diagram (i.e., more toward the center of the person's true being), there is an adverse implication for the person's health. To the extent that this center of gravity moves downward (i.e., more peripherally), there is progression toward greater health. This concept will be illustrated further in later chapters.

Mental Plane

The highest and most important level through which the human being functions is the mental and spiritual level. As a general definition for this plane, we can say: *The mental plane of an individual is that which registers changes in understanding or consciousness.* As discussed in the previous chapter, these changes are initiated by either internal or external stimuli, but they are registered on this plane of existence. It is on the mental level that an individual thinks, criticizes, compares, calculates, classifies, creates, synthesizes, conjectures, visualizes, plans, describes, communicates, etc. Disturbances of these functions in turn constitute symptoms of mental illness.

The mental level is the most crucial level for the human being. It is the mental and spiritual content of a person which is the true essence of that person. If the inner tools of attaining a higher consciousness are disturbed, the very central idea of the possibility of an evolution in consciousness is lost. Where then is the meaning of life?

A person can continue to live, be happy, and be of creative service to others and to himself, with a crippled body, the loss of limbs, or even the loss of sight or hearing. Many examples can be cited of people who were healthy on this level of existence, even though handicapped on more peripheral levels. There are well-known musicians today who are blind. Beethoven composed some of his most profound and powerful works after losing his hearing. One of the most revered and successful geniuses in astrophysics today is confined to a wheelchair, virtually paralyzed by a neurological ailment, unable to pronounce words clearly; yet he has contributed an unprecedented amount of insights to his field since his affliction. Spiritual giants such as Ramana Maharishi and Ramakrishna had cancer without dimming their spiritual reality or the impact on their disciples.

On the other hand, if there is a disturbance on the mental/spiritual plane, the person's very existence is threatened. Such is seen in conditions such as senility, schizophrenia, and imbecility. Although the physical body is the medium through which higher faculties can manifest themselves in this material world, its maintenance in health cannot become an end in itself. It is doubtful that anyone would claim that people have come into this life just to eat, to enjoy sex, and to acquire money and possessions. Even the most primitive men see a higher goal in life, leading them to value faith (which is a degree of understanding) and love; take these away from even the most primitive person, and the will to live will be lost.

If it were possible to have an absolutely healthy mind, we would see people who live continually in spiritual bliss, daily revealing new creative ideas expressed in a very clear way, always of service to others. Such people would be living constantly in the clearness of light and never in the confusion of spiritual darkness. From this state of absolute mental health to a state of total confusion of mind, we can discern a steady gradation of increasing confusion on the various sublevels of the mental plane.

There is a hierarchy within mental functions. Assuming conditions of equal intensity, we can see that a disturbance of memory is not as serious as an equal disturbance in the ability to concentrate; this is not as serious as the inability to discriminate; and, in turn, this is not as serious as a disturbance in the ability to think.

Understanding clearly such gradations is crucial for determining the prognosis in a given case. If we have a patient who has undergone treatment and progresses from a slight degree of confusion to a greater degree, from a slight disturbance of thinking to a greater one, then the patient's health has declined, even though a particular physical symptom may have been relieved. Far from being a mere academic observation, the suppression that can result from such thoughtless therapy can lead to a generalized breakdown in the health of the entire human race. It can be shown that in ancient times the defense mechanism was better able to contain illness and repair injury than we see today. Nowadays, visits to doctors become commonplace at a young age; consequently, large proportions of our populations are exposed from youth to suppressive therapies. This may well be the reason for the alarming rise during the past few generations of chronic disease morbidity and mortality rates.[1] Even the spiritual chaos of our modern world may well be the result of this progression, created by continual suppressive treatments of an increasingly powerful nature. James Tyler Kent, an American physician, in his *Lesser Writings* summed up the tragedy in this way: *"Today no skin eruption is left to appear. Everything that appears on the skin is quickly suppressed. If that continues for long the human race will disappear from the face of the earth."*

How, then, when confronted with an actual patient, can we recognize clearly the degree of health or disease on the mental plane? We need to have a simple and obvious way of defining the qualities which describe the degree of mental health in an individual. As on all levels, health is not merely the absence of symptoms referring to particular mental functions. It is a state of being which can be described as having three fundamental *qualities,* each of which is indispensable for a true state of health. If any one of them is lacking, the mind may be functioning quite well in terms of mere functions but may nevertheless be quite sick. The three indispensable qualities that should accompany the different functions of the mind are:

1. Clarity
2. Rationality, coherence, and logical sequence
3. Creative service for the good of others as well as for the good of oneself.

All three of these qualities must be present, but the third is of prime importance. It is this quality of creative service which appears to be the least understood in modern allopathic medicine, yet the lack of this quality leads eventually to the worst states of insanity imaginable.

Let us discuss a few examples of how consideration of these mental qualities can provide the practitioner with a precise way of

---

1. See Bibliography following the Introduction to this book.

evaluating the mental health of the individual. First, we consider a person who can never express his thoughts clearly. He has great difficulty finding the right words. His thinking has become weak; we are seeing the beginning of disturbance which may eventually lead to a state of senility or imbecility.

Another individual may have clarity but lacks coherence of thinking. He cannot express his thoughts in a logical manner and is therefore not understood by others. He has lost his capacity for abstract thinking, but perhaps even more importantly, he has become subject to impulses; he has become irrational. He jumps from subject to subject, perhaps brilliantly, but so rapidly that others are left mystified. The stereotype of the absent-minded genius is a good example of someone disturbed in the quality of coherence. Such a person is deeply disturbed on the mental level.

The same applies to the master criminal who is highly intelligent and plans a theft or a murder with the utmost degree of clarity and rationality of thinking. Yet this person is ill in the deepest regions of his being, because he is pursuing selfish goals at the expense of other people. Such a mentality pervades our modern world to an extreme degree, and is a root cause of the problems of competition, violence, alcohol and drug abuse, poverty, and war.

We have all known individuals who are highly egotistical and intolerant of the views of other people. Such a person believes that he is always right, that no one knows better than he does; he therefore cannot accept any new ideas, even though they may be correct and beneficial. This leads to a state of mind which excludes the possibility of seeing the truth. In such an instance, the qualities of clarity and creative service are lacking and are preventing the full and proper use of his mental faculties. Progressively, such a person is prone to develop a state of delusion, a state in which the false appears to him to be true. In this way, the highly egotistical and selfish person paves the way for a state of confusion which may eventually lead to a state of actual insanity.

We can see a similar process in a highly acquisitive individual. This person has great belief in material values; nothing is more important than the possessions he desires to acquire—which may be objects or people. Such possessiveness may evolve into a driving desire so out of proportion to reality that the person may seek satisfaction at any cost. Exploitation of others, or even harm to others, will not be sufficient obstacles once the desire becomes obsessive. A person in this state has lost all idealistic and ethical values. What can be more insane than hurting or even killing fellow beings in order to attain some material gain? Besides, this eventually results in a state of great insecurity for the possessive person himself. If for some reason this person loses his possessions, the shock will be virtually unbearable. By contrast, a person who is more healthy in regard to this quality, upon losing his possessions, will suffer only temporarily and then move on harmoniously to make a new beginning.

As we can see from such examples, there is a very fine line between what psychiatrists judge to be mental health, and what they call mental illness. At what point in the above examples do these people cross the boundary between health and illness? Rather, there is a continuous gradation of mental degeneration starting from selfishness and possessiveness and leading into what can eventually be clearly defined as insanity.

Finally, let us consider the basic sources of mental and emotional suffering which enable the initiation of psychosomatic illness in the first place. Psychosomatic perspectives have practically become a modern fad. We are aware, as are all modern physicians, that disturbing thoughts or feelings can disrupt very deeply the health of a person. A sudden grief, a sudden fear, a sudden communication of bad news can throw the organism into extreme suffering that can unbalance the organism for the rest of its life. Why is it that some people can experience such shock for a brief time, but others degenerate into a chronic and deteriorating state of health? What are the qualities on the mental level which lead to this difference in susceptibility?

If we meditate upon the source of mental or emotional suffering, it gradually becomes clear that such suffering arises from two basic sources: broken ambitions and broken attachments. These in turn are another way of saying selfishness and acquisitiveness.

Anyone who believes strongly in many selfish ambitions is setting himself up for a lot of suffering. As soon as it becomes clear that an overly inflated ambition is unreachable, the person will experience grief proportional to the degree of his original belief in it. The same applies to a person driven by acquisitiveness. The degree of suffering resulting from loss of a possession is proportional to the degree of attachment to that possession.

Thus, the conclusion can be drawn that if a person wishes to avoid mental and emotional suffering, he should cultivate selfless, humble, and altruistic qualities. This does not mean, however, that a person should become ascetic, refusing to meet the necessary needs required by every individual. The best policy to follow for maximizing health is "the way of the golden mean" of the ancient Greeks: neither too much nor too little. No excess. Such moderation applies equally to all three levels of human existence.

Emotional Plane

The level of human existence of next importance to the mental level is the emotional level. By this, we include all grades and shades of emotions from the most primitive to the most sublime. This level of existence acts as the defense mechanism's receptor of emotional stimuli from the environment, and also functions as the vehicle of expression for feelings, actions, and emotional disturbances occurring in the individual. The following is a definition of the emotional plane of existence: *that level of human existence which registers changes in emotional states.* The range of emotional expression can vary widely: love/hatred, joy/sadness, calmness/anxiety, trust/anger, courage/fear, etc. Thus it is this level which is very close to the core of daily existence of every individual.

Feelings as to their *quality* can be defined as positive or negative. Positive feelings are those tending to draw the individual toward a state of happiness; negative feelings are those tending to draw the individual toward a state of unhappiness. The more an individual feels or experiences negative feelings, the more unhealthy he or she is on this level. To measure the degree of emotional disturbance of a person is to find out how much, in his waking state, he is occupied with negative feelings such as apathy, irritability, anxiety, anguish, depression, suicidal thoughts, jealousy, hatred, envy, etc.

The most healthy and emotionally evolved people experience some of the most profound states known to mankind: mystical experiences, ecstasy, pure love, religious devotion, and a wide range of sublime feelings difficult to describe, and in our era limited to only a small number of rare beings. As a generalization, it can be said that imbalances on the emotional plane manifest themselves as heightened sensitivity to the sense of ourselves as vulnerable beings separate from the rest of creation; emotionally disturbed states tend to revolve around issues of personal comfort, personal survival, and personal expression. On the other hand, the most evolved emotional states tend to involve feelings of the Oneness of ourselves with all creation—love, bliss, devotion, etc. Thus positive feelings in an individual will always tend to create a sense of unification with the outside world; on the contrary, negative feelings will tend to produce a sense of isolation and separation from the outside world.

As we saw on the mental level, upon which a person can suffer from negative thoughts, so also on the emotional level a person can have negative feelings which create inner disturbance and disharmony within the environment. Positive feelings, on the contrary, strengthen the inner emotional state and create positive conditions in the environment which enhance communication with people and thereby serve the community. When someone expresses trust to another, this very act elevates both and creates a greater psychic equilibrium. By contrast, an expression of anger or mistrust creates a disharmonious emotional state in everyone's psyche, and in this way adds to the deterioration of community. Someone who lives with feelings of inner calm, joy, euphoria, etc., provides for himself and others the best possible emotional nourishment, which can only enhance the level of emotional health. A person, on the other hand, who lives continually with anxiety, sadness, or fear provides poisonous food which eventually leads to degeneration of health in himself and others.

As on the other two levels, there is a hierarchy of emotional disturbances which can be graded according to the extent that they reach deeply into the individual or remain relatively on the periphery. The current approximation of this hierarchy is listed in Figure 2 (page 24). Again, this is a rough approximation developed from past clinical experience and will undoubtedly be altered and refined by careful observers the world over. At the boundaries of the emotional plane with the mental and physical planes, there is a certain amount of "overlap" as described in Figure 3 (page 46). Still, within the emotional hierarchy itself we see a gradation of symptoms which again is useful in determining whether a given patient's progress is improving or declining. For example, considering each symptom at equivalent degrees of intensity, depression can be seen to be more seriously limiting to the life of the patient than anxiety, and anxiety more severe than irritability.

Comprehending the gradation of symptoms is helpful to the practitioner in determining in which direction the patient's progress is headed, but a quick guideline is needed with which to judge the degree of health or disease in an individual immediately at the first interview. At the highest state of emotional health, the individual experiences an absolute dynamic calmness combined

31

with love for self, others, and the environment. This is a state of serenity which is actively involved with people and the environment; it is not merely a lack of emotional feeling generated as a protection against emotional vulnerability. On the other hand, a person at the worst extreme of emotional health suffers severe internal anguish or depression of such intensity that all interest in life is lost and there is an active desire for death. In between these extremes, there are wide variations and individual modes of expression.

In modern times, weakness on the emotional plane has become one of our major existing health problems. Whether because of lack of understanding of the laws of nature, or because of continuous "therapeutic" suppression of relatively peripheral ailments into the core of human existence, many of the problems of today's world can be seen as arising from emotions which are imbalanced, misdirected, and destructive. Modern problems of indiscriminate warfare, random violence and terrorism in the cities, mass murders, racial oppression, and child abuse are all examples of mismanaged emotional states, both on individual and societal levels.

As described earlier, the human being both affects and is affected by the environment. On the emotional level, one of the major environmental influences is the almost complete failure of our educational systems to provide emotional training for young people. As a result, the emotional part in us remains undernourished and cachectic, becoming easy prey to disease conditions. Throughout Western history, and especially in the present-day materialistic and technological era, education has focused almost exclusively on athletics (physical level) and intellectual training (mental level). The primary heroes of young people are athletically or intellectually successful classmates. Sensitive, artistic, musical, or poetic young people are rarely glorified or given encouragement. In modern life, the major source of emotional education appears to be television, which involves the viewer only passively and emphasizes exaggerated or fantasized perspectives on life.

Education should follow a more natural procedure based on known stages of maturation. The *emphasis* of education should be placed on development of the physical body between the ages of 7 and 12, of the emotions between the ages of 12 and 17, and of the mental level between the ages of 17 and 22. Instead, our education is haphazard and random, often governed by political influences more than by recognition of the natural stages of development of the students. The result is the creation of graduates from school who are imbalanced and weakened on the emotional level. Although it is beyond the purpose of this book to fully delineate recommendations for changing the educational system, it is nevertheless important to the practitioner to understand the profound influence which this education inadequacy has on the health of the emotional plane of the individual.

Between the ages of 12 and 17, the human being experiences a natural awakening of the sexual instincts and also of the highest emotional feelings—appreciation of love, freedom, justice, etc. Because there is no programmed education to mobilize and develop these feelings, they get channeled into experiences which are bewildering, frustrating, and often humiliating to the young person. Early attempts to express and act upon these emotions are labeled by teachers and parents alike as "rebellious," "dreaming," "overly idealistic," or even "irrational." Healthy emotional expressions are downgraded and criticized, while the educational emphasis is on conformity, "normality," and success in competition with others. Usually what then happens is that young people channel all their emotional experiences into sex and immediate gratification of pleasure, which in turn often lead to experiences which are called illicit or degrading.

The final result is that young people go through strongly disappointing experiences which harden their emotions or sometimes deaden them completely. The need for emotional expression then becomes channeled into distorted goals. In this way, we witness eventually the emergence of the hard-headed, competitive businessman who is ruthless and indifferent to other people's feelings. People with inadequate emotional training enter marriages for which they are unprepared, a situation leading to our high divorce rate. Parents, faced with the unexpectedly great responsibility of having children, see them as objects or as projections of their own frustrated goals in life. Consequently, we end up with a society made up of people who are out of touch with their feelings and incapable of handling them maturely whenever they do erupt. From the emotional standpoint, we can say that we have today a society of people dead at 25, though living to 75.

Education should recognize the need for idealistic and esthetic feelings which emerge naturally at school age. When love, friendship and companionship, altruistic feelings, and sacrifice are expressed, they should be praised, encouraged, and channeled into

33

mature directions, rather than being either ignored or criticized. Natural inclinations toward music, poetry, and art should be specifically rewarded and developed under discriminating direction. Excursions to spots of natural beauty should be commonplace. Even religious and spiritual discussions should be available to students, and meditation techniques of various types should be offered to students with such interests. Between the ages of 12 and 17, the emphasis in education should be on creativity rather than conformity, esthetic rather than merely intellectual values, and inspirational rather than solely practical development.

If education were to be improved in this way, the result would be people who are mature and balanced on the emotional level, and therefore much less susceptible to diseases on this level. Marriage and family life would become stabilized and fulfilling rather than stressful and morbific. Stresses of life and the environment would then not so easily gravitate toward weakness of the defense mechanism on the emotional plane, thus preventing the modern epidemics of nervousness, insecurity, violence, anxiety, fear, and depression.

Physical Plane

The physical level of existence is the part of the human organism with which medicine has traditionally occupied itself. It has been researched in depth through anatomy, physiology, pathology, biochemistry, molecular biology, etc. However, there is a singular fact which appears to have not become evident to most physicians despite all this research—that the human body in its complexity maintains a hierarchy of importance of its organs and systems. One can only conjecture as to why this concept of hierarchy has been ignored in allopathic literature, but it would seem likely that the primary reason is that such a concept is not needed in the allopathic approach to treating disease. Nevertheless, a full comprehension of this perspective is absolutely necessary for the practitioner dealing with the patient as a totality.

As always, in considering the gradation of systems in the physical body, we first must recognize the tentative nature of the precision of the details until confirmed by further observation. The following principles will help us to elucidate the hierarchy:

1. If a given system contains an organ of central importance for maintaining a full sense of well-being, that system should be

graded according to the importance of that organ to the entire organism.

2. The relative grading of importance of an organ can be measured by the degree of damage to the organism produced by a particular amount of injury to that organ. For example, a scar on the brain will have a more damaging effect than an equal-sized scar on the heart or on the skin.

Following is a list of systems under consideration, and their organs, listed approximately in order of importance to the organism:

1. *The nervous system,* which includes brain, spinal cord, ganglia and plexuses, and peripheral nerve fibers.
2. *The circulatory system,* which includes heart, blood vessels, the blood itself, lymphatic vessels, and the lymph.
3. *The endocrine system,* which includes pituitary gland, thyroid and parathyroid glands, adrenal glands, islets of Langerhans, ovaries and testes, and pineal gland.
4. *The digestive system,* which consists of liver, pancreas, and alimentary canal with its accessory glands.
5. *The respiratory system,* which consists of lungs, bronchi, trachea, pharynx, and nose.
6. *The excretory system,* which consists of kidneys, ureters, bladder, urethra.
7. *The reproductive system,* which consists of the testes, seminal vesicles, penis, urethra, prostate, and bulbourethral glands in the male; and the ovaries, Fallopian tubes, uterus, vagina, and vulva in the female.
8. *The skeletal system,* which includes bones, connective tissues, and joints.
9. *The muscular system,* which consists of striated muscles and nonstriated muscles.

In this classification, we see that the first four systems listed contain one organ each which is vitally important to maintain life: first the brain, then the heart, the pituitary gland, and the liver. In these systems, there is one organ that is predominant and whose function cannot be duplicated by another equal or similar organ. As we look further down the list, we see systems which have two equally efficient organs, each capable of functioning for both: two lungs, two kidneys, and two reproductive organs in both male and female. Still further down in the hierarchy, we find the skeletal system, the central part of which is the vertebral column consisting of many vertebrae; several of these can be damaged without causing death. The same is true of the muscular system, listed last.

The hierarchy of physical systems can be considered in a different light by asking the question: How much damage to a particular organ or system is required to impair life? On the muscular level, it would require a systemic myopathy affecting nearly all of the muscles to impair life significantly; somewhat less damage, but still quite extensive, would have to be done to the vertebral column to destroy life. As we go higher in the hierarchy, we see that it requires progressively smaller and smaller amounts of destruction to the primary organ of each system to endanger the life of the organism. Of the organs most vital to the organism, quite small areas of damage are required to create very serious problems; an area of ischemia on the heart produces more damage to health than a similar area in the liver or kidney, but is still less threatening than similar damage in the brain.

From these observations, we can construct a hierarchy of organs in the physical body based on their importance to the organism:

1. Brain (1)
2. Heart (1)
3. Pituitary gland (1)
4. Liver (1)
5. Lungs (2)
6. Kidneys (2)
7. Testes/ovaries (2)
8. Vertebrae (28)
9. Muscles (many)

Understanding this hierarchy is not a mere academic exercise; it enables the practitioner to recognize the direction of progression of illness. If disease is progressing upwards in the hierarchy—from kidneys, lung, pituitary, heart, and finally brain—it is clear that progress is going in an adverse direction. On the contrary, if the progression is downward from brain toward muscles, there is clearly improvement occurring in the general health.

If a modern physician observes a particular patient progressing, for example, from eczema to bronchial asthma, he is likely to explain this to the patient in one of two ways: either it is the natural course of the disease in allergic individuals, or the asthma is an unfortunate, but coincidental, second ailment added to the eczema. If a patient who has suffered from rheumatoid arthritis later has a heart attack, the doctor will consider both events as separate and coincidental, and will treat them separately. Even more unfortunately, the deeper the organ involved, the more likely the physician will be to give a more toxic drug to control the symptoms (if indeed one has yet been invented); the patient with rheumatoid arthritis will likely be given aspirin or butazolidine, and after the heart attack he may receive digitalis, quinidine, propranolol, or anticoagulants as well. It is not considered possible by the allopathic profession that progressively more serious ailments may be the result of suppression of symptoms of less serious ailments. Regardless of whether the method of therapy being used is "artificial" or so-called "natural," if an adverse direction in the hierarchy occurs after the treatment, it must be suspected that the therapy is doing harm, and it should be either discontinued or changed.

The Definition and Measure of Health

Thus far we have tried to consider in some detail the human organism in its setting of environmental influences and on its three levels of function. Necessarily, this approach presents a somewhat fragmented picture of the human being. In fact, of course, the human organism is a completely integrated totality, always acting with innate intelligence to maintain homeostasis with varying degrees of success. Now we will attempt to pull together this fragmented image and illustrate with examples how these concepts can be used by practitioners to precisely evaluate the state of health of a given individual.

As we have seen, there is a hierarchical gradation of functions and disturbances within the human organism which tends to maintain order. This hierarchy is not merely limited to living entities; it is a characteristic of the structure and function of the universe itself. For instance, a sudden disturbance in the laws of attraction and repulsion, or of electromagnetic fields, would create unimaginable destruction in the Cosmos. A fundamental, even momentary, change in the activity of the sun would profoundly disrupt life on the Earth. Even small changes in the temperature range of the planet drastically alter the balance of life forms. On a lesser scale, the gravitational force of the moon affects life, as do humidity, wind, and local climatic conditions. In all of these phenomena, we can discern a hierarchy of functions and the laws governing their interactions. If a central process of fundamental importance is disturbed even slightly, the effect upon the whole system is much greater than would occur if a lesser process were disturbed to the same degree. As we have already seen, such a hierarchy is evident in the human organism as well, so that a small area of damage to the brain has far more effect on the organism than a similar area of damage on the skin.

The idea of hierarchy is actually the idea of the Oneness from which all else has been created. All entities and all levels are connected throughout the universe by this concept; therefore it can be considered a universal law.

The concept of hierarchy gains tremendous practical importance to the clinician upon consideration of the center of gravity of action or disturbance in the organism. In our era, it can be said from a practical point of view that every individual (viewed as a totality) at every moment of his life is ill to some degree. The extent of the disease is determined by the totality of the disturbance existing as symptoms on all three levels. A visible disturbance on one level, no matter how minute, simultaneously affects other levels as well, though to a greater or lesser degree. Nevertheless, when the greatest part of symptoms is on one level, we can say that the center of gravity of the disturbance at that moment is on that level. This is a highly dynamic state, of course, but the practitioner can in general discern a basic center of gravity of disturbance upon taking a careful history which includes all three levels of the individual.

Let us take as an example a patient who suffers with bronchial asthma and chronic constipation as the chief complaints in his physical body. After taking a careful history at all levels, it becomes clear that he is also quite irritable, he has a fear of the dark, a fear of disease, and anxiety about his future. Upon even further inquiry, he admits that he has lived for some time with the fact that his power of concentration has diminished. At this moment, as determined by the intensity of the chief complaint, the clinician perceives that the center of gravity of symptoms is on the physical plane.

The practitioner prescribes a course of therapy (whether allopathic medicine, psychotherapy, naturopathic treatments), and on the return visit discovers that the asthma and constipation have been ameliorated satisfactorily, while the symptoms of irritability and anxiety have increased. The patient complains of sadness, and his mental state exhibits further deterioration in his power to concentrate; his ability to perform creative work for himself or others is lessened to a noticeable degree. The orthodox allopathic doctor, focused by training on the physical level, would be likely to feel gratified by the results since the asthma and constipation have improved, and then refer the patient to a psychiatrist to handle the "new" psychological problems. A practitioner who understands the principles of the totality of the patient, however, would immediately see that the center of gravity of disturbance has moved from the physical to the emotional level, thus signifying a deterioration of health in general, despite the fact that the original physical complaints may have been 90% ameliorated.

During a real cure, the exact opposite sequence of events is likely to occur. At first, the physical symptoms may remain unchanged or perhaps grow slightly worse, while the power of concentration is improved and emotional symptoms are diminished. This would mean that the center of gravity is gradually lowering in the hierarchy and concentrating somewhat on the physical plane. The wise clinician would simply do nothing at this point, and on subsequent visits it will be observed that all of the symptoms, including the physical ones, have gradually disappeared. Thus by understanding the hierarchy of symptoms and observing the change in the center of gravity, we have a highly practical method of evaluating progress, a method which is based moreover on the actual workings of the defense mechanism of the organism.

Throughout the presentation thus far, we have mentioned two factors for consideration: the location in the hierarchy of the symptoms and their intensity. For example, two patients can have a spectrum of symptoms identical to those of the above patient, both with the same center of gravity, yet one may experience only slight impairment of his health, while the other may be severely crippled by disease. Such a difference results from the difference in intensity of symptoms. For this reason, we need a device for measuring readily both the overall degree of health of the individual, as well as a measure of the intensity of individual symptoms. Such a measure arises from the fundamental definition of health.

According to what has so far been said, it is easy to define the state of health of an individual. A comprehensive definition must fit the entire scope of the human being as a spiritual being. People throughout their lifetimes do little else than to free themselves from the bondage that pain creates in the body, that passions create in the emotions, and that selfishness creates in the spirit. The clinician who understands the objective of the healer's mission must try to lead the patient toward greater freedom from these three limitations.

Every pain, every discomfort, every weakness appearing in the body inevitably limits whatever freedom existed before the symptoms appeared. Therefore, the state of disease is bondage, a slavery of the body. Nearly everyone, however, at least for a brief moment in life, has experienced complete freedom of body function, when none of the organs are limited and when there is no sense of negative awareness of the body. Thus the state of physical health can be defined as follows: health in the physical body is freedom from pain, having attained a state of well-being.

On the emotional or psychic level, as long as a person is serene and calm, he can proceed without restriction in creative work both for himself and for others. From the moment passion appears and takes hold of the individual, there occur anxiety, anger, anguish, fear, fanaticism, etc. Such passion tends to enslave the emotional part of an individual, and it prevents free functioning in other realms. This is true even for idealistic passions which approach fanaticism in intensity, for any excessive passion tends to enslave; any passion prevents the person from being the master of himself. So, we can define the state of health on the emotional level in this way: health on the emotional level is a living state of freedom from passion, having as a result dynamic serenity. In this definition, it must be made very clear that the emphasis is on *dynamics.* This is not merely a condition of lack of feeling arising out of intellectual disciplines designed to control emotion; it is rather a state of being capable of freely feeling the full range of human emotions without being *enslaved* by them from moment to moment.

In an analogous manner, when there arise selfish tendencies and acquisitive desires, a state of pain is experienced. The selfish person is one who is diseased in the deepest strata of being, in proportion to the intensity of the egotism. All of us have known highly selfish people, who are easily hurt by events which run counter to their wishes. To the degree that a person is governed by selfish ambition and acquisitiveness, he or she approaches a state of mental illness that can end in total confusion. Hence this definition: health on the mental plane is freedom from selfishness, having as a state complete unification of the person with the divine, or with truth, and whose actions are dedicated to creative service.

In this way, we summarize the definition of health of the whole being as follows: *health is freedom from pain in the physical body, having attained a state of well-being; freedom from passion on the emotional level, having as a result a dynamic state of serenity and calm; and freedom from selfishness in the mental sphere, having as a result total unification with Truth.*

The question naturally arises at this point: How do we measure the comparative degree of health of any individual at any given moment? What is the parameter that defines, for instance, whether an individual with rheumatoid arthritis is in better health than another one suffering with depression?

The parameter which enables such measurement of health is *creativity*. By creativity, I mean all those acts and functions which promote for the individual himself and for others their main goal in life: continuous and unconditional happiness. To the extent that an individual is limited in the exercise of his creativity, to that degree he is ill. If the rheumatoid arthritis patient is crippled to the extent that his ailment prevents him from being creative more than the patient with depression, then the rheumatoid arthritis patient is more seriously ill than the depressed one, even though the center of gravity is on a lower hierarchical level.

Having the idea of creativity in mind, one can always deduce the degree of health or disease of an individual at any given moment.

Summary of Chapter 2

Summary of Mental Plane Section

1. The mental level of being is the most crucial for the individual's existence and maintains within itself a hierarchy very useful for evaluating the progress of a patient.

2. A healthy mind should be characterized in its functions from the following three qualities: clarity, coherence, and creativity. To the extent that any or all of these qualities are reduced or missing, the person is ill at the corresponding level.

3. Confusion, disunity, and distraction constitute the qualities of a completely diseased mind.

4. The practice of selfishness and acquisitiveness are the primary factors that derange the mind. Freedom from selfishness and acquisitiveness will naturally lead to a healthy state of mind.

Summary of Emotional Plane Section

1. The emotional plane of the human being is next in importance to the mental one. This plane is ill to the extent that the person maintains within himself, is trapped by, and expresses negative feelings, as envy, jealousy, anguish, fanaticism, sadness. If the individual can free himself from such "passions," then he can be healthy on this level.

2. On this level arise anxiety, anguish, irritability, fears and phobias, and depression, so common in our times. Our educational and political systems have never systematically developed the emotional plane which is generally weak, undernourished, and therefore vulnerable.

3. There is a hierarchy of symptoms within this level that is useful as a measure of progress during therapy.

Summary of Physical Plane Section

1. The physical body and its organs constitute the least important plane of the human being; the body also maintains a hierarchy of importance as to its organs and functions. An infarct of the brain will be of more importance than an infarct of the heart, and this in turn is of more importance than a thrombosis of an artery in the leg.

2. The organism will always try to keep disturbances away from important organs.

3. A disturbance that progresses during any treatment from less important organs to more important ones signifies a deterioration in general health. An opposite direction of progress indicates progress toward a better state of health.

Annotated Bibliography for Chapter 2

1. Janssens, Paul A., *Paleopathology* (London: John Baker, 1970), p. 150. *"Reactions to disease have remained unchanged since the time vertebrates appeared. That is completely contradictory to MacCallum's opinion, that spontaneous defensive reactions of man have developed and improved over the centuries. This is not*

so: Man has, perhaps, managed to protect himself against disease through external means, more than through internal ones or through immunity. The latter certainly existed in earlier times and may even have been more efficient then: the more primitive a being, the more efficient its defensive and recovery mechanisms seem to be."

2. Lilienfeld and Gifford, eds., *Chronic Disease and Public Health* (Baltimore: Johns Hopkins Press, 1966). Quotes an excellent study in Baltimore showing the percentage of people with one or more chronic conditions at different age levels. The "substantial chronic conditions" rose directly with age from 17.4% in the group under 15, to 85.2% for the group 65 and over.

3. Hinkle and Wolfe, "The Nature of Man's Adaptation to His Total Environment, and the Relation of This to Illness," *Archives of Internal Medicine* 99: 442 (1957). An excellent review of three major studies on the incidence of chronic disease symptoms in population groups which are not selected according to complaint, with emphasis on psychosomatic correlations. A total of 4500 people were included.
Conclusions:

1) Members of otherwise homogeneous populations have differences in susceptibility to illness.

2) Those with high susceptibility are susceptible to *all* types of illness. There are more organs involved, more accidents, more disturbances of mood, thought, and behavior.

3) Illness is not randomly distributed through life, but *clustered* in periods of a few years.

4) Clusters occur at times when the person perceives himself as having difficulty adapting to the environment; a very direct correlation.

5) Susceptibility is related both to differences in adaptive capacities and actual environmental situations.

6) The *form* of susceptibility has little to do with social environment, but this does affect the time the clusters occur and their course.

4. Simeons, A.T.W., *Man's Presumptuous Brain* (London: Longmans, Green, 1960). An excellent description of psychosomatic personality types.

5. Hinkle and Wolfe, "The Nature of Man's Adaptation." A good description of specific personality states correlated with specific physical symptoms, as tested by hypnotic induction of the desired attitudes and later observation of physiological changes.

6. Eastwood, M., *The Relation Between Physical and Mental Illness* (Toronto: Univ. of Toronto Press, 1975). One of the most thorough literature

43

reviews of the entire field of psychosomatic medicine; studies quoted exhaustively, pp. 15–24.

7. Hinkle and Wolfe, "The Nature of Man's Adaptation." Diseases do not occur randomly throughout life, but at particular cluster points, determined by personal attitudes and environmental influences, particularly social influences.

Chapter 3

The Human Being Functioning as an Integrated Totality

In Chapter 2, an attempt is made to describe the three levels of an individual in terms of the hierarchical importance of functions in both health and disease. In this chapter, this concept will be discussed in greater complexity and depth in order to emphasize the interaction between levels as the organism functions as a totality. The astute reader undoubtedly has already raised questions about the interaction of the levels at their boundaries. For example, is it true that a loss of memory (mental plane) represents a lower state of health than depression (emotional plane)? Is a state of irritability more severe than injury to the brain (physical plane)? What about patients who seem to fluctuate back and forth from one level to the next? Do instances such as these represent an imprecision in the hierarchy as presented, or is there overlap of levels at their boundaries?

For the sake of simplicity, the hierarchy has thus far been presented as a one-dimensional, linear description (and in two dimensions, considering the concepts of central and peripheral layers of importance). In reality, the relationship between levels is more complex than this. Figure 3 illustrates a three-dimensional construction which represents different levels of an individual as concentric conical envelopes or sheaths. The most central is, of course, the mental/spiritual plane, while the most peripheral is the physical envelope. In turn, each of these can be broken down into hierarchical arrangements of envelopes within each plane.

45

On the physical level, these envelopes could be elaborated even further to represent organ systems, organs themselves, tissues, the hierarchy of cells within a tissue, and even hierarchies within cells themselves (DNA and RNA, nucleus, cytoplasmic organelles, and cell membrane—in decreasing order of importance). Another significant detail to notice about the diagram is that each envelope begins and ends at a somewhat higher level than the one just peripheral to it; thus it is evident that the overlap is not complete. Upon reflection, then, we see that the diagrams presented in Chapter 2 can be viewed as one- and two-dimensional reflections of a structure which is in reality three-dimensional.

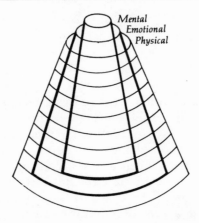

Figure 3: A diagram representing the three layers of human existence in three dimensions. The mental plane is the central conical envelope. The emotional level is shown as the next peripheral envelope, and the physical is the outermost sheath. Note that the tops and bottoms of each envelope do not correspond one to another.

At any given moment, the center of gravity will tend to rest at a particular location. With time, further morbific stimuli and/or treatment (either suppressive or beneficial) may change the center of gravity. The center of gravity may move higher or lower on the same plane, or it may move more centrally or more peripherally to higher or lower levels of correspondence.

In studying Figure 3, the center of gravity can be shown to move in two basic directions. On the one hand, each envelope has its own linear hierarchy; and on the other hand, each level has *correspondences* with the other levels. The higher one goes on any given envelope, the deeper into the organism one reaches. Also, in changing from one sheath to a corresponding level on another, the more central direction represents degeneration of the overall health of the individual, while movement toward outer sheaths indicates an improvement in health. The most important region is at the pinnacle of the central mental/spiritual level, which has no correspondences on the emotional or physical planes. The least important region is at the bottom of the outer (physical) envelope, which has no correspondences on the emotional or mental levels. In this way, it can readily be seen that each level is reflected to some extent upon the others, and there is always a dynamic inter-action between all levels simultaneously. Any stimulus or any change on one level simultaneously affects the others to a greater or lesser degree, depending upon the center of gravity of the disturbance at any given moment.

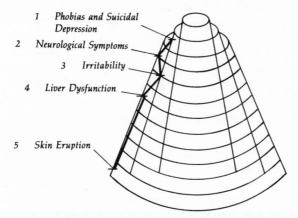

1   *Phobias and Suicidal Depression*

2   *Neurological Symptoms*

3   *Irritability*

4   *Liver Dysfunction*

5   *Skin Eruption*

Figure 4: Illustration of the change in center of gravity in a case involving alternating correspondences of emotional and physical levels. At point 1, the patient presents the prescriber with a totality of symptoms with center of gravity on the emotional level. After treatment, the center of gravity moves to the physical level at point 2. With further treatment, the center of gravity again shifts back to the emotional level, point 3, but at a lower level of correspondence. Then, as treatment progresses, the center of gravity again moves peripherally to point 4 and finally point 5 before the patient is fully cured.

To clarify this concept, let us take a detailed case example (Figure 4). If we have a psychotic patient who complains of a great

47

many fears and suicidal depression, we see that the center of gravity of disturbance is on the emotional plane. In taking the case history, it becomes evident that there are other symptoms affecting the physical level as well, but to a much lesser degree. The patient is treated successfully, and the psychotic state diminishes considerably. After six to nine months, however, neurological symptoms such as diplopia, muscular twitching and weakness, and areas of numbness develop. If it were possible to construct the diagram with precise accuracy, we would see that the center of gravity of disturbance has moved toward the periphery (toward the physical) but on a level which is nevertheless just below the corresponding level of the previous emotional symptoms. With further treatment, the neurological symptoms subside, but the patient, though still no longer psychotic, becomes very irritable and difficult to live with; the center of gravity has moved again toward the center (emotional plane), but at a still lower level of correspondence compared to the initial totality of symptoms. With further treatment, the irritability subsides, and the patient then develops a liver dysfunction of moderate intensity. Finally, after still more treatment, the liver problem disappears, and a skin eruption manifests itself, remains a few months, and then disappears. After such a progression, the practitioner can confidently expect the patient to remain cured for quite a long time, if there are no extreme shocks to the system or interferences by inappropriate therapies.

In this example, if viewed by the diagrams presented in Chapter 2, the practitioner might well have become confused at the point in the case when irritability replaced the neurological symptoms; this might have been interpreted as a degeneration of health, and drastic measures might have been taken to try to correct the problem. Utilizing his three-dimensional construction, however, it is possible to see that progress in this case was always in a positive direction when viewed with knowledge of correspondences from one level to another.

Although this construction appears complex and requires a tremendous amount of confirmation by clinicians all over the world, it is nevertheless a useful image to keep in mind while evaluating cases. Such an image helps the practitioner to sort through the morass of seemingly random and confusing changes with some confidence as to what is actually occurring in the patient. In future decades, systematic observations by careful interviewers will refine the details of these correspondences and hierarchies so that future clinicians will have a precise tool for evaluating clinical progress, with even greater accuracy than laboratory tests—a tool derived solely from symptoms given by the patient.

Modern physiology and psychosomatic medicine have documented quite well the fact that correspondences exist between the emotional and physical planes. EEG and biofeedback studies confirm that intense mental concentration or meditation increase circulation to the brain while producing relaxation of the musculature and lowering of the blood pressure. A state of fear creates palpitations, dry mouth, slowed peristalsis, perspiration of the palms, pupillary dilatation, etc. A pleasant emotion such as love between two people creates peripheral dilation of blood vessels, blushing, palpitations of the heart, and emotional and mental excitement. Every stimulus, every emotion, and every thought has a corresponding effect to some degree on all levels of the body simultaneously and instantaneously.

Clinically, the most obvious correspondences are those relating particular organs to specific emotional states. Every thought and emotion has a corresponding site it "favors" on the physical body. This area is positively or negatively affected depending on the nature of the thought or emotion corresponding ot it. A man undergoing the stress of breaking up a cherished love affair is likely to suffer heart symptoms; another person experiencing difficulty in business is liable to develop a peptic ulcer. A negative thought or emotion will retard the functioning of the corresponding organ or system, whereas a positive thought or feeling will strengthen the function of the corresponding organ.

To illustrate the interaction of corresponding levels in an organism, let us present a few clinical examples which are likely to be seen daily by any general physician:

CASE 1: A woman was brought up by her highly religious parents to consider sex a horrifying affair which ought to be shut out of her thoughts at any cost. She came to the doctor complaining that there was excessive growth of hair on unusual parts of the body such as chest, abdomen, and back, while there was loss of hair on the head almost to the extent of baldness; also, after delayed menarche, she experienced painful and irregular menses which were often late. When she eventually married, she developed severe headaches. In this case, suppression of the sexual instinct from the mental level led to a testosterone/estrogen im-

49

balance, resulting in a masculinized hair distribution. Eventually, this suppression evolved into another symptom on the mental level—aversion to sex. Marriage inevitably produced further stress on this already weakened level, causing changes on the corresponding emotional and physical levels—a feeling of dissatisfaction in her marriage, along with crippling headaches (replacing the hair loss). Originally, the defense mechanism was able to establish an equilibrium by limiting symptoms to the endocrine level, but the added stress of marriage broke down this defense and forced the defense mechanism to reestablish symptoms at a somewhat deeper, and more crippling, level.

CASE 2: Another woman, also raised with a strict upbringing, developed hair loss. At the age of 22, she fell in love and developed a very healthy emotional relationship in marriage. From the moment she entered this relationship, the hair loss subsided, and the patient felt a great sense of well-being, yet the amount of hair on her head remained much less than normal and did not increase in thickness. In this instance, the same degree of mental suppression produced a similar endocrine imbalance, but the healthy emotional stimulus was able to strengthen her defense mechanism enough to establish a new equilibrium of minor significance in terms of her freedom to live happily and creatively. Thus, although the hair on her head was not normal, the patient was advised that the defense mechanism had established a very acceptable balance which should not be interfered with.

CASE 3: A young man of 19 years developed excessive stiffness in the back of the neck while preparing for entrance to the university. The course of study he had decided upon was very arduous, and he felt great anxiety about his ability to complete the work successfully. As a generalization, it can be said that there are two centers on the physical body which correspond most closely to the emotional and mental levels of the human being—the heart and the brain. In this case, the young man decided mentally upon a course of study about which he felt great uncertainty on the emotional plane. The neck seems to be the main pathway connecting the brain and the heart on the physical level, so the reflected mental/emotional conflict created physical pain in the region of this pathway.

From these and other case examples, we observe that the defense mechanism always attempts to create a wall of defense, which is manifest as signs and sympoms at the most peripheral level possible. There are three factors which determine or alter the center of gravity of disturbance:

1. The *hereditary* strength or weakness of the defense mechanism in the first place; this is a major factor which will be discussed at great length in subsequent chapters. If the defense mechanism is weak, the center of gravity of symptoms will tend to affect the deepest mental and emotional levels quite readily; if the defense mechanism is strong, the symptoms will be contained on the least vital physical organs.

2. The *intensity* of the morbific stimuli, which are received on mental, emotional, or physical levels. If the shock to the system is very severe, even the strongest defense mechanism may not be able to maintain equilibrium at an unimportant level; if the morbific stimulus is weak (say, a cold virus of weak virulence), then even a relatively weak constitutional state can handle the stimulus with minimal disturbance.

3. The degree of interference by *treatments* which are not capable of strengthening the defense mechanism as a totality. If the body has established a defense at a particular level, symptoms will be manifest and will tend to remain stable at that level. If an allopathic drug is used to relieve the pain or allay the anxiety, the point of defense is removed, and the defense mechanism must then create a new barrier. This new barrier will inevitably be on a level more vital to the health of the organism, because the original equilibrium was the *best possible* that the defense mechanism could produce; in this way, allopathic medicines, or therapies of any kind which focus upon specific symptoms while ignoring the total picture, actually weaken the defense mechanism and eventually cause a deterioration of health into ever more serious chronic diseases.

These three factors affect both the best level of defense of the organism possible at any given moment, as well as the direction of change of the center of gravity when the person's health is altered. If these three factors combine in such a way as to result in deterioration of health, there are two possible directions in which the center of gravity can move:

1. It may change in a linear manner within the hierarchy of *one level,* with only minimal corresponding changes on other levels. If, for example, the symptoms move from one level on the physical

51

plane to a higher level on the same plane, it can be said that the defense mechanism on the mental and emotional planes was healthy enough to restrict the effect of the morbific stimulus to the physical level alone.

2. The symptoms may *jump* from a peripheral envelope to a more central envelope. This could occur if the defense mechanism is weak, if a severe shock occurs, or if a powerful suppressive therapy is employed. As general rule, progression to more central regions has a worse prognosis than linear progression within a single hierarchy.

To illustrate these factors and the interactions of correspondences and hierarchies, let us consider three patients suffering from eczema:

1. A woman suffering from eczema for many years is given cortisone ointments which she faithfully applies for three years. The eczema is controlled as long as the ointments are applied, but the patient notices a gradual increase in sulkiness and irritability, and a desire to limit her social contacts to just a few friends. The center of gravity has moved from the physical to the emotional level at this point; therefore, the treatment was suppressive. Eventually, she begins a beneficial form of meditation practice, but over a period of months begins to suffer from allergic rhinitis. This symptom represents progression again to the physical plane, but on a deeper level than the skin—i.e., the mucous membranes. The sulkiness and irritability are alleviated, but she now suffers from an annoying allergic rhinitis with occasional acute episodes of sinusitis. If the rhinitis is further suppressed by antihistamines, allergy shots, antibiotics, or even intranasal cortisone injections, this patient will again experience either deterioration on the emotional plane more marked than previously, or deterioration on the physical level, developing bronchial asthma. Thus there may occur a linear degeneration of health on the same level, or the center of gravity may jump back to the emotional level—a sign indicating a more discouraging prognosis.

2. Another woman has had eczema for many years, but is suspicious of mere palliative treatment and therefore refuses the cortisone ointments. The eczema persists, although without getting worse. Then she experiences the sudden loss of her husband in an automobile accident. This sudden shock weakens her on the emotional plane; the eczema disappears, but she now develops

anxiety, nervousness, fears, or delusions. If this patient is given tranquilizers to calm the emotional symptoms, and if they happen to act curatively, then the eczema will reappear as the emotional symptoms subside. If the tranquilizers act suppressively, however, deterioration may occur in one of two directions, depending on the strength or weakness of her constitutional defense mechanism. If it is relatively strong, she would be likely to develop allergic rhinitis or bronchial asthma (a return to the physical plane, but on a deeper level than the skin). If it is not strong enough to cope with the suppressive influence of the tranquilizers, a deterioration on the deeper emotional or the mental level would ensue.

3. Another patient with long-standing eczema is treated by a homeopathic remedy prescribed on the totality of symptoms, and the eczema moves first from the face and torso out to the extremities, and finally leaves altogether. From what has been said thus far, this is obviously a curative direction, and the long-term prognosis is excellent.

In these examples, we see correspondences between the physical and emotional planes, and also a predictable sequence of conditions on the physical level—from eczema, to allergic rhinitis, and to bronchial asthma. Each case proceeds differently depending upon the strength and the nature of the treatments given.

Such cases also highlight the observation that there are quite predictable pathways which are followed in degenerating cases. Along these pathways, there are "stations" representing progressively deeper lines of defense created by the defense mechanism. These stations are crucial; otherwise, a morbific stimulus would rapidly penetrate to the deepest levels of the organism and quickly result in death.

The relationship of stations along a pathway has long been known by orthodox medicine, at least on the physical level of symptomatology. Cancers of different types have characteristic organs to which they metastasize: breast cancers to regional lymph nodes, lung, bones, and brain; prostate cancer to the lymphatic system and bones of the pelvis, and then to the spine; lung cancer to local nodes, the central nervous system, the long bones, kidneys, the adrenal glands, and the skin. Autoimmune disorders characteristically affect certain tissues to the exclusion of others: rheumatic fever and rheumatic disorders of other types produce streptococcal pharyngitis, heart valve degeneration, glomerular nephritis, rheumatoid arthritis, etc.; lupus erythematosus produces characteristic skin eruptions, nephritis, colitis, arthritis, hepatomegaly and splenomegaly, and pericarditis. Reiter's syndrome includes gonococcal urethritis, monoarticular arthritis, and uveitis. The burgeoning field of psychosomatic medicine has noticed many correspondences between emotional states and physical ailments: melancholy corresponds to liver dysfunction, suppressed irritability correlates with peptic ulcer, suppressed anxiety is commonly seen in ulcerative colitis, anal-retentive personality types tend to suffer from constipation and hemorrhoids, "type A" personalities have a particular blood type and increased incidence of hypertension and early myocardial infarctions, and compulsive personalities with suppressed anger tend to be cancer-prone.

Such correlations are known, but precisely what determines the pathways of these correspondences? In some instances, speculation centers naturally on the nervous system or the circulatory system as pathways for metastasis. Chinese medicine, based upon centuries of observation, has developed quite specific correlations between particular acupuncture points and particular organs, as well as correlations between specific organs and corresponding mental and emotional states, but it does not explain the origins of these correspondences.

Another perspective is derived from the modern science of embryology. Upon further research, it may well be found that many of the pathways arise from embryological primordial tissues. Each person begins life as a single cell. This cell gradually develops in an orderly fashion into an enormous number of cells through progressive cell division. As this process advances, three different layers of cells develop and become the primordial structures from which the rest of the organism grows. These three levels are called: ectoderm, mesoderm, and endoderm. From each layer, specific organs and systems develop, as follows:

Ectoderm

The skin and its appendages. (Specifically, the epithelium of skin, hair, nails, epithelial cells of sweat, sebaceous glands, and mammary glands.)

Epithelium of the beginning and end of the gastrointestinal tract. (Specifically, epithelium and glands of lips, cheeks, gums, part of the floor of the mouth and of the palate, and mucous membranes of nasal cavities and paranasal sinuses, as well as epithelium of the lower part of the anal canal, and terminal parts of the genital and urinary tracts.)

Tissues of the nervous system. (Specifically, the entire central nervous system including the retina; the peripheral nervous system, including sympathetic nerve cells and fibers, the medulla of the adrenal gland, and the neurilemmal sheath cells; and the sensory epithelium of the olfactory and auditory organs.)

Anterior part of the pituitary.

Lense of the eye, anterior epithelium layer of the cornea, muscles of the iris, and the outer layer of the eardrum.

Endoderm

Epithelium of the gastrointestinal tract, except its terminal parts, and the parenchyma of glands derived from it (liver, pancreas, thyroid, parathyroid, and thymus).

The lining epithelium of the Eustachian tube and of middle ear cavity, including inner layer of eardrum and lining of the mastoid air cells.

Lining epithelium of the larynx, trachea, bronchi, and alveoli.

Epithelium of the bladder, of most of the female urethra, and part of the male urethra, plus the glands derived from them (e.g., prostate), and lower part of the vagina.

Mesoderm

Epithelial derivatives:
Visceral and parietal linings of the peritoneal, pleural, and pericardial cavities.

Cortex of the adrenal gland.

Mesenchymal derivatives:
Connective tissue, cartilage and bone, including dentine. Myocardium and visceral musculature, including blood vessels. Endocardium and endothelium of blood vessels.

Lymph glands, lymph vessels, and spleen.

Blood cells.

Connective tissue sheaths of muscles, tendons, and nerve endings, and the synovial membranes of joints and bursae.

From this classification, it is clear that different organs and systems have a specific affinity for each other due to their common origin in one of the three primordial tissue layers. These affinities may eventually be found to be important factors governing the predictable direction of symptoms into ever deeper regions of the body as health degenerates.

Summary of Chapter 3

1. The human organism works as a totality always, whether performing its normal functions or defending itself from morbific stimuli.

2. Signs and symptoms of a morbific stimulus can be seen on one or more of the three levels of existence.

3. The organism always maintains a hierarchical importance of these three levels, and within each level. This can be represented by a three-dimensional diagram of cones.

4. The defense mechanism creates the best defense possible at any given moment, always attempting to limit symptoms to the most peripheral levels.

5. Three factors affect changes in the center of gravity of disturbance: hereditary strength or weakness of the defense mechanism, intensity of the morbific stimuli, and degree of interference by suppressive treatments.

6. The center of gravity of disturbance may change in one of two directions: up or down within a single plane, or from one plane to another.

7. There exist predictable pathways, with intermediate "stations" of defense, along which symptoms progress as general health deteriorates. These may be affected, in part, by affinities arising out of known embryological layers of development.

Annotated Bibliography for Chapter 3

1. Simeons, A.T.W., *Man's Presumptuous Brain* (London: Longmans, Green, 1960). An excellent and thorough description of the personality correlations to physical ailments. Mostly provides personality descriptions useful to a clinician; does not list research data supporting the observation.

2. Hinkle and Wolfe, "The Nature of Man's Adaptation to His Total Environment and the Relation of This to Illness," *Archives of Internal Medicine* 99: 442 (1957). A good survey of psychosomatic correlates to physical states. Does provide research data on subjects in whom attitudes were induced by hypnosis.

3. Eastwood, M., *The Relation Between Physical and Mental Illness* (Toronto: Univ. of Toronto Press, 1975). An up-to-date and extremely thorough review of research done in the entire field of psychosomatic medicine. Quotes both physiological and epidemiological studies.

4. World Health Organization, *Psychosomatic Disorders*, WHO Technical Report Series No. 275 (Geneva: WHO, 1964). An overview, and a reasonable perspective on correlates.

5. Raven, R. W., ed., *Cancer*, Vol. 4 (London: Butterworth, 1958). Describes direction of metastasis for individual types of cancers: p. 227 for breast cancer, p. 201 for prostate cancer, and p. 308 for lung cancer.

6. Cann and Cann, eds., *Current Diagnosis* (Philadelphia: W.B. Saunders, 1971).

7. Harvey, A.M., and Bordley, J., *Differential Diagnosis* (Philadelphia: W.B. Saunders, 1970).

8. Simeons, *Man's Presumptuous Brain.*

9. Hamilton, Boyd, and Mossman, *Human Embryology* (Baltimore: Williams & Wilkins, 1972), Chapter 7, p. 162.

Chapter 4

Vital Force as Seen by Modern Science

To this point, we have discussed at length the defense mechanism and some of the dynamics of its action, but we have not yet offered a precise definition of it. What is it? How can it be perceived? What precisely are the qualities which define its function in various circumstances?

From the cases so far discussed, it can be readily understood that the defense mechanism is not confined merely to the physical processes known so well by physiologists: the immune system, the reticuloendothelial system, the endocrine system, the sympathetic and parasympathetic nervous systems, or other mechanisms. These are indeed important functions of the defense mechanism on the physical plane, but they are not the only levels of its functioning. As we know, the defense mechanism acts on mental and emotional levels as well, in a highly systematic and orderly fashion. It functions as a totality, as an integrated whole, always defending the organism in the best possible manner at any given moment. Its function, insofar as possible, is to defend the inner and higher spiritual regions of the organism against the progression of disease.

What is this mechanism? This question has intrigued philosophers and healers throughout the ages. Centuries ago, the predominant point of view centered on the philosophy of "vitalism," which postulated the presence of a vital force possessing the intelligence and power to govern the myriads of processes involved in both health and disease. It seemed obvious to them that some force animates the human body, because the human organism is more than a mere sum of its physical components. Some animating force or principle enters the organism at the time of conception, guides all the functions of life, and then leaves at the time of death. What does occur at the moment of death? The organism is structurally intact, cells are busily functioning, chemical reactions are still proceeding, yet a sudden change occurs and the body begins to decompose! Reflection upon this fact renders the concept of "vital forces" not only understandable, but appealing.

The vital force idea has been described throughout history with remarkable similarity from writer to writer. The basic qualities ascribed to it are described in the following quote from Ostrander and Schroeder:

> The prime question for all the Westerners who've come up against this vital, or psychometric energy, for the past five hundred years is, what does it do?
>
> Paracelsus, the Renaissance alchemist and physician, reported this energy radiated from one person to another and could act at a distance. He believed it could purify the body and restore health, or could poison the body and cause disease. Dr. van Helmont, the seventeenth-century Flemish chemist and physician, believed the energy could enable one person to affect another at a distance. The famous German chemist, Baron von Reichenbach, said the energy could be stored and that substances could be charged with it. Unknown to Reichenbach, the Polynesian practitioners of Huna agreed that the vital energy could be transferred from humans to objects.[1]

The vital force is an influence which directs all aspects of life in the organism. It adapts to environmental influences, it animates the emotional life of the individual, it provides thoughts and creativity, and it conducts spiritual inspiration. The vitalistic school of thought believed, in fact, that this vital force connects the individual with the ultimate Unity of the universe. Clearly, the vital force includes a wide variety of functions, and that *aspect* of the vital force which establishes balance in states of disease we call the "defense mechanism." It is an integral part of the vital force, but it is only one of many functions; the defense mechanism, acting on all three levels of the organism, can be viewed as a tool of the vital force acting in the context of disease.

During the past 250 years, a materialistic view of the universe gained steadily in the thinking of industrialized societies, and the vitalistic concept consequently fell into disrepute. The world

---

1. S. Ostrander and L. Schroeder, *Psychic Discoveries Behind the Iron Curtain* (Englewood Cliffs, N.J.: Prentice-Hall, 1970), p. 69.

came to be viewed by science as being completely explainable in purely mechanical terms. Biological sciences also adopted this viewpoint; thus vast amounts of information regarding physical and chemical functioning of the human body have been amassed. These data are true and correct. They do not contradict the idea of the vital force at all. Physical and chemical mechanisms are merely tools of the vital force acting upon the physical plane of the organism.

In this century, vast changes have occurred in all endeavors of human life; perhaps the most dramatic were the advent of radically new concepts in the field of physics. Previously, Newtonian physics offered reproducible and predictable explanations of the mechanics underlying phenomena visible to our physical senses. Newtonian laws, although still applicable to the perceptual world, failed to explain observations in the atomic and subatomic realms of existence. New theories and laws had to be developed to explain phenomena on these levels. Einstein, Heisenberg, and others elucidated these phenomena by developing the new concepts now known as field theory, quantum theory, and relativity theory. The revolutionary effect that these concepts have had on modern thinking is described superbly by Fritjof Capra in *The Tao of Physics*:

> The classical, mechanistic world view was based on the notion of solid, indestructible particles moving in the void. Modern physics has brought about a radical revision of this picture. It has led not only to a completely new notion of particles, but has also transformed the classical concept of the void in a profound way. This transformation took place in the so-called field theories . . .
>
> The field concept was introduced in the nineteenth century by Faraday and Maxwell in their description of the forces between electric charges and currents. An electric field is a condition in the space around a charged body which will produce a force on any other charge in that space. Electric fields are thus created by charged bodies and their effects can only be felt by charged bodies. Magnetic fields are produced by charges in motion, i.e. by electric currents, and the magnetic forces resulting from them can be felt by other moving charges. In classical electrodynamics, the theory constructed by Faraday and Maxwell, the fields are primary physical entities which can be studied without any reference to material bodies. Vibrating electric and magnetic fields can travel through space in the form of radio waves, light waves, or other kinds of electromagnetic radiation.
>
> Relativity theory has made the structure of electrodynamics much more elegant by unifying the concepts of both charges and currents and electric and magnetic fields. Since all motion is relative, every charge can also appear as a current—in a frame of reference where it moves with respect to the observer—and consequently, its electric field can also appear as a magnetic field. In the relativistic formulation of

electrodynamics, the two fields are thus unified into a single electromagnetic field . . .

Matter and empty space—the full and the void—were the two fundamentally distinct concepts on which the atomism of Democritus and of Newton was based. In general relativity, these two concepts can no longer be separated . . .

Thus modern physics shows us once again that material objects are not distinct entities, but are inseparably linked to their environment; that their properties can only be understood in terms of their interaction with the rest of the world. According to Mach's principle, this interaction reaches out to the universe at large, to the distant stars and galaxies. The basic unity of the cosmos manifests itself, therefore, not only in the world of the very small but also in the world of the very large; a fact which is increasingly acknowledged in modern astrophysics and cosmology . . .

The unity and interrelation between a material object and its environment, which is manifest on the macroscopic scale in the general theory of relativity, appears in an even more striking form at the subatomic level. Here, the ideas of classical field theory are combined with those of quantum theory to describe the interactions between subatomic particles. Such a combination has not yet been possible for the gravitational interaction because of the complicated mathematical form of Einstein's theory of gravity; but the other classical field theory, electrodynamics, has been merged with quantum theory into a theory called 'quantum electrodynamics' which describes all electromagnetic interactions between sub-atomic particles. This theory incorporates both quantum theory and relativity theory. It was the first quantum-relativistic model of modern physics and is still the most successful.

The striking new feature of quantum electrodynamics arises from the combination of two concepts; that of the electromagnetic field, and that of photons as the particle manifestations of electromagnetic waves. Since photons are also electromagnetic waves, and since these waves are vibrating fields, the photons must be manifestations of electromagnetic fields. Hence the concept of a quantum field, that is, of a field which can take the form of quanta, or particles. This is indeed an entirely new concept which has been extended to describe all subatomic particles and their interactions, each type of particle corresponding to a different field. In these 'quantum field theories,' the classical contrast between the solid paticles and the space surrounding them is completely overcome. The quantum field is seen as the fundamental physical entity; a continuous medium which is present everywhere in space. Particles are merely local condensations of the field; concentrations of energy which come and go, thereby losing their individual character and dissolving into the underlying field. In the words of Albert Einstein:

"We may therefore regard matter as being constituted by the regions of space in which the field is extremely intense . . . There is no place in this new kind of physics both for the field and matter, for the field is the only reality." [2] (Emphasis mine.)

These new concepts in physics have changed our entire outlook on reality. If matter and energy are interchangeable, and indeed

---

2. Fritjof Capra, *The Tao of Physics* (New York: Bantam, 1977), pp. 207-211.

continuously and rapidly interchanging in the context of fields of varying intensity, whole new vistas open up for mankind. On the one hand, there is the possibility of using these new insights in previously unimagined ways for the benefit of the human race, or improper use of such energies may well lead to the destruction of the human race.

Despite the radical advances in physics, biological sciences have been slow to incorporate such concepts into their view of the human body. The body is still viewed as conforming to mechanistic physical and chemical laws, as in the Newtonian era of physics. In very recent years, however, scientists in Russia and the United States are beginning to investigate the electrodynamic fields involved in the human organism. This research is as yet quite tentative and preliminary, but its validity has aroused enough interest to motivate increasing numbers of scientists of very high caliber to enter the field. Thus there is a kind of return to the ancient vitalistic concept of living organisms, but this time with technology to measure precisely biological electrodynamic fields and their actions. Let us skim lightly over the exciting new information arising from this New Biology for what insights into the vital force it may provide.

The first striking evidence of electromagnetic fields associated with the human body came not from research but from observations of unusual cases in which the field was exaggerated beyond normal experience.

The first recorded case dates back to 1879. A nineteen-year-old girl, living in Ontario, Canada, after recovering from an unknown illness symptomized by convulsions, not only discharged electricity but also appeared to have electromagnetic properties. Any metal objects which she picked up would adhere to her open hand and would have to be forcibly pried away from her by another individual.

Nine years later, in Maryland, a sixteen-year-old boy with similar electromagnetic properties came to the attention of scientists at the Maryland College of Pharmacy because of his ability to suspend iron and steel rods, half an inch in diameter and twelve inches in length, from his fingertips. The boy could also lift a beaker of water filled with iron fillings merely by pressing three fingers against the side of the container. An audible clicking would occur when he pulled one of his fingers away.

Perhaps the most impressive of these cases was that of a fourteen-year-old girl in Missouri who, in 1895, suddenly seemed to turn into an electrical dynamo. When reaching for metal objects such as a pump handle her fingertips gave off sparks of such high voltage that she actually experienced pain. So strong was the electricity coursing through her body that a doctor who attempted to examine her was actually knocked onto his back, where he remained unconscious for several seconds. To the young lady's relief, her ability to shock eventually began to diminish and had vanished completely by the time she was twenty.[3]

One area of considerable interest involves research into the effects of electromagnetic fields upon the human organism; vast amounts of data have been accumulated, and a precise understanding of these effects is emerging. Even without referring directly to such research, however, we can look to our own experience and that of our friends and neighbors to recognize that electromagnetic fields have definite effects on us on all levels of existence. "Dr. A. Podshibyakin discovered that in the presence of close-to-the-ground magnetic storms the electrical potential of the skin rises. Some people seem to experience a foreboding of these invisible whirlwinds in varying degrees. Some experience these sensations twenty-four hours before the storm, others up to three or four days even before it registers on physical instruments."[4] Such environmental electromagnetic influences may be considered indirect evidence for the presence of a receptive electrodynamic field intimately connected with the human organism.

One of the most systematic researchers in the field of measuring bio-electric fields was Harold Saxton Burr, M.D., of Yale University. Using a high-impedance vacuum tube apparatus based on a Wheatstone bridge, Burr developed an electrode which could be inserted into living tissue for the purpose of measuring electrical potential, without significantly disturbing the electromagnetic field of the organism. Over a period of thirty years, he systematically studied organisms of progressively increasing complexity, from single cells to trees to human beings. Eventually it was possible to place the electrodes very near the surface of the organism without actually penetrating it, while continuing to get meaningful results. The story of this research is presented in Dr. Burr's book *The Fields of Life*, which is highly recommended for readers wishing to go more deeply into the details. Here is a brief description of his initial observations:

With our "navigational instruments"—a high impedance amplified and silver-silver chloride electrodes working through salt bridge in contact with living systems—we have been able to develop a technique which gives reliable results. With

---

3. S. Krippner and D. Rubin, eds., *The Kirlian Aura* (New York: Anchor, 1974), p. 29.
4. Ibid., p. 147.

this it soon became clear that every living system possesses an electrical field of great complexity. *This can be measured with considerable certainty and accuracy and shown to have correlations with growth and development,* degeneration and regeneration, *and the orientation of component parts in the whole system. Perhaps more interesting than any one thing, this field exhibits remarkable stability through the growth and development of an egg.*[5] (Emphasis mine.)

Dr. Leonard Ravitz, a close colleague of Dr. Burr's, corroborates and expands upon the implications of his research in this statement:

As Dr. Burr has described in the preceding pages, instruments have found what he and Dr. Northrop postulated over thirty years ago. Countless experiments have demonstrated that the electric fields they discovered serve basic functions, controlling growth and morphogenesis, maintenance and repair of living things. Naturally, these differ from the alternating-current electric output of the brain and heart, as well as from the epiphenomenal skin-resistance, serving rather as an electronic matrix to keep the corporeal form in shape.

Obviously such studies throw a wet blanket on scientific dogmas currently in vogue, which still assert that the special human body is principally a chemical product deriving from mystical activities of the DNA molecule. However disquieting, chemistry represents a scalar property—the downhill flow of energy—requiring some vector force to give it direction. According to Dr. Henry Margenau, Eugene Higgins Professor of Physics and Natural Philosophy at Yale University, of all the known forces it is only electro-magnetic, or electro-dynamic, fields which can act as signposts to direct continuous chemical, metabolic, or molecular transformations in the system—fields which, in fact, appear to underwrite the development of structure even prior to any known chemical reactions.[6]

After thirty years of painstaking, systematic research into the subject, these are the conclusions of Dr. Burr:

The following theory may then be formulated. The pattern or organization of any biological system is established by a complex electro-dynamic field which is in part determined by its atomic physio-chemical components and which in part determines the behavior and orientation of those components. This field is electrical in the physical sense and by its properties relates the entities of the biological system in a characteristic pattern and is itself, in part, a result of the existence of those entities. It determines and is determined by the components.

More than establishing pattern, it must maintain pattern in the midst of a physio-chemical flux. Therefore, it must regulate and control living things. It must be the mechanism, the outcome of whose activity is wholeness, organization, and continuity.[7] (Emphasis Dr. Burr's.)

---

5. H.S. Burr, *The Fields of Life* (New York: Ballantine, 1972), p. 43.

6. Ibid., p. 174.

7. Ibid., p. 29.

While Dr. Burr was doing his work on bio-electric fields, a husband-wife team of scientists in Russia, Semyon and Valentina Kirlian, were developing another technique. The electrodynamic field permeating and surrounding all objects, whether living or nonliving, could be visualized photographically by exposing film to the object in the midst of a high intensity electromagnetic field. This method, known variously as "Kirlian photography" or "high-voltage photography," has probably done more than any other observations to spark an incredible amount of investigation on the bioelectromagnetic field the world over, especially in the United States.

The work of the Kirlians first became widely known in the United States because of the graphic description given in Ostrander and Schroeder's *Psychic Discoveries Behind the Iron Curtain:*

> Basically, photography with high frequency electrical fields involves a specially constructed high frequency spark generator or oscillator that generated 75,000 to 200,000 electrical oscillations per second. The generator can be connected to various clamps, plates, optical instruments, microscopes, or electron microscopes. The object to be investigated (finger, leaf, etc.) is inserted between the clamps along with photo paper. The generator is switched on and a high frequency field is created between the clamps which apparently causes the object to radiate some sort of bio-luminescence onto the photo paper. A camera isn't necessary for the photography process.
>
> The very first photographs were a "window on the unknown," say the Kirlians. A leaf torn from a tree, when placed in the field of a high frequency current, revealed a world of myriad dots of energy. Around the edges of the leaf there were turquoise and reddish-yellow patterns of flares coming out of specific channels of the leaf. A human finger placed in the high frequency field and photographed, showed up like a complex topographical map. There were lines, points, craters of light and flares. Some parts of the finger looked like a carved jack-o'-lantern with a glowing light inside.
>
> But the photographs only showed static images. Soon the Kirlians had developed a special optical instrument so they could directly observe the phenomenon in motion. Kirlian held his hand under the lens and switched on the current. And then, a fantastic world of the unseen opened before the husband and wife team.
>
> The hand itself looked like the Milky Way in a starry sky. Against a background of blue an gold, something was taking place in the hand that looked like a firework display. Multi-colored flares lit up, then sparks, twinkles, flashes. Some lights glowed steadily like Roman candles, others flashed out then dimmed . . .[8]

The dramatic beauty of the photographs taken by this technique excited researchers everywhere and many visits were made to Russia to acquire blueprints and technical information on the

---

8. Ostrander and Schroeder, *Psychic Discoveries*, p. 199.

equipment involved. Since then, masses of photographs produced in laboratories of the United States have found their way into journals and popular magazines to such an extent that nearly everyone is familiar with them. The question naturally arose, what do these lights and colors really represent? Are they actual images of the "human aura," as some wish to believe, or are they merely artifactual phenomena of no significance? One of the most careful researchers in the field is William A. Tiller, Professor in the Materials Science and Engineering Department at Stanford University, who systemically defined the parameters of the observations from his detailed knowledge of materials science and came to the following conclusions about the phenomenon:

> One has only to casually read the work of Loeb to realize that we are dealing here with the corona discharge phenomena called streamers. In this process, a few electrons are first produced in the interelectrode space either by cosmic ray events, U.V. radiation, or field emission from the cathode. These electrons are accelerated by the field and ionize the air molecules yielding an exponential growth in the number of electrons and positive ions, i.e., an avalanche. The electrons sweep quickly toward the anode (positive side) and the cluster of positive ions moves somewhat more slowly towards the cathode (negative side). When the positive ion cluster in the air gap reaches a critical density, it strongly attracts the electrons so that a large number of recombination events occur and photons of light are generated to such a degree that the cluster of positive ions is brightly luminous and travels at speeds about 1% the speed of light (about 10^7 to 10^8 cm/sec) . . .
>
> As a result of the driving field on the electrode, we should anticipate some type of energy coupling with the cells of the object. This, in turn, may lead to energy emissions from the cells which could influence the ionization properties of the gas and thus alter the quantitative details of the electron avalanche process. Since skin is strongly piezoelectric, an electrical stimulus will generate a mechanical resonance and vice versa. We do hear mechanical noise in the high audio range during the discharge. Conventional secondary emission events due to impacting photons, ions and electrons will lead to photoelectron and secondary electron emission. Changes in mental or emotional states should change the electron state population in the finger and thus reveal itself via altered emission processes.[9] (Emphasis mine.)

In the course of research by several workers, many common parameters which might be expected to cause these discharges were ruled out. Fingers were photographed in varying states of vasodilation (confirmed by plethysmography), varying tempera-

---

9. W.A. Tiller, "Proceedings of the A.R.E. Medical Symposium on New Horizons in Healing," Phoenix, Arizona, Jan. 1974, pp. 6 and 12.

tures (confirmed by thermisters), varying states of skin conductance (confirmed by GSR measurements), and varying degrees of sweat. All such parameters were found to have no effect on the Kirlian discharges.

The Kirlian technique, of course, sparked many similar devices and studies in the Soviet Union, and interesting observations were demonstrated to further amplify knowledge of the effect:

Research on force field detectors is being done in Leningrad at the Laboratory for Biological Cybernetics in the University of Leningrad Physiology Department. The research group led by Dr. Vasiliev's successor, Dr. Pavel Gulyaiev, uses extremely sensitive high-resistance detection electrodes to chart the force field or "electrical aura," as they call it.

The Soviets report that muscular reactions which accompany even a thought can be detected and measured and that the signals in the electrical aura reveal a great deal about the state of the organism. Dr. Gulyaiev feels that this force field may be the means by which communication between fish, insects, and animals occurs.

The Soviet research is directed toward using the force field detectors for medical diagnosis and PK. The signals generated by a thought could be picked up at a distance, amplified, and used to move objects.

Dr. Gulyaiev's "electro-auragram" device is so sensitive it can measure the electrical field of a nerve. The nerves of a frog, for instance, have an electrical field of twenty-four centimeters. A nerve from the human heart has a field of ten centimeters. The electrical emanations around the body change according to health, mood, character. The distance at which this field can be measured depends on the amount of tension generated. (See Parapsychology Newsletter, *Jan.-Feb. 1969, May-June 1969).*

The Sergeyev detectors apparently measure the human force field at a distance of four yards from the body.[10]

Another fascinating aspect of the Soviet research involves observations on acupuncture points. Acupuncture is believed by the Chinese to be a technique whereby the flow of vital force through the body can be modified, channeled, and balanced by the insertion of needles at specific points. It is considered to be a therapy directly affecting the field of the vital force, and therefore the Soviet observations, though still preliminary, offer interesting speculations for further research:

There remains one last area of preliminary study to be reported: the possibility of a correlation between radiation photography and acupuncture. This is a subject discussed by T.C. Inyushin (1969) at length in a recent symposium. This research

---

10. Ostrander and Schroeder, *Psychic Discoveries*, p. 393.

suggests that acupuncture points become visible through Kirlian photography. Using our apparatus, we have reached no final conclusions regarding this claim. However, in working with a skilled acupuncturist, we have observed dramatic differences in the corona before and after treatment in which a needle, or needles, were inserted into one or more acupuncture points. But, again, this is not an invariable effect; rather, it depends on the specific acupuncture point being treated. With certain points, pierced with a needle, there is no discernible change in the aura, but with other points (usually related to specific physical complaints), an increased brightness and clarity of the corona is obtained. Thus, although our research has only begun, we have learned that the insertion of the needle—with the ensuing pain—does not necessarily cause a change in the photographed emanations. This seems to rule out pain as a possible answer to the question as to what these photographs reveal.[11]

Now that some techniques have been developed to observe the electrodynamic field of the body, and some of the parameters of the field are beginning to be elucidated, the logical question for our purpose arises: What connection does this field have to health and disease, and especially to the workings of the vital force in its function as defense mechanism? Fortunately, there are some beginning observations bearing on this question; thus far the research seems to confirm a correlation between changes in the electrodynamic field and changes in emotional and physical states in both health and disease.

Again, the Russians have made some intriguing observations which tend to indicate that the phenomena they are measuring do indeed produce effects similar to what we have discussed in previous chapters. Following is an account of the Kirlian experience with diagnosing illness in leaves of plants; after testing some leaves provided by the chairman of a major scientific institute, the Kirlians thought something was wrong with their equipment because they could not get certain of the leaves to conform to the usual pattern seen in the others, so they worked through the night to correct the problem, only to be told later:

In the morning, weary and worried, they showed their troubling results to their celebrated scientist guest. To their surprise, his face lit up with delight. "You've found it!" he said excitedly.

The two exhausted inventors forgot their fatigue as the botanist explained, "Both leaves were torn from the same species of plant all right. But one of these plants had already been contaminated with a serious plant disease. You've found this out immediately! There is absolutely nothing on the plant or this leaf to indicate

---

11. Krippner and Rubin, *The Kirlian Aura*, p. 70.

that it has been infected and will soon die. No tests on the actual plant or the leaf show anything wrong with it. With high-frequency photography you've diagnosed illness in the plant ahead of time! . . ."

Soon institutes were bringing the Kirlians hundreds of "green patients"—leaves of grapevines, apple trees, tobacco and so on. In every case, the Kirlians could establish whether or not the plant was ill long before there were any physical pathological changes in the leaves or the plants, by studying the leaf's energy counterpart body in high frequency photos.[12]

On another occasion, this effect was observed on Semyon Kirlian himself. While calibrating his equipment, he tested his own hand in the machine, but he was unable to get the usual pattern of emanations no matter how hard he tried. His wife, however, was able to get the machine to work perfectly. Shortly thereafter, Semyon fell ill with an acute ailment and realized that he had seen the change in his electrodynamic field prior to the actual onset of the illness. Since then, further studies have confirmed this observation:

Kirlian and Kirlian (1959) note that when a person is in poor mental and or physical health, the photographs taken of that person reflect changes in his field (e.g., in diameter, in color, in regularity). This finding related to Presman's statement (1970:6) that, in the living organism, systems that handle information are ordinarily shielded from interference from external electromagnetic fields, but in pathological states the barriers break down and more of an influence is exerted by the external forces (e.g., solar flares, lightning discharges).

Lewin (1951) has noted that the ordinary boundaries do not function well in pathological states.[13]

They have found that a withered leaf showed almost no flares and that the clots barely move. As the leaf gradually dies, its self-emissions also decrease correspondingly until there is no emission from the dead leaf. Likewise, the finger of a human body, dead for several days, exhibits no distinctive self-emissions. The self-emission of living things seems to be a direct measure of the life processes occurring within their system.[14]

Working with Harold Saxton Burr's technique, Louis Langman, M.D., of the Department of Obstetrics and Gynecology, New York University College of Medicine and Bellevue Hospital, studied large numbers of women in the outpatient clinics by inserting electrodes near the cervix and on the external abdominal wall, and recording the potential differences. This data was then

---

12. Ostrander and Schroeder, *Psychic Discoveries*, p. 202.

13. Krippner and Rubin, *The Kirlian Aura*, p. 90.

14. Ibid., p. 102.

correlated with the subsequent clinical course of the patients, with the following results:

In the more recent paper, the electro-metric observations in 428 women were reported. In 75 patients with known cancer of the female generative tract, 98.7% showed the cervix to be consistently electro-negative to the ventral abdominal wall. *In 353 patients suffering from* non-malignant *conditions 289 showed the cervix to be positive with respect to the abdomen (81.9%)* . . .[15]

The findings in patients who have had follow-up electro-metric studies indicate that a reversal in polarity from negative to positive occurs after total hysterectomy for intra-epithelial carcinoma of the cervix. This reversal is not found in cases with more advanced stages of cervical carcinoma (Stages II and III), who have had either a radical operation or radium and X-ray therapy. Following a total hysterectomy, women in whom a diagnosis of squamous metaplasia of the cervix had been made pre-operatively, show a similar reversal in polarity.

These findings suggest that the electro-metric correlates result from causes inherent in the tissue involved and if the involved tissue can be removed in its entirety reversal in potential occurs. Conversely reversal does not occur when all the tissue involved is not removed by operation.[16] (Emphasis Dr. Langman's.)

Leonard Ravitz, M.D., a distinguished American psychiatrist affiliated with several universities and professional societies, also worked closely with Dr. Burr on several clinical studies. Psychotic patients were observed during their excited states, during quiescent states, and after successful treatment. Very striking results were consistently obtained on large numbers of patients. Particularly interesting to us were results correlating changes on the mental plane with changes in the electrodynamic field:

With regard to human experimental studies in which subjects serve as their own controls, one of the initial approaches compared shifts in individual states before and after hypnosis along with effects of hypnosis as recorded and studied. Hypnotic and posthypnotic changes were then compared with corresponding field alterations. Disquietudes of all sorts induced in so doing have been studied electrometrically and compared with those arising spontaneously both in waking and in hypnotic states. Further, changes have been measured before, during, and after various drugs and placebos, and proper dosages to achieve effects correlated with field intensities and polarities at given times. Similar experiments have likewise been conducted on effects of subjecting controls and patients to several therapeutic procedures.

In brief, subjects in trance states, induced or spontaneous, show a smoothing of the field recording and usually a slow decrease, although sometimes an increase, in

---

15. Burr, *The Fields of Life*, p. 153.

16. Burr, *The Fields of Life*, p. 159.

intensity. At trance termination dramatic voltage shifts occur, the time before the record returns to that of the waking state depending on the rapidity with which the subject returns to the waking state. Subjects who have been aroused from trance states, but who actually are only partially aroused or return to the trance state though superficially appearing "awake," show field correlates with such state changes, either by using pen-writing photo-electric recorders or cathode-ray oscillographs attached to the millivolt-meters, now commercially manufactured. (This was first publicly demonstrated at the Second Annual Scientific Assembly of the American Society of Clinical Hypnosis in 1959.) Waking states show almost continuous, slow variations, usually at higher intensities than during hypnosis.

It follows that hypnotic depth can now be defined electro-metrically, the "depth," however, having nothing whatever to do with abilities to develop various complex hypnotic phenomena.[17] (Emphasis mine.)

William A. Tiller of Stanford University has also used systematic Kirlian photography studies to demonstrate the relationship between mental and emotional changes and the electromagnetic field emanations. Here, he describes results of others and himself:

These investigators have been using a technique similar to that of Moss and have been studying the manifested energy changes on Kirlian photographs both before and after treatment of a group of schizophrenics and a group of alcoholics. They have observed that, before treatment, both of these groups show a marked spatial fragmentation or annihilation of large portions of the normal emission from the finger pad. In addition, the pattern of emission from the contact portion of the finger pad appears quite chaotic. As a result of successful treatment, as indicated by conventional psychiatric criteria, one observes (a) the filling in of the emission pattern around the finger pad, (b) an enhancement of manifested energy intensity and (c) a more orderly and coherent fingerprint pattern on the contact portion of the photographs. They have also noted marked pattern changes associated with respiratory infections . . .

In one recent experiment, we studied a subject's finger pad while he changed his mental state. He changed state every two minutes, and we took a high-voltage picture with him consciously trying to maintain constant finger pressure on the transparent electrode. The sequence was (a) normal, (b) State 1, (c) State 2, (d) State 3, (e) rest, and repeat sequence again and again. The results indicate that, indeed, the change in mental state manifests as a change in emission pattern. Since the rest state result corresponds more closely to the normal state result than that of either States 1, 2, or 3, and since two minutes does not seem like a long enough time for skin surface chemical changes to have occurred, we can deduce that other physiological effects are not important here and that we are monitoring a real internal state change.[18]

17. Ibid., p. 176.
18. Tiller, "A.R.E. Medical Symposium," p. 17.

71

So, it can be seen that some very exciting observations are being made by modern biological scientists, that the results are intriguing enough to entice many researchers into the field, and that the results thus far seem to confirm the statements about the vital force and the defense mechanism presented herein.

The point of this quick survey of research is not to try to prove the existence and functioning of the vital force in detail, for the research is still too preliminary and unsophisticated for the purposes of a clinician. Nevertheless, these observations point to a direction which may be analogous to the changes which occurred in physics earlier in this century; if progress in such research continues as it seems to promise, we may well see the dawning of a new era in medicine—an era of *energy medicine*.

Let us conclude this chapter by returning to the very astute observations of a homeopathic physician of the nineteenth century, J.T. Kent. Dr. Kent describes the qualities of the vital force, which he terms "simple substance," in profound detail. His thoughtful insights are liable to be confirmed and reconfirmed by research for many decades to come.

A) Simple substance is endowed with formative intelligence, *i.e., it intelligently operates and forms the economy of the whole animal, vegetable and mineral kingdoms . . . The "simple substance" gives to everything its own type of life, gives it distinction, gives it identity whereby it differs from all other things. The crystal of the earth has its own association, its own identity; it is endowed with a simple substance that will establish its identity from everything in the animal kingdom, everything in the mineral kingdom. This is due to the formative intelligence of simple substance . . . Plants grow in fixed forms. So it is with man from his beginning to his end; there is a continuous influx into man from his cause. Hence, man and all forms are subject to the laws of influx . . .*

B) This substance is subject to changes; *in other words, it may be flowing in order or disorder, may be sick or normal . . .*

C) It pervades the entire material substance without disturbing or replacing it . . .

D) It dominates and controls the body it occupies . . . By it are kept in order all functions and the perpetuation of the forms and proportions of every animal, plant, and mineral. All operation that is possible is due to the simple substance and by it the very universe itself is kept in order. It not only operates every material substance, but it is the cause of cooperation of all things . . .

72

E) The simple substance may exist as simple, compound, or com-
plex... *In considering simple substance we cannot think of time, place or
space because we are not in the realm of mathematics, nor the restricted
measurements of the world of space and time, we are in the realm of simple
substance. It is only finite to think of place and time.* Quantity *cannot be
predicated of simple substance, only* quality in degrees of fineness.

F) The simple substance also has adaptation... *That the individual
has an adaptation to his environment is not questioned... The dead body
cannot. When we reason from within out we see that the simple substance
adapts itself to its surroundings... and thus the human body is kept in a
state of order, in the cold or in the heat, in the wet and damp, and under all
circumstances.*

G) We see also that this vital substance when in a natural state is
constructive; *it keeps the body continuously constructed and reconstructed.
But when the opposite is true, when the vital force from any cause with-
draws from the body, we see that the forces that are in the body being
turned loose are destructive.*[19]

These words of an American physician, expressed twenty
years before the promulgation of Einstein's field theories, are
truly an amazing feat of deduction and insight. It is doubtful if a
more complete and concise description of the elemental qualities
of the vital force (and therefore of the defense mechanism) has
ever been written.

To summarize what we have discovered thus far it can be
stated with confidence that there is a vital force animating all
levels of the human organism, one aspect of which is the defense
mechanism, and that this vital force possesses all of the qualities
being discovered by modern research into biological electrodynamic fields—and more!

Summary of Chapter 4

1. The defense mechanism, acting on all levels of the organism, functions as an integrated whole and systematically defends
the inner and spiritual regions in the best possible manner.

2. The known physiological and chemical mechanisms of the
body are tools of the defense mechanism.

3. The human organism is more than the mere sum of its

---

19. J. T. Kent, *Lectures on Homeopathic Philosophy* (Richmond, California: North Atlantic
Books, 1979), Chapter 8.

physical components, a fact most dramatically evident at the moments of conception and death. From this is surmised the presence of an intelligent "vital force" which animates, guides, and balances the organism on all levels in both health and disease.

4. The defense mechanism is that aspect of the vital force responding specifically in the diseased state.

5. New concepts in physics are beginning to be reflected in biological science, particularly in the study of electrodynamic fields of the human body. Instruments now exist that can directly measure the electromagnetic field of the body, and these measurements are clinically useful in diagnosing cancer, infectious diseases, and in staging levels of hypnotic trance.

6. Kirlian photography is a dramatic technique whereby the electromagnetic field can be directly visualized. This phenomenon has also been demonstrated to be not merely artifactual in nature. Characteristic changes can be seen in altered mental or emotional states, and in health and disease.

7. Despite the advances being made in bio-electromagnetic field research, existing evidence has a long way to go before it can be considered "proof" of the actions of the vital force.

8. J.T. Kent's lucid description of the vital force ("simple substance") characterizes it as having formative intelligence, being subject to changes, pervading the material substance without replacing it, creating order in the body, belonging to the realm of quality rather than quantity (the realm of degrees of fineness), being adaptable, and being constructive.

Chapter 5

The Vital Force in Disease

THE IDEA that there is an intelligent vital force animating the human organism, and that this vital force may be a field simiar or analogous to the electromagnetic field, opens new possibilities for therapeutics which can truly lead toward an era of Energy Medicine. Understanding the laws and principles involved in such an idea can be of vast usefulness to practitioners and the patients being served by them. In this chapter, I shall present the hypothesis that the vital force behaves in an analogous way to the electromagnetic fields and perhaps conforms to standard concepts in physics pertaining to those fields. I shall then attempt to describe the implications of such an idea in the therapeutic context.

Basic Concepts of Physics

To begin with, some basic terminology used in standard physics must be presented. This terminology will be described only briefly; for further details, one needs merely to refer to any standard textbook of physics.

As described by Fritjof Capra in the previous chapter, particles and waves are completely interchangeable at the atomic and subatomic levels. The electrodynamic field is the interrelationship of particles which are affecting each other through charge and movement. These relationships are definable in terms of oscillations or vibrations. As electrons move around the nucleus of an atom, for instance, the motion can be described as a "wave," from the point of view of an external observer. As it circles around the nucleus, the electron appears to an outside observer first to move in one direction, then it appears to move back to its original location. In Figure 5, we see a typical waveform characterized first by motion in a "positive" direction, then in a "negative" direction. One complete wave is called a *cycle*.

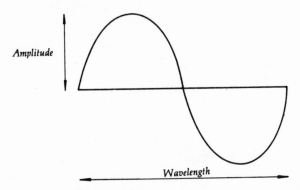

Figure 5: A diagram representing one complete cycle. The height is called the "amplitude" and is one measure of the force of the wave. The horizontal length is called the "wavelength." Because the speed of propagation is constant, wavelength and frequency are interchangeable terms.

The concept of waves is familiar to all of us. In water, a wave is characterized by motion of molecules upward (to a crest) and downward (to a trough), and back again. A piece of paper floating on the surface will remain in the same spot as the wave passes, yet the wave itself moves on. A pebble thrown into a pond transmits force to the water which results in a wave radiating outward from the point of impact. The piece of paper remains stationary, while the force of the wave is nevertheless radiated throughout the pond. Another familiar example is sound waves; sound waves cause air molecules to move back and forth in relation to each other, thus propagating the force of the sound over a distance. Electromagnetic waves transmit force as well, but these waves can be transmitted even in a vacuum and over great distances.

The speed of propagation of such waves is characteristic for the type of substance it is traveling in. Sound waves at sea level travel at a constant speed, the speed of sound. Electromagnetic waves travel at the speed of light.

There are three basic parameters defining a waveform: frequency (measured commonly in cycles per second), wavelength (measured commonly in centimeters or meters), and amplitude (measured in units of force).

The "frequency" of vibration is described as the number of waves, or "cycles," per unit of time. Thus we may see a vibration rate of one cycle/second, or a million cycles/second. Since the speed of propagation is constant, any given frequency has a corresponding "wavelength," the actual length of each individual wave. When physicists or electronic technicians talk about propagated waves, they use the terms "frequency" and "wavelengths" interchangeably.

The concept of different frequencies, or vibration rates, is immediately comprehensible to everyone in terms of music. Each note has a specific pitch, which is its frequency; when the frequency changes, the pitch changes. Vibration rates range from the very low (as seen in a bridge rumbling up and down during an earthquake) to the very high (as in light, X-rays, microwaves, etc). The human ear detects a certain range of frequencies, and the eye a different range.

The height of a wave is called "amplitude." Amplitude is one measure of the actual force contained within the wave. The higher the amplitude, the greater the force; the smaller the amplitude, the less force exists in the wave. This can be seen easily by the difference in the force of waves in water created by throwing a pebble into a pond, compared to throwing a boulder into a pond. The boulder transmits greater force to the water, and the amplitude of the wave is proportionately greater. Similarly, comparing two electromagnetic waves of equal frequency, the one with greater amplitude contains and transmits more force.

Conversely, of two electromagnetic waves with equal amplitude, the one with the higher frequency contains and transmits greater force. For this reason, microwaves are more powerful than lower frequency radio waves of the same amplitude. Therefore, as one lowers the frequency of a wave (without changing its amplitude), its energy level is diminished; if the frequency can be increased, more energy is packed into the wave.

Each substance has a characteristic frequency or range of frequencies at which it most easily vibrates. A homogeneous substance such as a crystal, or a metal tuning fork, will vibrate strongly at only one frequency, called its "resonant frequency," and less strongly at its harmonic frequencies. If we strike a middle C tuning fork across the room from another middle C tuning fork, the second will begin vibrating in resonance with the first. If we strike a high C tuning fork across the room from a middle C tuning fork, the second will vibrate at a reduced amplitude, but it will still vibrate. Thus we see that vibrations can have an effect at a distance and even at different vibration levels, but the effect will be harmonious only through the principle of *resonance* (see Figure 6).

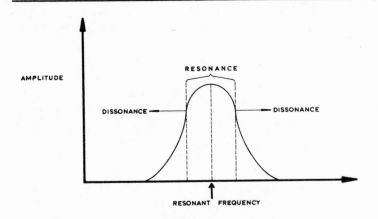

Figure 6: A graph demonstrating the relationships between the resonant frequency and harmony. At the resonant frequency, the energy or force of the system is maximized in a state of harmony. The farther one deviates from the resonant frequency, the more dissonance occurs with a simultaneous decrease of energy.

If a substance is nonhomogeneous, such as a rock, or an organ of the human body, then each component of it will tend to vibrate at its own resonant frequency, but the resulting activity of the whole will not be readily recognizable to our senses. This does not mean that outside vibrations are having no effect, but merely that the effect is not detectable to our senses.

Now, considering the vital force of the human organism in terms of electrodynamic vibrations obviously involves a tremendous degree of complexity. The resultant vibration of such a complex organism is undoubtedly highly complicated, changing from moment to moment not only in frequency but also in regularity of frequency and in amplitude as well. This is why the vital force level of the human organism is considered the *dynamic plane,* affecting all levels of the being at once and with varying degrees of harmony and strength. It is a highly complex, fluid, flexible, and energetic process, simultaneously responding to and affecting the surrounding environment. Despite this complexity, however, there are laws and principles governing both morbific and therapeutic influences on such a system—laws and principles which are grounded in concepts of resonance, harmony, reinforcement, and interference. The whole organism, and any component of it, can be strengthened or weakened depending upon the degree of harmony, resonance, and force of the morbific or therapeutic influence applied to it. Again, this is why it is so important for any practitioner of "energy medicine" to clearly comprehend the fundamental laws and principles involved in such influences.

The Defense Mechanism

When the organism is exposed to a stimulus, whether morbific or beneficial, the first event which occurs is an alteration of the vibration rate on the dynamic plane. For most routine stimuli, to which we all are exposed constantly, the dynamic plane is able to respond and adjust with no noticeable effect on the mental, emotional, or physical levels.

If, however, the strength of the stimulus is stronger than the strength of the vital force, the defense mechanism is called into play to counteract the stimulus. If this were not so, any powerful stimulus would alter the state of the entire organism without defense, and death would rapidly ensue. There is a certain threshold in any given individual below which the dynamic plane handles stimuli without visible changes, and above which the defense mechanism generates processes *which are perceived by the individual as symptoms on one or more levels.*

Before actual symptoms develop, there is a *latent period* during which the defense mechanism begins to adjust to the effect of the stimulus. The change on the dynamic plane, of course, is instantaneous, but varying amounts of time may pass before the defense mechanism generates symptoms expressed on physical, emotional, or mental levels. Depending on circumstances, this latent period may be hours, days, weeks, or even months. In an acute illness, the latent period is known as the "incubation period," which ranges from hours or days for influenzas and bacterial infections, to several weeks in gonorrhea, and up to three months for rabies and infectious hepatitis.[1] Less widely recog-

---

1. In the instance of latent periods of infectious disease, it might be argued that the time lapse is merely during the cultivation and growth of the microorganisms. This is correct, but it gives only a superficial explanation of the entire phenomenon. In reality, if the

nized is the occurrence of a latent period in chronic disease. A person may undergo an emotional stress and then develop asthma after six months, or cancer after an even longer period of time.

The initial instantaneous change in vibration level also alters the person's susceptibility to further noxious influences of the same type. For example, if a person is exposed to a virus, the vibration rate is immediately altered, and the person will then not be susceptible to invasion by other viruses of similar type and virulence; symptoms may not emerge until the latent period has passed, but the organism nevertheless is "immune" to other similar viruses during the latent period. This phenomenon occurs because the resonant frequency has been changed by the initial stimulus, rendering the organism susceptible only to new morbific influences on the new resonant frequency.

Such a change in susceptibility can occur, of course, not only by exposure to viruses and bacteria, but also by emotional shocks, changes in environmental temperature or humidity, and especially by treatment with allopathic drugs.

The best way to illustrate this principle is to present a case example which is very common in the practice of any physician. Let us consider a patient who has contracted a staphylococcal infection in the lungs. From the moment of onset of the infection, the vibration rate (the "resonant frequency") changes somewhat, and the patient is "immune" to invasion by other similar organisms. The defense mechanism calls into action the normal mechanisms of fever, cough, chills, prostration, etc., and the patient goes to the doctor. Tests are done and reveal an elevated white blood cell count, antibody production against staphylococcus, an abscess on X-ray, and a culture which grows Staphylococcus sensitive to a wide variety of antibiotics. The patient is given one of these antibiotics, and promptly the fever decreases, the energy begins to return, and the quality of sputum improves.

If this patient's defense mechanism is strong, it eventually reestablishes an equilibrium and corrects the changes in vibration rate caused by the bacteria and the antibiotic. If, on the other hand, the defense mechanism is not quite strong enough, a different course of events occurs. The vibration rate does not return to normal and is altered even more deeply by the antibiotic. After a week or so, there occurs a pleural reaction with pain and effusion.

organism does not maintain a susceptibility to the microorganism, it will not be allowed to thrive in the body.

The doctors recognize that a "complication" has occurred, and draw out of the pleural space some fluid which now reveals a new bacteria, Proteus, which is sensitive to fewer antibiotics than was the Staphylococcus. The reason this occurred is that the new resonant frequency of the patient enabled susceptibility to a new and more serious organism.

A second antibiotic is then given, again altering the vibration rate of the defense mechanism. Gradually the patient feels a little better, the pain subsides somewhat, and it appears that recovery will ensue. Still, however, nothing has been done to appreciably strengthen the defense mechanism. On the contrary, two bacterial infections and two courses of antibiotics have weakened it. Finally, the effusion increases again, and it is found that an even more serious organism, Bacillus pyocyanaeus, is present and that it is insensitive to all known antibiotics. To the allopathic physician, the only alternative left is surgical drainage and perhaps lobectomy; the case is now considered very serious and likely to die in any event.

Such cases as this are far from rare; every physician has a wealth of experience of cases which progress in exactly this way. When referring such a patient to a specialist, it is commonplace to comment on the predilection of such a patient to develop "complications"; even allopathic physicians talk in terms of systemic weakness in such cases, and by experience they have learned to expect the worst.

Since the problem is fundamentally not one of a particular microorganism but rather a weakness of the defense mechanism of the patient, antibiotic therapy cannot be expected to work in such a case. The antibiotic is a further noxious stimulus with which the defense mechanism must cope, and the vibratory level inevitably progresses deeper and deeper. Instead, a therapy must be applied which strengthens the resonant frequency of the entire organism. Once this occurs, the defense mechanism can function effectively, and progress will proceed in reverse order through previous vibratory levels; i.e., the cultures will show Bacillus pyocyanaeus, then Proteus, and then Staphylococcus before the patient can be discharged from the hospital feeling well. Such is the experience of homeopathic physicians who are wise enough not to give antibiotics with each new microbe, but instead allow the strengthened defense mechanism to complete its process.

As has been mentioned, the continued suppression (by inappropriate therapies) of the defense mechanisms of large numbers

81

of our populations leads to progressive weakness. It is for this reason that we see an increasing incidence of heart disease, neurological disorders, cancer, psychosis, and violence in society; it is also the reason why we see an upsurge in microbial epidemics such as Legionnaire's disease and others which are insensitive to all known antibiotics. This is not merely a matter of bacterial mutation, but a consequence of progressive weakening of the defense mechanisms of people through inappropriate therapy.

The principle of resonance renders the organism susceptible to influence on basically only one level at any given moment. In Figure 7, we see a simplified diagram of a spectrum of resonant frequencies. Each level represents, for example, susceptibility to a particular range of diseases. If a person treated on Level B for gonorrhea receives antibiotics, his resonant frequency changes; over time, he will become susceptible to illnesses on, say, Level C. While experiencing symptoms of illness on this level, he will not acquire gonorrhea, even though he may be exposed. This is true also of people suffering from long-term chronic diseases. If, however, such a person were to be treated homeopathically, the vibration rate would again move back down the scale, and the patient may well become susceptible to gonorrhea once again. To the superficial observer, this renewed susceptibility to gonorrhea might seem to be a sign of deteriorating health, whereas in fact it is a sign of progress!

Thus a person can be "immune" to illness on Level B for two reasons: either he is *too sick*, with a vibration rate corresponding to the deeper levels of resonance; or he is *too healthy*, with a vibration rate at the very bottom of the diagram.

This principle of susceptibility also explains a phenomenon observed frequently by careful clinical observers. Schizophrenics get acute ailments only very rarely, even when exposed to very virulent organisms. The more psychotic a person is, the less likely he will be to acquire an acute ailment. This is because the resonant frequency is on a very deep mental level, and the defense mechanism simply does not have the force to react on more peripheral levels. If a person is only mildly psychotic, it is possible that he will acquire an acute infection; it has been observed that the psychotic symptoms then dramatically diminish during the acute illness, only to return upon recovery. Although allopathic physicians have been unable to offer an explanation for this phenomenon, it nevertheless became the basis for fever therapy, insulin shock therapy, and finally electroshock therapy. In addition, it is true that if a psychotic patient does acquire an acute infection, the infection is unusually severe and often fatal. This observation is readily explained by the principle of resonance when one realizes that the defense mechanism is weakened. Finally, if a psychotic patient is treated homeopathically with success, one sees a return of susceptibility to acute ailments; at first, these may be quite severe, but as homeopathic treatment proceeds, the ability to throw off such ailments becomes strengthened.

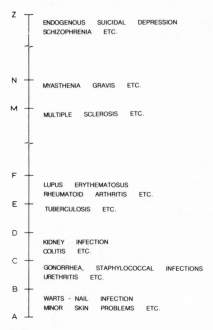

Z — ENDOGENOUS   SUICIDAL   DEPRESSION
SCHIZOPHRENIA   ETC.

N — MYASTHENIA   GRAVIS   ETC.

M — MULTIPLE   SCLEROSIS   ETC.

F — LUPUS   ERYTHEMATOSUS
RHEUMATOID   ARTHRITIS   ETC.

E — TUBERCULOSIS   ETC.

D — KIDNEY   INFECTION
COLITIS   ETC.

C — GONORRHEA,   STAPHYLOCOCCAL   INFECTIONS
URETHRITIS   ETC.

B — WARTS - NAIL   INFECTION
MINOR   SKIN   PROBLEMS   ETC.

A

Figure 7: A diagram showing different vibration rates of susceptibility to diseases. Each level represents a spectrum of diseases, the least serious being depicted at the bottom of the scale and the most serious at the top. Of course, the disease clusters listed are merely hypothetical, given merely for the purpose of illustration, and should not be considered factual. Once an individual's vibration rate is established on a given level, the person will be relatively immune to ailments on other levels.

Within a given level, susceptibility can fluctuate readily, depending on such factors as fatigue, diet, weather, etc. A person cannot, however, jump from one level to another on his own; such major leaps require influences such as powerful therapies or extreme emotional shocks.

Once a state of illness is established at a particular level, the person will be relatively resistant to disease on other levels, but stimuli on the same level of resonance can still produce changes in the vibratory rate. Again, these stimuli may be due to drugs, emotional shocks, or environmental influences, but the stimuli must resonate with the vibratory rate of the organism in order to produce an effect. For example, suppose we have a patient with heart disease. If he receives news that his child has died—an emotional shock affecting the vibrational level corresponding to the heart—it is likely that the patient will develop a psychosis. Meanwhile, the symptoms of the heart dysfunction will disappear. The same could occur if the patient were to be treated by a powerful drug acting on the level of the heart.

Conversely, it is true that a *beneficial* stimulus matched to the correct resonant frequency alters the vibration rate toward a direction of greater health. Such beneficial influence can occur by virtually any mode of therapy, but with most therapies, it occurs by accident, because principles are not followed by which the resonant frequency of the therapeutic agent is matched to that of the illness. For example, electroshock usually relieves psychotic depression only temporarily, and certainly it has its own damaging effects on central nervous system function; yet, in rare instances, such cases experience permanent relief. This occurs because, by accident, the vibratory rate of the electroshock matches the resonant frequency of susceptibility closely enough that the defense mechanism is strengthened. Unfortunately, physicians handling such cases do not realize what has happened and are then likely to use suppressive drugs whenever corresponding illnesses on the physical plane emerge, thus all too often throwing the patient back into a psychotic state.

Virtually any therapy can produce occasional curative responses in exactly this accidental manner. Psychotherapists or encounter groups may produce powerful benefits at a moment when the patient is receptive to such influences, and, if left alone, the benefit can be very lasting. Unfortunately, the tendency of therapists is to probe still further instead of letting well enough alone; if by this process an emotional upset occurs on the new vibratory level, it may have a morbific influence and thereby result in a relapse to the previous state—or often to one even worse. The same is true of herbal treatments, acupuncture, polarity massage, etc. All can produce benefit when the therapeutic stimulus matches the level of receptivity of the organism, and this benefit can then be lasting if progress is allowed to proceed undisturbed, despite the development of new symptoms on more peripheral levels.

In homeopathy, we at last see a scientific system which is based upon clear principles, which aims to stimulate the organism beneficially at precisely the resonant frequency, and which then allows the strengthened defense mechanism to complete its work in proper order. As we shall see in subsequent chapters, each homeopathic prescription is supposed to be based upon the totality of the expressions of the defense mechanism; in this way it is matched to the resonant frequency. Even so, it is true even in homeopathy that an incorrect remedy based only on a partial image of the patient's symptomatology can be given; such a prescription can also drive the vibrational level deeper and result in deterioration of the general health of the patient. Similarly, even a homeopathic remedy, if improperly given at a time when the defense mechanism is already proceeding efficiently in the proper direction, can disrupt the progress and unnecessarily delay recovery.

Summary of Chapter 5

Summary of Physics Section

1. One can hypothesize that the vital force is synonymous with the electrodynamic field of the body and therefore conforms to known principles of physics.

2. Matter and energy interchange in the electrodynamic field; this field is measurable in terms of waveforms, composed of frequency, wavelength, and amplitude.

3. The force or energy of the wave or field is proportional to both amplitude and frequency.

4. Every substance has a particular resonant frequency at which it will vibrate with greater force when stimulated by a wave of similar frequency. This resonant frequency may be easily discernible, as in a homogeneous object, or difficult to perceive, as in a nonhomogeneous object such as the human body.

5. The electromagnetic field of the human body can be considered its "dynamic plane"—a plane of inconceivable complexity which nevertheless conforms to laws and principles grounded in electromagnetic concepts of resonance, harmony, reinforcement, and interference. These laws and principles, therefore, are the basis for the new "energy medicine."

Summary of Defense Mechanism Section

1. Most morbific stimuli are managed successfully by the vital force without producing symptoms. If the morbific stimulus is stronger than the defense mechanism, the initial response is a change in the resonant frequency of the organism.

2. There is a latent period before actual symptoms are produced, even though the vibration rate of the organism is changed immediately by the stimulus.

3. Once the resonant frequency has changed, the susceptibility of the organism to disease has also changed; there is a new spectrum of diseases to which the person is susceptible. This changed susceptibility explains the numerous known cases in which the patient seems to acquire a series of infections of increasing virulence and decreasing responsiveness to antibiotics.

4. The principle of resonance renders the organism susceptible to morbific influence on basically only one level at any given moment. Thus a person can be "immune" to gonorrhea for two reasons: he is too sick, or he is too healthy to resonate with the level of the gonorrhea influence.

5. Beneficial influences also are subject to the principle of resonance. If a curative action occurs, by any therapy, it is because the treatment resonates with the level of susceptibility of the organism at that moment. Such an occurrence is rare, and occurs by accident because the laws and principles of cure are not understood. Most such cases are later suppressed by inappropriate therapeutic manipulations.

Annotated Bibliography for Chapter 5

Beaty, N.N., and Petersdorf, R.G., "Iatrogenic Factors in Infectious Disease," *Annals of Internal Medicine* 65: 641–656 (Oct. 1966). An extensive review of the literature, including 39 references. Studies the prevalence of iatrogenic illness in hospitalized populations. Particularly focuses on antibiotic therapy. *"If the sputum flora of the patient under treatment for pneumonia is followed throughout treatment, colonization by an organism resistant to the antibiotic employed can be documented frequently. Usually this constitutes bacterial superinfection without clinical disease, but in a significant number of instances this ecological change in flora is accompanied by an exacerbation of signs and symptoms. These infections are often refractory to treatment because the superinfecting organism is resistant to most antibiotics."*

Chapter 6

The Fundamental Law of Cure

THE *dynamic plane* is the plane of the essence of life, the plane on which disease originates, as well as the plane of origin of the defense mechanism. It is not as if the dynamic plane is a separate fourth level of the organism. Rather, it permeates all levels, is prior to them, and interacts with them. It has exactly the same relationship to the physical body as electromagnetic fields have to matter. This concept is illustrated in Figure 8, which is a simplification of the construction presented in Chapter 3. As the arrows indicate, the vital force or dynamic plane interacts intimately with all three levels. Whenever an organism receives a stimulus through one of its three levels of reception, the effect is responded to initially by the electrodynamic field (or vital force) and is then distributed to the three levels according to the strength of the stimulus and the degree of resistance of the organism.

Modern concepts of cybernetics demonstrate a fundamental principle which applies to the human organism as well as to other systems: *any highly organized system reacts to stress always by producing the best possible response of which it is capable in the moment.* In the human being, this means that the defense mechanism makes the best possible response to the morbific stimulus, given the state of health in the moment and the intensity of the stress.

When disease occurs, the first disturbance occurs on the dynamic electromagnetic field of the body, which then brings into play the defense mechanism. This concept was first enunciated

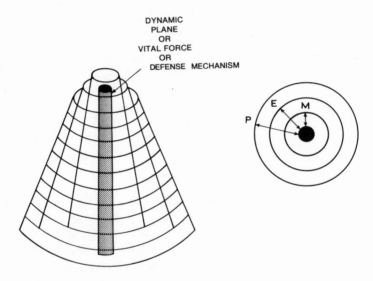

DYNAMIC
PLANE
OR
VITAL FORCE
OR
DEFENSE MECHANISM

Figure 8: A diagram illustrating the interaction of mental, emotional, and physical planes as governed by the dynamic plane. The dynamic plane permeates the entire organism on all levels; it is the intelligent mediator of all three levels, creating the best possible response of the entire organism once a stimulus is received on one of the receptor levels.

Note that the arrows connecting each level point in both directions. Also note that there are no arrows connecting directly the mental, emotional, and physical levels.

definitively as the basis for therapeutics by Samuel Hahnemann, the nineteenth-century German physician who discovered and developed the science of homeopathy. In Aphorism 11 of his monumental masterpiece, *The Organon of Medicine*, Hahnemann writes: *"This vital force is the one which is primarily deranged by dynamic influences upon it of a morbific agent."* [1]

For any therapy to be effective, it is obvious that the practitioner must cooperate with this process and must not deviate from it at all. Since the defense mechanism is already responding with the best possible response, any deviation from the direction of its action must inevitably be of a lesser degree of effectiveness. This is why therapies which are based upon intellectual theories and partial comprehension of the totality can only inhibit the process of cure, and often produce actual harm to the organism through suppression.

Since the activity of the defense mechanism originates on the dynamic plane, the most logical therapeutic approach would be one which enhances and strengthens this level, thus increasing the effectiveness of the organism's own healing process. In general, therapeutic measures can accomplish this in two ways:

1. The therapeutic agent can affect primarily one of the three levels, and through the mediation of the dynamic plane *indirectly* affect all of the other levels. Since this approach carries the risk of being focused only on a partial resonance, the results will be likely to be disappointing. Even so, cures can be produced by this approach if by accident the effect causes a strengthening of the defense mechanism as a totality.

2. The therapeutic agent can act *directly* upon the electrodynamic field as a totality and thereby directly strengthen the defense mechanism. The result of such an action, because it automatically relies upon the intelligence of the defense mechanism itself, can only be beneficial and will result in a high rate of cure of disease, not only on one level but of the entire person.

Of these two therapeutic strategies, the second would seem to be the best, even considering the difficulty in finding agents which can act directly upon the dynamic plane. In the world today, there are only three widely known therapies which can act directly

---

1. Samuel Hahnemann, *Organon of Medicine*, Sixth Edition, translated by William Boericke (New Delhi: B. Jain Publishers, 1974).

upon the dynamic plane. Acupuncture is one such therapy which also has a deep comprehension of the laws and principles of healing. The ancient form of acupuncture, practiced by dedicated and experienced masters, is a highly curative method. Unfortunately, however, even in modern China the influence of technological thinking has caused such masters to become rare indeed. Acupuncture, of course, is currently sweeping across the world, but its form of practice is generally a superficial reflection of the ancient form.[2] To do acupuncture to the highest standard of effectiveness is said to require many years of intensive supervised training and experience. The form which is commonly practiced today is being done by practitioners with often only one- or two-week seminar training, or at most two or three years of training. Alas, the true masters of acupuncture are becoming very rare, and it seems unlikely that very many people in our modern world will undergo the necessary years of training to become highly qualified acupuncturists.

The "laying on of hands" by a highly evolved spiritual individual is another therapy which can directly affect the plane of the electrodynamic field. By this is *not* meant the common psychic healing, faith healing, or massage practices, which affect the vital force only indirectly through one of the three levels. "Laying on of hands" by a spiritually evolved person who is in fact a channel for universal energies can directly strengthen the defense mechanism and thereby bring about a lasting cure. The drawback to this is that there will always be too few people of such spiritual evolution to effectively deal with the health problems of our age.

The third therapy which directly stimulates the dynamic plane is the administration of the homeopathically "potentized" remedy. The homeopathic science of therapeutics has demonstrated again and again extremely effective curative results in high percentages of cases, with long-lasting benefit. It is based on readily comprehensible principles, and it can be learned by any dedicated student in approximately the same amount of time required for allopathic medical training. Thus it is a therapy which carries the possibility of producing a large number of qualified prescribers to meet the health needs of our populations.

---

2. M. Duke, *Acupuncture* (London: Constable, 1973), p. 12. Since interference by the government of Chiang Kai-Shek in the examination procedures, the ancient traditions have become diluted. The classical learning methods and examinations were destroyed, and promptly multitudes of quacks began practicing in China. Many of these diluted forms of teaching have subsequently been exported outside of China.

In homeopathy, then, or indeed in any therapy acting on the dynamic plane, how do we discover the therapeutic agent which can directly resonate with the resultant frequency of the organism on the dynamic plane? We appear to be decades away from possessing technology refined enough to actually measure this frequency, so how exactly do we go about selecting the therapeutic agent which can stimulate powerfully the dynamic plane?

To begin with, it must be recalled that the dynamic plane in a relatively good state of health does not manifest itself; it balances and adjusts the organism without the person having to focus awareness on its action. In disease, however, once a certain threshold has been crossed, the defense mechanism is called into play and eventually produces symptoms as the manifestation of its action.

Symptoms and signs are the only way we have of perceiving the workings of the defense mechanism. It is acting in the best possible manner for the benefit of the organism; for this reason, the symptoms and signs produced are actually attempts on the part of the organism to heal itself. This is undoubtedly a paradoxical concept to many readers, but reflection upon what has thus far been said will make this idea clear and logical.

Fever, malaise, loss of appetite, pain, emotional reactions, mental confusion as well as more refined and individualistic responses of each person are not problems in themselves but are rather the defense mechanism's best possible attempt to produce cure of a disturbance which originated upon the dynamic plane. Again, it is Samuel Hahnemann who first and most clearly stated this concept, in his Aphorism 7: *"The totality of the symptoms must be the principal, indeed the only thing the physician has to make note of in every case of disease and to remove by means of his art, in order that the disease shall be cured and transformed into health."*

To affect directly the dynamic plane, we must find a substance similar enough to the resultant frequency of the dynamic plane to produce resonance. Since the defense mechanism's only manifestation perceptible to our senses is the symptoms and signs of the person, it follows that we must seek a substance which can produce in the human organism a similar totality of symptoms and signs. If a substance is capable of producing a similar symptom picture in a healthy organism, then the likelihood of its vibration rate being very close to the resultant frequency of the diseased organism is good, and therefore a powerful strengthening of the defense mechanism can occur—through the principle of resonance.

91

It is this insight which is the fundamental pillar of the science of homeopathy: *Similia Similibus Curentur,* as it was coined by Hahnemann.—*"Like Cures Like." Any substance which can produce a totality of symptoms in a healthy human being can cure that totality of symptoms in a sick human being.*

Of course, this is a startling new principle in therapeutics. Throughout history, symptoms or groups of symptoms have been viewed as problems which must be eradicated immediately, and medical thought has focused all its attention on agents which can get rid of particular symptoms or syndromes. If a person has a runny nose, give a decongestant. If a person has a pain, give an analgesic. If constipation, give a laxative. For nervousness, give a tranquilizer. This approach is based merely upon the symptom manifestation itself, rather than upon the original disturbance on the dynamic level. It does not respect the symptom as an attempt of the body to heal, and therefore its therapeutics are not designed to strengthen the defense mechanism of the organism.

On the other hand, homeopathy (from *homeo,* meaning "similar," and *pathos,* meaning "suffering") recognizes symptoms as the defense mechanism's best attempt to heal and endeavors to cooperate with it via the Law of Similars, which is a method arising out of the principle of resonance. How precisely this is done, of course, is the subject of the rest of this textbook, but we can give a simplified example to demonstrate what we mean.

Suppose your healthy, robust child suddenly develops a high fever, a flushed face, glassy eyes with dilated pupils, dry mouth without thirst, a dry raw sore throat, swollen submaxillary glands which are more marked on the right side, and a wild kind of delirium causing him to try to climb the walls. The allopathic physician interprets these symptoms and signs as evidence of a viral or bacterial infection and takes a culture of the throat in the hope of finding an organism which responds to antibiotics; this approach assumes that the "cause" is the microbe. The homeopathic practitioner, on the other hand, is relatively uninterested in the nature of the microbe. He sees the symptoms as a manifestation of disturbance on the dynamic plane which can never be "cultured." The homeopath, therefore, studies carefully the symptoms themselves in their totality, especially searching for individualizing traits which represent the "resonant frequency" that can be used for cure. He searches for a substance which reflects as closely as possible the total picture of symptoms. In this example, such a substance is belladonna; the patient is given belladonna in a single, minute dose, the fever drops rapidly to normal, and the child falls into a peaceful sleep. By morning, the child is completely well, and any throat culture taken at that time may well show disappearance of whatever microbe had been found. This story may seem difficult to believe, but every homeopath can cite innumerable such cases from routine daily practice.

In the above description, it should be noted that the symptoms described were not merely gross descriptions of "fever, sore throat, adenopathy, and delirium." The symptoms of importance to the homeopath are those which are the most highly individualized to that patient. Ten people with "strep throat" are likely to show ten different pictures of the totality of symptoms, once the individualizing qualities are determined. Often, in homeopathic practice, the most valuable symptoms of all are what are called *strange, rare, and peculiar* symptoms. It is obvious why this is so, because only by such refinement is it possible to approach with precision the true resonant frequency which can lead to cure.

The principle of resonance is also the basis for the insistence of homeopathy upon the *totality* of symptoms. If only a partial image of the total symptom picture is acquired, the effect of the therapeutic substance on the organism will be limited only to that vibrational level. If a patient comes to the homeopath complaining of arthritis, for instance, and the only symptoms noted are those relating to the joints while ignoring the rest of the physical plane, the emotional plane, and the mental plane, the prescription can be expected only to act on the joints. Such a procedure is unlikely to produce a cure, and moreover may well result in degeneration on deeper levels.

To find the resonant frequency of the entire organism and therefore strengthen the entire dynamic plane of action, one must record the totality of all deviations from normal on all three levels, in all details of their individualizing character. As an example, the following are just a small sample of the types of questions the homeopathic practitioner must put to the patient: all influences which alter the major complaint presented by the patient, tolerance to heat and cold in the environment, effect of humidity and weather changes, time of day or night in which the patient feels worse in general, effects of all natural foods, any strong food cravings or aversions, the position and degree of comfort in sleep, any anxieties or phobias the patient may suffer, whether there is irritability and under what circumstances, how the mind functions in various situations, etc. All of these questions and many more must be explored in great detail in order to elucidate the totality of individualizing symptoms which indicate in every particular the direction and form that the defense mechanism has decided upon as best to take.

The symptom areas of most importance to the homeopath are those having to do with basic functions which occupy the attention of the person. Everyone of necessity pays considerable attention to things having to do with environmental comfort, food, sex, sleep, relationships with loved ones, financial issues, and influences of occupation or housework. These areas of human existence are of much more fundamental importance to the homeopathic prescriber than the actual clinical details of the patient's heart disease, lupus erythematosus, migraines, etc. Of course, clinical knowledge does play a role in choosing the therapeutic agent, but its role is much less significant in homeopathy than it is in allopathic medicine.

Samuel Hahnemann

Before proceeding farther, it would be useful to pause a moment to examine the life of Samuel Hahnemann, the remarkable genius who discovered, developed, and systematized the fundamental laws of cure which are producing such revolutionary changes in thinking about health and disease. Hahnemann's story is one of the most singular sagas of discovery in the history of medicine.

Commenting about the Law of Similars, Hahnemann was the first to admit that the concept had been put forward by others throughout Western history, beginning with Hippocrates himself. Despite previous speculations about it, however, no one prior to Hahnemann had recognized its true importance, much less proceeded to systematize it into the basis of an entire science of therapeutics.

Hahnemann was born in 1755 in a small town in Germany and from an early age demonstrated remarkable abilities. His father recognized his abilities and taught him discipline from an early age; he used to lock young Samuel up in a room with "thinking exercises"—problems he was required to solve by himself, for "the boy must learn to think." Hahnemann had a great talent for languages, and even by the age of twelve his instructor had him teaching Greek to other pupils.

Hahnemann studied medicine at the Universities of Leipzig, Vienna, and Erlangen, qualifying in 1779, and soon became highly respected in professional circles for his papers on both medicine and chemistry. Even so, Hahnemann was greatly disturbed by the lack of fundamental thinking underlying the therapeutics of the day, which consisted of bloodletting, cathartics, leeches, and the use of toxic chemicals. Hahnemann wrote to one of his friends:

It was agony for me to walk always in darkness, when I had to heal the sick, and to prescribe, according to such or such an hypothesis concerning diseases, substances which owed their place in the materia medica to an arbitrary decision . . . Soon after my marriage, I renounced the practice of medicine, that I might no longer incur the risk of doing injury, and I engaged exclusively in chemistry, and in literary occupations. But I became a father, serious diseases threatened my beloved children . . . My scruples redoubled when I saw that I could afford them no certain relief. [3]

He returned to the profession of translating medical works, but his inquiring mind was always searching for the fundamental principles upon which therapeutics should be based. It was while translating Cullen's edition of the *materia medica* that he came upon the idea which led to his revolutionary discovery. Cullen was a professor of medicine at Edinburgh University and had devoted twenty pages of his *materia medica* to the therapeutic indications of Peruvian bark; and he attributed its success in the treatment of malarias to the fact that it was bitter. Hahnemann was dissatisfied with this explanation so much that he decided to test it upon himself, an act which was completely out of the realm of thinking of the time. He says:

I took by way of experiment, twice a day, four drachms of good China. My feet, finger ends, etc., at first became cold; I grew languid and drowsy; then my heart began to palpitate, and my pulse grew hard and small; intolerable anxiety, trembling, prostration throughout all my limbs; then pulsation in the head, redness of my cheeks, thirst, and, in short, all these symptoms, which are ordinarily characteristic of intermittent fever, made their appearance, one after the other, yet without the peculiar chilly, shivering rigor.

Briefly, even those symptoms which are of regular occurrence and especially characteristic—as the stupidity of mind, the kind of rigidity in all the limbs, but above all the numb, disagreeable sensation, which seems to have its seat in the

---

3. Thomas L. Bradford, *Life and Letters of Dr. Samuel Hahnemann* (Philadelphia: Boericke and Tafel, 1895).

periosteum, over every bone in the body—all these make their appearance. This paroxysm lasted two or three hours each time, and recurred if I repeated this dose, not otherwise; I discontinued it, and was in good health.[4]

Thus Hahnemann came upon the idea that a substance which can produce symptoms in a normal person can cure them in a sick person. Even more fundamentally, perhaps, he recognized the necessity for human experimentation in order to delineate the curative indications of therapeutic agents. So he and some other like-minded physicians began systematically testing substances upon themselves and recording their observations in minute detail. This continued for a period of six years, during which Hahnemann also compiled an exhaustive list of poisonings recorded by different doctors in different countries through centuries of medical history.

He and his colleagues began to try the Law of Similars on clinical cases and immediately began to see astounding results which far transcended the allopathic results of the time. In Aphorism 19 of the *Organon*, written after he had become very experienced and widely known for his results, Hahnemann summarizes the fundamental importance of the discovery:

Now, as diseases are nothing more than alterations in the state of health of the healthy individual which express themselves by morbid signs, and the cure is also only possible by a change to the healthy condition of the state of health of the diseased individual, it is very evident that medicines could never cure diseases if they did not possess the power of altering man's state of health which depends on sensations and functions; indeed, that their curative power must be owing solely to this power they possess of altering man's state of health.

The systematic procedure of testing substances on healthy human beings in order to elucidate the symptoms reflecting the action of the substance is called "proving." Hahnemann developed specific procedures for conducting a proving, and procedures which fit modern conditions and circumstances will be provided later in this book. Provings have continued since Hahnemann's time and have become the basis upon which a given remedy is chosen for a given patient. In this way, the symptom manifestation of the patient and the symptom manifestation of the remedy are matched, thus enabling the principles of resonance to excite and strengthen the defense mechanism of the patient and bring about cure.

---

4. Ibid., pp. 36–37.

The Proving of Remedies

During a proving, we introduce into the organism a substance sufficiently high in concentration to disturb the organism and mobilize its defense mechanism. The defense mechanism produces a spectrum of symptoms on all three levels of the organism; this spectrum of symptoms then characterizes the peculiar and unique nature of the substance. In a similar way, we note down the symptoms of the patient, recording the peculiar way in which his organism reacted to the morbific stimulus on the dynamic plane. In both cases, the exciting cause must be strong enough to mobilize the defense mechanism, so that symptoms are produced. This occurs only if the agent is strong enough, or if the person is sufficiently sensitive to the vibratory frequency of the substance.

Fortunately for the science of therapeutics, it happens that the symptom pictures of remedies match quite accurately the symptom pictures of virtually all illnesses in existence, in all their variety. Today, there are hundreds of remedies which have been proved in this way and which cover the major part of all possible disturbances in the human being.

In order to be able to say that a drug has been fully proved, however, it should first be tried on the healthy person in toxic, hypotoxic, and highly diluted and potentized doses (potentization will be discussed in the next chapter). Second, the symptoms produced by the drug on all three levels must be noted down. Third, the substance's action must be completed by observing the symptoms which have disappeared from the patient after the remedy has produced a cure.

If the symptoms of a proving are recorded only on the physical level, the proving is still incomplete. It is for this reason that simple toxicology described in medical schools is insufficient. The symptoms have been recorded in too gross a form, without adequate individualizing information, and they record almost exclusively actions on the physical level.

In Chapter 10, further elaboration will be provided on the specific techniques for conducting a proving, and one of Hahnemann's original provings will be presented as an example of the specific detail with which the action of substances is considered.

Summary of Chapter 6

1. The dynamic plane permeates all levels of the organism just as the electromagnetic field permeates matter, and it is the origin

of all actions of the body in health and disease. A highly organized system reacts to stress by always producing the best possible response of which it is capable.

2. Therapeutic measures utilizing the dynamic plane may act either indirectly through a single level, or directly on the dynamic plane itself.

3. Three modes of therapy are capable of acting directly on the dynamic plane: acupuncture, "laying on of hands" by a spiritually evolved individual, and homeopathy.

4. The Law of Similars matches the symptom manifestated on the dynamic plane in a patient with the analogous symptom of a therapeutic substance manifested in a healthy individual to establish resonance between patient and remedy.

5. The Law of Similars states: any substance which can produce a totality of symptoms in a healthy human being can cure that totality of symptoms in a sick human being.

6. The Law of Similars was a basic contribution of Samuel Hahnemann, a German medical doctor dissatisfied with the crude practices of his day. Hahnemann systematized this law by doing "provings," or systematic recordings of symptoms produced by substances on healthy human beings.

7. To be complete, a proving must be tested in a full range of doses (or potencies), the symptoms recorded must include all three levels of the individual, and symptoms cured in sick patients after administration of the remedy must be included.

Chapter 7

The Therapeutic Agent
on the Dynamic Plane

Thus we have presented the concept of the electromagnetic dynamic plane and the Law of Similars which enables us to utilize the principle of resonance to stimulate it. The next logical step is to develop therapeutic agents which themselves are on the dynamic plane and are capable of affecting this realm of the human organism. The purpose of this chapter is to demonstrate specifically how the science of homeopathy has achieved this object through Hahnemann's technique of *potentization*.

If we reflect upon the fact that every substance has an electromagnetic field (from simple organisms to even the entire planet), it can be said that any substance administered to a person has at least the potential to affect the organism in two ways. On the one hand, the substance may have a *chemical* effect, such as we see with foods, vitamins, drugs, tobacco, coffee, etc. And on the other hand, there may be an effect on the *electromagnetic* field of the body caused by the corresponding electromagnetic field of the substance, especially if vibration levels are close enough to resonate with one another. Ordinarily, of course, the electrodynamic effect of a crude substance is liable to be too weak to be noticed, but it may nevertheless play a role in such circumstances as mineral baths, sea bathing, poultices, etc.

In regard to the human organism, substances can be readily classified as being biologically inert or biologically active. Biologically *inert* substances such as gold, silica, metallic iron, platinum, cellulose, etc., are chemically and energetically "closed" to inter-action with the human body. They merely pass through the intes-tinal tract with nothing more than mechanical effect. Even their electromagnetic influence on the organism is so small as to be undetectable.

A biologically *active* substance is one in which the chemical or other energies are "open" to interaction with the body; there is a chemical affinity between the substance and the organism. If one eats a food, takes a vitamin pill, or ingests an aspirin tablet, there immediately occur complex chemical reactions which create ef-fects on many organs of the body. Biologically active substances may have beneficial effects, as with food, or they may have highly toxic effects, as with sufficient doses of arsenic, mercury, or al-lopathic drugs. Such toxic substances will have some effect on virtually anyone who takes them, but the degree of toxicity of a given dose will vary from one individual to another. Someone with a very high degree of sensitivity, or "affinity," may react so violently that death can occur, whereas another person with less sensitivity to that substance may experience only a mild reaction. As Hahnemann discovered by his studies of the symptomatology of poisonings, the very sensitivity of a person to a given substance can be an expression of resonance between the person and the substance; in homeopathy, this resonance is utilized as a thera-peutic principle.

It is possible for a cure of disease to occur by a biologically active agent even in crude form if the resonance or affinity of the person matches closely enough the vibration of the substance. This is likely the explanation for the benefit some people receive from bathing in mineral baths. Not everyone experiences a benefi-cial effect, of course; a few may feel aggravated after exposure to such a bath, most experience relatively little effect at all, and per-haps 15-20% experience a relief of symptoms and a general in-crease in vitality. Very likely, those who experience benefit (and in an obverse way, those who experience aggravations) are reso-nating closely in their electromagnetic planes with one of the many minerals present in the bath. Such benefit may well last 6 to 9 months; then there is a relapse. If the person returns to the bath, it is then observed that the second exposure produces benefit for a lesser period, say, 3 months. By the third or fourth exposure, there may be no benefit at all. Whatever therapeutic stimulus to the dynamic plane had occurred from the mineral in crude form originally has finally become too weak to affect the defense mechanism of the person any further.

The same observation is commonly seen with administration of herbal remedies. If by chance one of the herbs in a particular formula prescribed by an herbalist resonates with the dynamic plane of the patient, there may be a benefit which can last quite some time. If the weakness of the defense mechanism of the patient is severe enough, however, there will be a relapse. It will then be found that administration of the same herb will produce a less intense effect, or will last less long, than the original prescription. This is because the dynamic action of the herb has not been intensified, whereas the defense mechanism may well have been weakened even further than originally. As mentioned before, similar observations can be made with accidental curative effects from acupuncture, allopathic drugs, and other therapies.

In order to produce lasting curative results, it is necessary to increase the intensity of the electrodynamic field of the therapeutic agent, or in other words, we must liberate the energy contained within the substance in such a way as to make it more available to interaction with the dynamic plane of the organism. This is the point at which Samuel Hahnemann made his second ingenious contribution to medicine by devising the technique of *potentization*. It is as yet unknown exactly how Hahnemann came upon this technique, whether it arose from his background in chemistry or by sheer divine inspiration. In any case, he developed a very simple method of extracting the therapeutic energy of a substance without altering its vibration rate. Thus the resulting "homeopathic remedy" is a form of intensified energy which can still be administered according to the basic resonance principle of the Law of Similars, but now with enhanced ability to affect the dynamic plane of the organism and thereby produce a lasting cure of the total organism.

As described in the previous chapter, Hahnemann's first great discovery was the importance of "proving" substances on healthy human volunteers in order to acquire a complete description of the symptomatology of the substance. Unfortunately, however, most potentially useful substances are highly toxic in their biological action—substances such as arsenic, mercury, belladonna, snake venoms, etc. Some information was available from poisonings with these substances, but the symptomatology was not as refined as Hahnemann needed for homeopathic prescribing. It

101

was in the process of struggling with this problem that Hahnemann made his discovery.

At first, Hahnemann tried to simply dilute the substances. This, of course, succeeded in reducing the toxicity of the agents, but it also proportionately reduced the therapeutic effect. Somehow, Hahnemann then hit upon the technique of adding kinetic energy to the dilutions through shaking, or "succussion." This combination of succussion and serial dilution Hahnemann called "potentization" or "dynamization." The crucial observation was that *the more the substance is succussed and diluted, the greater the therapeutic effect while simultaneously nullifying the toxic effect.*

Let us now describe how homeopathic pharmacies prepare their homeopathic medicines. Detailed descriptions will be provided in Chapter 11, but it is important here to give a brief description for the sake of clarity. Initially, the substance is dissolved in an alchohol/water solution in a standard chemical or botanical manner. One drop of this "tincture" is then diluted into 9 or 99 drops of 40% alcohol/water solution. This dilution is then succussed with great force 100 times. One drop of the succussed dilution is then added to 9 or 99 drops of fresh solvent; this is then sucussed 100 times again, and diluted as before. This process can be carried out literally forever, always increasing the therapeutic power while nullifying the toxic properties.

In homeopathy, there is a specific nomenclature for each "potency" or dilution. If the serial dilutions are done on the basis of 1/10, the scale is called the "decimal" scale, and the resulting potency numbers are designated by "x"; e.g., the first 1/10 dilution is called a 1x potency, the second a 2x potency, the thirtieth dilution 30x. If the dilutions are made 1/100, the scale is called the "centesimal" scale, designated by a "c"; the first 1/100 dilution is then called a 1c, the thirtieth dilution 30c, and the thousandth dilution 1000c.

According to the laws of chemistry, there is a limit to how many serial dilutions can be made without losing the original substance altogether. This limit is called Avogadro's number, and it roughly corresponds to a homeopathic potency of 24x (which is equivalent to 12c). Thus any potency beyond 24x or 12c has virtually no chance of containing even one molecule of the original substance. One would think that further potentization would cease to be effective at this point, but in actual fact potencies ranging far beyond this "limit" continue to increase in power. Thus far, there has not been found any limit whatsoever, even though homeopaths often successfully use potencies over 100,000c! To give the reader some idea of how extremely dilute such a potency is, let us describe the dilutions in terms of a numerical fraction; Avogadro's number would correspond roughly to a dilution represented by 1/1000 . . . to a total of 24 zeroes. A potency of 100,000c would be represented by a dilution of 1/100,000 . . . to a total of *100,000 zeroes*—inconceivably far beyond the point at which not one molecule of original substance is left!

How do we actually know that the therapeutic power of potencies truly increases with further dilution and succussion? This is confirmed by the frequent clinical observations of all homeopaths. Once the correct remedy is selected according to the Law of Similars, it is true that it will act even in crude form. For example, a patient with a belladonna fever (with all the individualizing homeopathic symptoms found in the provings of belladonna), will respond to even just a few drops of belladonna tincture. The response may be minimal, however, and short-acting. If a 12x potency of belladonna is given, the relief will likely be more dramatic. If, however, we administer a 10,000c potency, the response will likely be a complete disappearance of all symptoms within a matter of hours, with no relapse whatsoever.

We also see other types of cases in which the crude form of the substance, as well as low potencies up to 30c, do not act at all. Once the correct potency is reached, however, if it be as high as 100,000c, a dramatic and lasting cure follows.

The assertion that by mere succussion and serial dilution the therapeutic power of a substance can be increased without limit while nullifying toxicity certainly seems to violate our usual understanding of physics and chemistry. The clinical results of homeopaths the world over, routinely using potencies beyond Avogadro's number, cannot be denied, but what then is actually occurring during the process of potentization?

We know that dilution alone is not sufficient to produce the phenomenon. Succussion adds kinetic energy to the solution, which is crucial. If one merely succusses a solution without diluting it further, a raise in level of only one potency occurs, regardless of how many times it is succussed; therefore, *both* succussion and dilution are required. We also know that the more there is succussion and dilution, the more the therapeutic power is increased, even beyond the point of there being even one molecule of the original substance remaining.

As far as is yet known, there is no available explanation in modern physics or chemistry for this phenomenon. It appears that some new form of energy is released by this technique. The energy which is contained in a limited form in the original substance is somehow released and transmitted to the molecules of the solvent. Once the original substance is no longer present, the remaining energy in the solvent can be continually enhanced *ad infinitum.* The solvent molecules have taken on the dynamic energy of the original substance. We know from clinical results that the therapeutic energy still retains the "vibrational frequency" of the original substance, but the energy has been enhanced to such a degree that it is capable of stimulating the dynamic plane of the patient sufficiently to produce a cure.

Hahnemann's discoveries of the process of potentization and the Law of Similars have truly revolutionized the scientific potential of therapeutics. On the one hand, the principle of the Law of Similars provides us with a method of matching resonant vibrations of virtually any substance in the environment with that of the patient. As we have seen in instances of temporary relief, through administration of crude therapeutic agents, the crude form often possesses insufficient intensity to produce permanent cure. On the other hand, with Hahnemann's discovery of a technique to increase therapeutic intensity on the dynamic plane indefinitely, we now possess a way to stimulate the defense mechanism of the patient with whatever intensity is needed to overpower the force of the disease.

It will have to be left to physicists and chemists to discover precisely how energy is transferred to the solvent by this technique. There are a few clues perhaps which can be found within the empirical experience of homeopaths. One definite property of homeopathic remedies is great susceptibility to exposure to the rays of the sun. If a remedy is exposed directly to the sun, all therapeutic power is lost. It also appears to be true that remedies can be inactivated by exposure to heat above 110–120° F. Many homeopaths report in addition that at least some remedies are inactivated by exposure to strongly aromatic substances, especially camphor. Why it is that exposures so readily inactivate remedies is as yet unknown, but we can at least hope that these clues arising out of experience will someday provide leads for researchers trying to find the exact nature of this energy.

As homeopathy becomes increasingly respected for its astounding effectiveness in diseases of all types, whether acute or chronic, we can hope that researchers will begin to investigate the nature of homeopathic remedies. Once we know more about their properties, it will become possible to refine our techniques of matching remedies and potencies to individual patients with even greater precision than is presently possible. That possibility alone should motivate investigators to enter this field; it is an area of research with wide open vistas both for profound theoretical discoveries and for practical application to benefit mankind.

Summary of Chapter 7

1. Every substance, animate or inanimate, has an electromagnetic field.

2. Any substance can affect the human organism in one of two ways: by direct chemical action, or through interaction of electromagnetic fields, if the frequencies are close enough to resonate.

3. Biologically inert substances are chemically and energetically "closed" to interaction with the human body.

4. Biologically active substances are capable of acting on the tissues of the body chemically. The specific reaction of the organism depends upon the degree of susceptibility or "affinity" for the substance.

5. If the sensitivity is close enough, even the crude form of a biologically active substance can be therapeutic, although generally the effect lasts only temporarily.

6. To get curative results that are lasting, it is necessary to increase the intensity of the electromagnetic field of the substance. This is done through potentization, which is succussion and dilution. Neither succussion alone nor dilution alone are effective.

7. There is no limit to the degree of potentization possible, even when Avogadro's number is exceeded and no molecule of the original substance is present.

8. As yet, there is no available explanation for this phenomenon, although its validity has become undeniable. Somehow, the force of the electromagnetic field of the original substance is transferred to the solvent molecules, yet without changing the resonant frequency.

9. Remedies have properties which may be useful clues for future research into the phenomenon of potentization: they are inactivated by direct sunlight, heat in excess of 110–120°F., and perhaps by aromatic substances such as camphor.

Chapter 8

Dynamic Interaction of Disease

THUS FAR in the text, we have depicted the human organism as being an integrated totality responding to external morbific stimuli first by a change in vibration rate on the dynamic electromagnetic level. If the defense mechanism is weak, or if the stimulus is very powerful in relation to it, the vibration rate will remain altered, and the organism will be unable to return to the original state on its own. For this reason, we potentize substances that can then act to strengthen the dynamic level, and we prescribe them according to the Law of Similars, in order to take advantage of the principle of resonance between the therapeutic agent and the resultant vibration level of the organism. Stimuli which are capable of altering the resonant frequency of the organism may be weak and transient, as in changes in humidity or barometric pressure, or they may be very powerful, such as deep emotional shocks or prolonged and severe stress. In this chapter, we shall examine further a few of the most powerful influences which can deeply and chronically alter the health of an individual. In homeopathic experience, three such powerful influences which must be taken into account during a patient's history are powerful acute illnesses, suppressive therapies, and vaccinations. All three of these, when the organism is weakened and vibrating on a susceptible level, can be major turning points in the health history of an individual.

106

Acute Disease Influence

As we discussed in the Introduction, virtually everyone has some degree of chronic disease tendency influencing his or her health throughout life. In some people, the constitution is relatively strong, while in others it is quite weak. In the absence of curative therapy or major shocks to the system, the vibration rate in a given individual will vary within a certain range of disease susceptibilities. Depending on nutrition, amount of rest and sleep, emotional stress, environmental stimuli, etc., there will be variation from hour to hour and day to day within a certain spectrum of susceptibility, but the organism will not jump *major* levels upward or downward without the impact of powerful influences. Thus a person may vary in susceptibility to colds, minor skin eruptions, and transient moodiness; but the same person is very unlikely to jump major levels and become suddenly psychotic. Or conversely, a psychotic individual is unlikely to spontaneously become mentally and emotionally clear, and then maintain symptoms on more peripheral levels only.

One of the major influences which can adversely alter the health of an individual is the acquisition of an acute illness to which the individual is at that moment very susceptible. Every experienced clinician has encountered patients who complain of arthritis for many years after suffering from a severe influenza, who develop chronic relapsing bronchitis after a severe pneumonia, or who never quite regain the same level of vitality experienced prior to mononucleosis or hepatitis. Major changes in health would not occur by minor illnesses to which the patient is only transiently susceptible, but when the system has been weakened at a particular level of susceptibility, such major changes can occur, and then the individual will not be able to return unaided to the original level. Such are circumstances in which homeopathy produces very dramatic results.

Samuel Hahnemann was a particularly astute observer of the interactions which can occur between different disease states. Suppose a person has a given chronic disease predilection, and then acquires another disease to which he is strongly susceptible. What will be the result of such an interaction for the health of the individual? Hahnemann describes the possibilities in the following aphorisms:

107

Aph. 36: I. *If the two* dissimilar *diseases meeting together in the human being be of equal strength, or still more if the* older one be the stronger, *the* new disease will be repelled by the old one from the body and not allowed to affect it. A patient suffering from a severe chronic disease will not be infected by a moderate autumnal dysentery or other epidemic disease ... Those suffering from pulmonary consumption are not liable to be attacked by epidemic fevers of a not very violent character.*

Aph. 38: II. *Or* the new dissimilar disease is the stronger. *In this case the disease under which the patient originally labored, being the weaker, will be kept back and suspended by the accession of the stronger one, until the latter shall have run its course or been cured, and then the old one reappears* uncured. *Two children affected with a kind of epilepsy remained free from epileptic attacks after infection with ringworm (tinea); but as soon as the eruption on the head was gone the epilepsy returned just as before ... So also the pulmonary phthisis remained stationary when the patient was attacked by a violent typhus, but went on again after the latter had run its course. If mania occur in a consumptive patient, the phthisis with all its symptoms is removed by the former; but if that go off, the phthisis returns immediately and proves fatal ... And* thus it is with all dissimilar diseases; the stronger suspends the weaker *(when they do not complicate one another, which is seldom the case with acute diseases),* but they never cure one another.

Aph. 40: III. *Or* the new disease, *after having long acted on the organism, at length joins the old one that is dissimilar to it, and forms with it a* complex *disease, so that each of them occupies a particular locality in the organism, namely, the organs peculiarly adapted for it, and, as it were, only the place specially belonging to it, whilst it leaves the rest to the other disease that is dissimilar to it ...* As two diseases dissimilar to each other, they cannot remove, cannot cure one another. .... *When two dissimilar acute infectious diseases meet, as, for example smallpox and measles, the one usually suspends the other, as has been before observed; yet there have also been severe epidemics of this kind, where, in rare cases, two dissimilar acute diseases occurred simultaneously in one and the same body, and for a short time combined, as it were, with each other.*

Aph. 43: *Totally different, however, is the result when* two similar *diseases meet together in the organism, that is to say, when to the disease already present a stronger similar one is added. In such cases we see how a cure can be effected by the operations of nature, and we get a lesson as to how man ought to cure.*

Aph. 44: *Two similar diseases can neither (as is asserted of dissimilar diseases in I) repel one another, nor (as has been shown of dissimilar* diseases in II) suspend *one another, so that the old one shall return after the new one has run its course; and just as little can two* similar *diseases (as has been demonstrated in III respecting dissimilar affections)* exist beside each other *in the same organism, or together form a* double *complex disease.*

Aph. 45: *No. Two diseases, differing, it is true, in kind, but very similar in their phenomena and effects and in the sufferings and symptoms they severally produce, invariably annihilate one another whenever they meet together in the organism; the stronger disease, namely, annihilates the weaker, and that for this simple reason, because the stronger morbific power when it invades the system, by reason of its similarity of action involves precisely the same parts of the organism that were previously affected by the weaker morbid irritation, which, consequently, can no longer act on these parts, but is extinguished, or (in other words), the new similar but stronger morbific potency controls the feelings of the patient and hence the life principle on account of its peculiarity, can no longer feel the weaker similar which becomes extinguished—exists no longer—for it was never anything material, but a dynamic—spirit-like—(conceptual) affection. The life principle henceforth is affected only and this but temporarily by the new, similar but stronger morbific potency.*

Hahnemann's descriptions can be readily understood in terms of the model considered in this book. When he is speaking of two dissimilar diseases, he refers to two diseases in the same approximate spectrum which are close enough to resonate to some degree with the organism, but which are not quite close enough to annihilate each other. In such a circumstance, the *strength* of the disease is the crucial factor. If two diseases are similar enough (possess almost the identical resonance), they will stimulate the defense mechanism in such a manner as to annihilate one another completely; in this instance, the crucial factor lies more in the similarity than in the strength of the diseases. Of course, if one is exposed to a disease of extreme dissimilarity as to be on a different level altogether, the organism will simply not respond. All of us are exposed every day to potentially morbific agents, but we only occasionally actually contract the disease—depending upon our level of vibrational susceptibility and the degree of weakness of the defense mechanism at the moment.

In the next chapter, we will see how important the above concepts of disease interaction are to health. If enough powerful disease influences occur in the life of an individual, the defense mechanism becomes progressively weakened in layers. These layers of predisposition are called in homeopathy "miasms," and they become important factors to any clinician dealing with chronic diseases.

Suppressive Therapies

I have commented throughout the book on the dangers of prescribing therapeutic agents based solely on local symptoms, while ignoring the totality of the symptom expression. Allopathic medicine in particular has developed an entire methodology of therapeutics based on the concept of counteracting specific symptoms and syndromes. Allopathic drugs themselves are morbific shocks to the organism, and therefore stimulate reaction on the part of the defense mechanism. Such response on the part of the defense mechanism consists of symptoms which are usually called "side-effects" in the allopathic profession. On the contrary, these symptoms are themselves signs of sensitivity on the part of the organism; they are the best possible response of the defense mechanism to counteract the morbific stimulus of the drug. In this way, drugs can be seen to be diseases in themselves, following the same dynamics as described by Hahnemann in the above aphorisms.

Hahnemann specifically comments on the effect of allopathic drugs in Aphorism 76:

Only for natural diseases has the beneficent Deity granted us, in Homeopathy, the means of affording relief; but those devastations and maimings of the human organism exteriorly and interiorly, effected by years frequently, of the unsparing exercise of a false art, with its hurtful drugs and treatment, must be remedied by the vital force itself (appropriate aid being given for the eradication of any chronic miasm that may happen to be lurking in the background), if it has not already been too much weakened by such mischievous acts, and can devote several years to this huge operation undisturbed. A human healing art, for the restoration to the normal state of those innumerable abnormal conditions so often produced by the allopathic non-healing art, there is not and cannot be.

Even more concisely, in Aphorism 75, Hahnemann states:

These inroads on human health effected by the allopathic non-healing art (more particularly in recent times) are of all chronic diseases the most deplorable, the most incurable; and I regret to add that it is apparently impossible to discover or to hit upon any remedies for their cure when they have reached any considerable height.

If this was true in Hahnemann's time, how much more true it is today! Modern science has developed chemicals which are even more potent that those in Hahnemann's time. Drugs of all types, of course, are damaging, but in my experience the most disturbing to the organism are antibiotics, tranquilizers, contraceptive pills, cortisone, and other hormones. In any specific individual, however, literally *any* drug or foreign substance can be disruptive if the person is susceptible to it. Thus we see people having even fatal anaphylactic reactions to very minute doses of drugs such as penicillin, aspirin, and other supposedly mild drugs.

Since allopathic drugs are never selected according to the Law of Similars, they inevitably superimpose upon the organism a new drug disease which then must be counteracted by the organism. Furthermore, if the drug has been successful in removing symptoms on a peripheral level, the defense mechanism is then forced to reestablish a new state of equilibrium at a deeper level. In this way, the vibration rate of the organism is disturbed and weakened by two mechanisms: 1) by the influence of the drug itself and 2) by interference with the best possible response of the defense mechanism. Consequently, if the drug is powerful enough, or if drug therapy is continued long enough, the organism may jump to a deeper level in its susceptibility to disease. The real tragedy of such a consequence is that the defense mechanism of the individual cannot then reestablish the original equilibrium on its own; even with homeopathic treatment of very high quality, it may take many years to return to the original level, much less to make any progress on the original ailment.

It is a strange but true paradox that people who have been weakened by allopathic drugging become relatively "protected" from certain infections and epidemics. This, of course, occurs because the center of gravity of susceptibility has moved into more vital regions of the organism that there is not enough susceptibility on superficial levels to produce a symptomatic reaction. In such an instance, this not a sign of improvement in health, but rather a sign of degeneration.

Let us consider the example of a person infected with syphilis. He develops a chancre on the penis, which is then treated by high doses of penicillin over a period of two weeks. The chancre disappears, and the patient is considered cured. Research and clinical experience have shown that such a patient cannot re-acquire a chancre. Such apparent "immunity" is not a sign of improved health but rather an indication of further degeneration in the ability of the defense mechanism to maintain the symptoms on more peripheral levels of the organism. From the homeopathic point of

111

view, this is considered a suppression. The organism as a whole is suffering even more than during the initial stage of the chancre. After three to six months, however, the secondary stage of syphilis emerges as a skin eruption elsewhere on the body. Then, after many years, the tertiary stage manifests as central nervous system degeneration and perhaps insanity. During the development of these later stages, it is also true that the patient is "immune" to further re-infection with syphilis. Clearly, such immunity is not a sign of improved health but rather of further degeneration in the ability of the defense mechanism to maintain the symptoms on more peripheral levels of the organism.

Therefore, because of the severe suppressive effects on drugs, every clinician should be as aware as possible of the therapeutic history of the patient. *Drug diseases* can then be recognized, and the major suppressive influences in the life of the patient can be determined.

In a more general sense, it is also important to realize the effect that such massive and systematic suppressive therapies have on entire populations. As described so well by Ivan Illich in *Medical Nemesis* [1] and Allen Klass in *There's Gold in Them Thar Pills*,[2] the entire medical establishment has built-in structural commitments to maintaining the current model of disease and therapy. Statistics demonstrate quite clearly that the threat of acute diseases has diminished in this century, although not because of therapeutic effectiveness, and that there is a corresponding increase in crippling chronic diseases,[3] cancer, heart disease,[4] strokes,[5] neurological disorders and epilepsy,[6] violence, and insanity.[7] Such is the inevitable result when the processes of Nature are ignored. On the other hand, as we see increasing progress toward cooperation with the processes of Nature, statistics will demonstrate a decline in such problems. As a matter of fact, within the past few years, the

---

1. Ivan Illich, *Medical Nemesis* (New York: Bantam, 1976). The first section gives specifics, while later sections discuss societal implications.

2. Allen Klass, *There's Gold in Them Thar Pills* (Baltimore: Penguin, 1975).

3. Lilienfeld and Gifford, eds., *Chronic Disease and Public Health* (Baltimore: Johns Hopkins Press, 1966), p. 8. Leading causes of death and their rates, comparing 1900-1960. A Baltimore study demonstrated the rise of chronic diseases with age.

4. Curriel et al., *Trends in the Study of Morbidity and Mortality*, Public Health Papers No. 27 (Geneva: WHO, 1965). Demonstrates increase in mortality rates for heart disease, stroke, and diabetes.

5. Ibid.; and Lilienfeld and Gifford, *Chronic Disease.*

6. M. Ferguson, *Brain Revolution* (New York: Taplinger, 1973).

7. Donald Jackson, ed., *The Etiology of Schizophrenia* (New York: Publisher's Basic Books, 1960).

increased interest in weight control, good nutrition, and exercise, has already resulted in a slight decline in heart disease and stroke for the first time in many decades. As more people are treated by homeopathy, we can expect even further progress.

Vaccination

Vaccination is cited by many as being an example of allopathic use of the Law of Similars; superficially, this would appear to be true because vaccines are small amounts of material which are capable of producing disease in normal people. Reflection on the principles enunciated in this book, however, will quickly clear up this point of confusion. Vaccines are administered to entire populations without any consideration of individuality. Each individual will have a unique degree of susceptibility to any vaccine, yet it is administered without regard to the uniqueness of each individual. Therefore, the concept of vaccination is almost the precise opposite of the principles of homeopathy; it is indiscriminate administration of a foreign substance to everyone, regardless of state of health or individual sensitivity.

What exactly does happen to the organism upon administration of a vaccine? Of course, modern studies in the field of immunology document very well the varieties of chemical and cellular mechanisms which are brought into play, but the further question can be asked: What happens on the dynamic plane upon administration of vaccine?

The experience of astute homeopathic observers has shown conclusively that in a high percentage of cases, vaccination has a profoundly disturbing effect on the health of an individual, particularly in relation to chronic disease.[8] Whenever a vaccine is administered, it tends to change the electromagnetic vibration rate in the same way that a severe illness or allopathic drug does. Depending upon the state of health of the individual, there are two basic types of responses which can occur after vaccination:

1. There may be no reaction to the vaccine at all.
2. The vaccination may "take," which means that some degree of reaction is produced.

In the first instance, the lack of reaction may indicate either: 1) a very healthy system or 2) a system with deep constitutional

---

8. J. Compton Burnett, *Vaccinosis* (London: Homeopathic Publishing Co., 1884).

weakness. This is analogous to the situation mentioned in Chapter 5 regarding susceptibility to gonorrhea. If a person's state of health is nearly perfect, i.e., at the bottom of the scale in Figure 7 (page 83) the organism is simply not sensitive to the vaccine, no resonance occurs, and there is no reaction. On the other hand, if the system is very weak, i.e., vibrating on a much deeper level of susceptibility, the defense mechanism is incapable of producing an immediate reaction to the vaccine. Of course, both individuals displaying no reaction would also acquire no illness if exposed to the epidemic for which the vaccine is intended, because both organisms are vibrating at levels far removed from that of the disease.

If the organism is capable of reacting to the vaccination, this signifies that the vibration rate of the vaccine is close enough to that of the patient to produce resonance. The reaction, then, is a sign of the defense mechanism responding to the morbific influence of the vaccine. Basically, there are three possible types of reactions, each representing a different intensity of response:

1. A mild reaction.
2. A strong reaction, with fever and other systemic symptoms.
3. A very strong reaction, with complications such as encephalitis, meningitis, paralysis, etc.

Let us consider the meaning of each of these possible reactions separately. In the first instance, a mild reaction indicates that the patient is indeed susceptible to the disease against which he is vaccinated, and consequently the defense mechanism creates a local inflammation, itching or pain, and perhaps a little pus. A mild reaction, however, indicates that the defense mechanism is not strong enough to fully deflect the effect of the vaccine. Its morbific influence then remains in the body, and the vibration rate of the entire organism is changed in proportion to the strength of the vaccine itself. If the vaccine is very powerful (e.g., smallpox vaccination) and resonates closely with the patient's level of susceptibility, the organism's vibration rate may change levels completely, and it will become incapable of returning to the prevaccination level without the aid of homeopathic treatment. Such a change in level of vibration is further confirmed by the fact that this patient will later be unlikely to react to further administrations of the same vaccine.

If the vaccine stimulates systemic symptoms such as fever,

malaise, anorexia, muscle aches, etc., then the defense mechanism is quite strong and may be able to successfully counteract the morbific influence of the vaccine. Such a strong reaction is commonly seen in children, whose defense mechanisms have not yet been seriously weakened by external morbific stimuli. Of course, if the defense mechanism is successful in this way, the person will remain unprotected against the disease. Unlike the very healthy person who possesses no susceptibility to either the vaccine or to the microbe, the person who demonstrates a strong systemic reaction is sensitive to the microbe and the vaccine, and may well contract the disease upon exposure, despite vaccination. Such cases are relatively rare, because few people have such a high degree of health in our modern world; thus, statistics show the "effectiveness" rate of vaccinated populations to be in the range of 10%-15% depending upon the particular type of immunization.[9,10] Unfortunately, such statistics are not truly measures of vaccine effectiveness; rather, they are measures of the low state of health of the population.

The third type of reaction is the very strong reaction with complications. This also indicates that the susceptibility of the organism to the disease is quite high, but in this case the defense mechanism is too weak to counteract the morbific stimulus of the vaccine, so a deep illness is produced. This is perhaps the most tragic circumstance, because if the patient survives the complication at all, his state of health may remain impaired for a very long time. It is in such cases that we see the development of chronic conditions of great severity, dating from the time of the vaccination. The weakening of the defense mechanism in such cases can be so severe that even careful homeopathic prescribing may require years to return the person to health. It is true that if such a sensitive person were to be exposed to the epidemic, the same complications would ensue; but who is to say that all of these people would be exposed at all?

In homeopathy, any chronic condition which can be traced to a vaccination is called *vaccinosis*. In his book *Vaccinosis*, J. Compton Burnett presents his very detailed cases which demonstrate clearly

---

9. V. Tudor and I. Stratt, *Smallpox: Cholera* (Turnbridge Wells, Kent: Abacus Press, 1977), p. 133.

10. P. Wright et al., "Safety and Antigenicity of Influenza A/Hong/Kong/ 68-ts-1 [E] (H3N3) Vaccine in Young Seronegative Children," *Journal of Pediatrics* 87: 1109-1116 (Dec. 1975).

that vaccinations can have profoundly disturbing and lasting influences on the health of susceptible individuals.[11] His cases involved administration of smallpox vaccination, but modern homeopaths see similar cases of vaccinosis occurring after rabies, measles, polio, influenza, typhoid, paratyphoid, and even tetanus vaccines.

The fact that vaccinosis is indeed due to vaccination and not merely coincidence is seen by the fact that many cases are dramatically benefitted by administration of a potentized preparation of the particular vaccine used. For example, suppose we see a case who has suffered for many years from chronic sinusitis since receiving a smallpox vaccination to which she had reacted mildly the first time; in such a case, Variolinum 1 M (a 1000c potency of the smallpox vaccine itself) may completely clear up the entire condition. In other cases, we see patients, who simply do not respond to well-selected homeopathic prescriptions; once the vaccine is identified, and the corresponding potentized preparation given, such cases then react nicely to their appropriate remedies.

One dramatic case which comes to mind is that of a 50-year-old woman who suffered from hay fever for many years. After homeopathic treatment, she was completely free of hay fever for over two years. Then, in preparation for a foreign trip, she received a smallpox vaccination. Her system reacted with only slight localized redness, and no systemic symptoms. Unfortunately, her hay fever returned immediately. She was then much more difficult to treat homeopathically; even the same remedies, although still indicated, did not act as effectively as before. Variolinum helped to reestablish order in the system, and the patient then responded again to the appropriate remedies.

Such cases can be quoted in great numbers by any homeopath who takes the time to elucidate the complete history of the patient. Thus even something as popular and widespread as vaccination—one of the so-called major "successes" of modern medicine—can be a large-scale factor in the degenerating health of our populations. A striking example in recent times was the major effort on the part of the United States government to vaccinate the entire population against an expected swine flu epidemic which was feared would be as severe as the 1918 influenza epidemic. As it turned out, the vaccine was not manufactured quickly enough to have much effect, but the epidemic never materialized anyway.

---

11. Burnett, *Vaccinosis.*

Of the 50 million Americans who were vaccinated, 581 developed Guillain-Barré syndrome, a paralytic neurological disorder. This incidence represents a sevenfold increase over that of the population at large. One could attribute this to some impurities in the preparation or to some other cause, but from the homeopathic point of view such consequences are predictable whenever a foreign substance is injected into large numbers of people without regard to individual susceptibility.

Summary for Chapter 8

Summary of Disease Influence Section

1. Virtually everyone has some degree of chronic disease tendency.

2. One cannot jump major levels of susceptibility on one's own; only powerful influences can produce such changes. One such major influence is a serious illness.

3. Of two dissimilar diseases, the strong one repels the weaker one, but they never cure one another.

4. Rarely, two dissimilar diseases may create a complex of diseases without curing either one.

5. Two similar diseases cure one another. Here, similarity is a more important factor than the strength of the disease.

6. Enough serious illnesses can engraft upon the constitution of the individual chronic disease predispositions that can persist throughout life and into subsequent generations.

Summary of Suppressive Therapy Section

1. Allopathic drugs themselves are morbific stimuli to the human body.

2. "Side-effects" are in fact signs of the defense mechanism reacting to this morbific influence.

3. Sufficient allopathic drugging can create such damage to the defense mechanism that the patient can become virtually incurable.

4. Since allopathic drugs are never prescribed according to the Law of Similars, they inevitably superimpose upon the organism a new drug-disease.

5. Drugs have two effects: a direct morbific influence, and the suppressive influence resulting from removal of the defense mechanism's best possible response.

6. Drug suppression is a major factor in the alarming increase in chronic diseases in our societies.

Summary of Vaccination Section

1. Vaccination is not really an example of the homeopathic principle, since it is an indiscriminate administration of a substance to an entire population without regard to individuality.

2. A vaccination is a morbific stimulus which changes the resonant frequency of the defense mechanism.

3. Lack of reaction to vaccination may represent either a very healthy system or a deep constitutional weakness, as in both instances the resonant frequency of the patient does not allow a response. In such case, the patient would be immune to the epidemic, even if not vaccinated.

4. A mild reaction—merely local inflammation—indicates a relatively weak defense mechanism, and the altered vibration rate may well persist for a long time, leading to chronic disease later in life. Such cases are unlikely to react to further administration of the vaccine, confirming the fact of the change in resonant frequency.

5. A systemic reaction with fever, malaise, etc, indicates a strong defensive reaction which is likely to be successful in throwing off the morbific influence of the vaccination. The patient then remains unprotected against the disease, despite having been vaccinated.

6. A systemic reaction with complications such as encephalitis and neurological disorders is the worst possible case, for the subsequent degeneration in health will be severe and prolonged.

7. In chronic cases of vaccinosis, the appropriate nosode frequently produces great benefit.

Annotated Bibliography for Chapter 8

1. Thomas, E.W. *Syphilis: Its Course and Management* (New York: Macmillan, 1949), p. 10. "*Within two years after infection, untreated syphilis produces immune changes in the host which, with rare exceptions, are permanent and make it impossible for the tissues to react to subsequent infection with the development of early syphilitic lesions.*" In fact, in the experience of the above author, only one exception was found in 2000 cases studied.

2. International Agency for Research on Cancer and John E. Fogarty International Center of the National Institutes of Health, USA, *Host En-*

vironment Interactions in the Etiology of Cancer in Man (Lyons: International Agency for Research on Cancer, 1973), p. 50. People in cancer families have a 300% increase in incidence of cancer compared to the general population. Leukemia in children shows a 400% family increase over the general population. There is also a high correlation between people with cancer and the incidence of chromosome-damage diseases in their families. In identical twins, one of which has leukemia, there is a 20% concordance in the remaining twin.

Chapter 9

Predisposition to Disease

IT SHOULD BE CLEAR that disease is a result of a morbific stimulus which resonates with the particular level of susceptibility of the organism. This stimulus is called the *exciting cause* and may be a microorganism, a foreign chemical, an emotional shock, an allopathic drug, a vaccination, or any one of many other influences. A strong susceptibility to the morbific agent is necessary for producing disease; this predisposition is called the *maintaining cause* because it is the weakness of the defense mechanism which maintains a lowered state of health, rather than a succession of exciting causes. In this chapter, we shall consider exactly what this predisposition is, what its characteristics are, how it is transmitted, and its importance in treatment.

As described in Chapter 5, the susceptibility of a given person tends to vary within a narrow spectrum of illnesses. Throughout life, a particular individual remains on a certain level of susceptibility unless a major influence (such as those discussed in Chapter 8) produces a jump in levels; even then, the organism will remain on the new level unless treated by homeopathy. *Within* a certain range of diseases, a person will vary according to such factors as the amount of sleep he gets, nutrition, sanitation, the degree of stress in his life, etc., but he will be *unable* to make changes from *one level to another* on his own.

How does a person acquire a predisposition to illness in the first place? How is the weakness on a given level established? As we know, powerful acute ailments, allopathic drugs, and vaccinations are major factors, but it is also clear that a considerable portion of predisposition is hereditary. It is well known that certain diseases such as heart disease, cancer, diabetes, Huntington's chorea, tuberculosis, alcoholism, schizophrenia, and many others tend to run in families. All clinicians have also observed frequently that there is a predisposition toward serious disease *per se* in certain families and not others. For example, a patient may develop symptoms of ulcerative colitis at a young age even though no one else in the family ever had colitis; on taking a family history, however, it will be found that many parents and grandparents were sick most of their lives with different ailments. It is quite rare for a person to acquire a very serious chronic disease at a young age if the ancestors were all healthy into an advanced age.

It is known that the genetic make-up, the DNA, of an individual plays a role in shaping the hereditary predisposition to disease, but this is not the whole story. As we shall see a bit later, it is possible for a parent to acquire an ailment during life whose influence can be transmitted to the children, even though no known change has occurred in the genetic structure of the parent. Taking into account the dynamic plane, it is quite easy to imagine how such a thing can occur. If the vital force is significantly weakened in the parents, the child's electrodynamic field can be correspondingly weakened at the moment of conception.

The clinical recognition of this "maintaining cause" for disease becomes apparent when we see a patient returning time and again for the same or similar complaint, even though the homeopathic remedies seemed to have acted quite well in each acute crisis. In such cases, it seems as if the remedies have affected the defense mechanism on an insufficiently deep level of predisposition. It was in frustration over such cases that Hahnemann devoted the last years of his life to searching for the causes of these deep predispositions. These investigations finally led to his third major contribution to medicine: the theory of *miasms*.

In Aphorism 72 of the *Organon*, Hahnemann describes his initial perceptions on this matter:

Diseases peculiar to mankind are of two classes. The first includes rapid, morbid processes caused by abnormal states and derangements of the vital force; such affections usually run their course within a brief period of variable duration, and are called acute diseases. The second class embraces diseases which often seem trifling and imperceptible in the beginning; but which, in a manner peculiar to

121

themselves, act deleteriously upon the living organism, dynamically deranging the latter, and insidiously undermining its health to such a degree, that the automatic energy of the vital force, designed for the preservation of life, can only make imperfect and ineffectual resistance to these diseases in their beginning, as well as during their progress. Unable to extinguish them without assistance, the vital force is powerless to prevent their growth or its own gradual deterioration, resulting in the final destruction of the organism. These are called chronic diseases.

Hahnemann's investigations into this problem occupied him for 12 years; he systematically questioned each case relentlessly, even inquiring into the ailments of parents and grandparents in his effort to elucidate the origin of the problem. Hahnemann's account of this investigation is described in *Chronic Diseases*. It is so lucid, and answers so many questions that will undoubtedly arise in the mind of the reader, that I quote him at some length here:

> The chronic diseases could, despite all efforts, be but little delayed in their progress by the Homeopathic physician and grew worse from year to year . . . Their beginning was promising, the continuation less favorable, the outcome hopeless . . . Nevertheless this teaching was founded upon the steadfast pillar of truth and will evermore be so . . . Homeopathy alone taught first of all how to heal the well-defined idiopathic diseases . . . by a few small doses of rightly selected homeopathic medicine.
>
> Whence then this less favorable, this unfavorable, result of the continued treatment of the non-venereal chronic diseases even by Homeopathy? What was the reason for the thousands of unsuccessful endeavors to heal the other diseases of a chronic nature so that lasting health might result? Might this be caused, perhaps, by the still too small number of Homeopathic remedies that have so far been proved as to their pure action? The followers of Homeopathy have hitherto thus consoled themselves; but this excuse, or so-called consolation, never satisfied the founder of Homeopathy—particularly because even the new additions of proved valuable medicines, increasing from year to year, have not advanced the healing of chronic (non-venereal) diseases by a single step, while acute diseases are not only passably removed, by means of a correct application of Homeopathic remedies, but with the assistance of the never-resting preservative vital force in our organism, find a speedy and complete cure.
>
> Why, then, cannot this vital force, efficiently affected through Homeopathic medicine, produce any true and lasting recovery in these chronic maladies even with the aid of the Homeopathic remedies which best cover their present symptoms; while this same force which is created for the restoration of our organism is nevertheless so indefatigably and successfully active in completing the recovery even in severe acute diseases? What is there to prevent this?
>
> To find out then the reason why all the medicines known to Homeopathy failed to bring a real cure in the above-mentioned diseases . . . occupied me since the year

1816, night and day; and behold! The Giver of all good things permitted me within this space of time to gradually solve this sublime problem through unremitting thought, indefatigable inquiry, faithful observation and the most accurate experiments made for the welfare of humanity.

It was a continually repeated fact that the non-venereal chronic diseases, after being time and again removed homeopathically, always returned in a more or less varied form and with new symptoms, or reappeared annually with an increase of complaints. This fact gave me the first clue that the Homeopathic physician with such a chronic (non-venereal) case, has not only to combat the disease presented before his eyes, and must not view and treat it as if it were a well-defined disease, to be speedily and permanently destroyed and healed by ordinary Homeopathic remedies, but that he had always to encounter some separate fragment of a more deep-seated original disease . . . He, therefore, must first find out as far as possible the whole extent of all the accidents and symptoms belonging to the unknown primitive malady before he can hope to discover one or more medicines which may homeopathically cover the whole of the original disease by means of its peculiar symptoms . . .

But that the original malady sought for must be also of a miasmatic chronic nature clearly appeared to me from this circumstance, that after it has once advanced and developed to a certain degree it can never be removed by the strength of any robust constitution, it can never be overcome by the most wholesome diet and order of life, nor will it die out of itself . . .

I had come thus far in my investigations and observations with such non-venereal patients, when I discovered, even in the beginning, that the obstacle to the cure of many cases which seemed delusively like specific, well-defined diseases, and yet could not be cured in a Homeopathic manner with the then proved medicines, seemed very often to lie in a former eruption of itch, which was not infrequently confessed; and the beginning of all the subsequent sufferings usually dated from that time. So also with similar chronic patients who did not confess such an infection, or, what was probably more frequent, who had, from inattention, not perceived it, or, at least, could not remember it. After a careful inquiry it usually turned out that little traces of it (small pustules of itch, herpes, etc.) had showed themselves with them from time to time, even if but rarely, as an indubitable sign of a former infection of this kind.

These circumstances, in connection with the fact that innumerable observations of physicians, and not infrequently my own experience, had shown that an eruption of itch suppressed by faulty practice or one which had disappeared from the skin through other means was evidently followed, in persons otherwise healthy, by the same or similar symptoms; these circumstances, I repeat, could leave no doubt in my mind as to the internal foe which I had to combat in my medical treatment of such cases . . . [1]

---

1. Samuel Hahnemann, *Chronic Diseases*, translated by Louis H. Tafel from the second enlarged German edition (Philadelphia: Boericke & Tafel, 1896; Calcutta: L. Ringer, 1975), pp. 19-22.

To most of us in the modern world, this concept may seem a bit simplistic. Nevertheless, it does fit what has thus far been said concerning suppression of symptoms from peripheral levels to deeper levels. This is a good example of the way in which the resonant frequency of the organism can be changed, thus creating susceptibility to deeper ailments. In *Chronic Diseases*, Hahnemann quotes a large number of cases which demonstrate this principle very convincingly:

A boy of 13 years having suffered from his childhood with Tinea Capitis *had his mother remove it for him, but he became very sick within eight or ten days, suffering with asthma, violent pains in the limbs, back and knee, which were not relieved until an eruption of* Itch *broke out over his whole body a month later. (Pelargus, [Storch] Obs. clin. Jahrg., 1722, p. 435)*

Tinea Capitis *in a little girl was driven away by purgatives and other medicines, but the child was attacked with oppression of the chest, cough and great lassitude. It was not until she stopped taking the medicines, and the* Tinea *broke out again, that she recovered her cheerfulness and this, indeed, quickly. (Pelargus,* Breslauer Sammlung v. Jahrg., 1727, p. 293)

A 3-year old girl had the Itch, *for several weeks; when this was driven out by an ointment she was seized the next day by a suffocating catarrh with snoring, and with numbness and coldness of the whole body, from which she did not recover until the* Itch *re-appeared. (Suffocating Catarrh, Ehrenfr. Hagendorn,* Hist. Med. Phys. Cent. I, hist. 8, 9)

A boy of 5 years suffered for a long time from Itch, *and when this was driven away by a salve it left behind a severe melancholy with a cough. (Riedlin,* Obs. Cent. II, obs. 90, Augsburg, 1691)

A girl of 12 years had the Itch *with which she had frequently suffered, driven away from the skin by an ointment, when she was seized with an acute fever with suffocative catarrh, asthma and swelling, and afterward with pleurisy. Six days afterward, having taken an internal medicine containing sulphur, the* Itch *again appeared and all the ailments, excepting the swelling, disappeared; but after twenty-four days the* Itch *again dried up, which was followed by a new inflammation in the chest with pleurisy and vomiting. (Pelargus,* Obs. clin. Jahrg., 1723, p. 15)

A girl of 9 years with the Tinea Capitis *had it driven away, when she was seized with a lingering fever, a general swelling and dyspnoea; when the* Tinea *broke out again she recovered. (Hagendorn,* Recueil d'observ. de Med., Tom. III, p. 308)

From Itch *expelled by external application there arose amaurosis, which passed away then the eruption re-appeared on the skin. (Amaurosis, Northof,* Diss. de Scabie, Gotting., 1792, p. 10)

A man who had driven off a frequently occurring eruption of Itch *with an ointment fell into epileptic convulsions, which disappeared again when the eruption reappeared on the skin. (Epilepsy, J.C. Carl in* Act. Nat. Cur. V., obs. 16)

Two children were freed from epilepsy by the breaking out of humid Tinea, *but the epilepsy returned when the* Tinea *was incautiously driven off. (Tulpius,* Obs. Lib. I., Cap. *8)* [2]

Eventually, Hahnemann described three basic miasms which he believed to be the underlying causes of chronic disease. In any given patient, there could be one miasm, or any combination of them. The first that he described was the *Psoric Miasm* (derived from the Greek word *psora,* meaning "itch"). Hahnemann considered this the earliest miasm affecting the human race, and thus the most fundamental underlying layer of weakness upon which the others have subsequently been built. Specific diseases which Hahnemann associated with Psora ranged from virtually all physical ailments including cancer, diabetes, arthritis, etc., to the most severe mental illnesses of epilepsy, schizophrenia, and imbecility.

The second miasm to affect the human race Hahnemann considered to be the *Syphilitic Miasm.* The specific disease syphilis was considered to be one of the manifestations of this predisposition, but it also was implicated in a wide range of other disorders found as well in late stages of other miasms as well. Hahnemann believed that patients suffering from the Syphilis Miasm acquired its influence by exposure to syphilis, or by inheritance from an infected ancestor—the trait then being transmitted from generation to generation.

The third Hahnemannian miasm was the *Sycosis Miasm* (from the Greek word *syco,* meaning "fig"). This miasm he considered to have arisen out of gonorrhea, either contracted by the patient or by one of the patient's ancestors.

It should be made clear that Hahnemann did not consider the actual microbes, the spirochete or the gonococcus, to be the specific cause of the venereal miasms. These microbes, as with all disease-causing agents, were considered to have morbific influences on the dynamic plane as well. If the patient is weakened by the Psoric Miasm and then ends up exposing himself to a venereal disease through illicit sexual conduct, this combination then leads to the illness and subsequent miasm. Not everyone who actually acquires the disease gonorrhea necessarily progresses into the Sycosis Miasm; only a relatively small percentage develop it, but once this "taint" becomes engrafted upon the dynamic plane of the organism, it will be passed on from generation to generation.

---

2. Ibid.

A common misunderstanding about the miasmatic theory is that specific pathological conditions result from specific miasms. For example, it is often said that eczema is a psoric disease, ulcers are syphilitic, and that cancer, psoriasis, and others result from a combination of all three miasms. In reality, however, all three miasms can result in any pathological change. Cancer, diabetes, insanity, imbecility, etc., can arise from the last stage of *any* of the miasms, or from any combination of them.

The degree of chronic weakness of the defense mechanism is a direct result of the intensity of the miasmatic influences. If we contrast two patients with leukemia, for example, the age at which the disease occurs is a measure of the number of miasms involved. If it were to develop at the age of 70 after a lifetime of good health, it is likely that only the Psoric Miasm is involved. If, on the other hand, it were to arise in childhood, very likely three or more are implicated. While evaluating any individual case, having an idea of the number of miasms involved has important prognostic significance; the more miasms are involved, the slower the response to treatment.

Since Hahnemann's time, the miasmatic theory has been largely misused or misunderstood by the homeopathic profession. Many homeopaths simply ignored the concept as being too simplistic or of little practical value. Many adopted the theory uncritically, simply as an act of faith in the Master who had made such massive contributions. Unfortunately, such blind faith prevented a real understanding of the idea and further elaboration of it in actual clinical practice. Consequently, there are presently two basic schools of thought in the homeopathic profession regarding miasms: one which ignores the idea altogether, and another which accepts it thoughtlessly and therefore adopts a routine of prescribing in an attempt to "clear" the case of miasms. The confusion and controversy which have resulted since Hahnemann's death have caused tremendous degrees of misunderstanding about the miasmatic concept; for this reason, in this book I will emphasize the term *predisposition* rather than "miasm." In addition, I will not describe the detailed clinical signs and symptoms associated with each miasm, in order to keep readers from being misled into the idea of prescribing specifically on the basis of the miasm alone.

A further confusion which has arisen since Hahnemann's time is that certain miasms are a complex *combination* of two or more of the original three miasms. The best known example of confusion over this issue is that the so-called Tuberculosis Miasm is actually

126

a combination of Psora and Syphilis. The known history of diseases on the planet clearly contradicts this theory. Tuberculosis is one of the earliest diseases known to mankind, found in skeletons of the earliest primitive humans. Syphilis, on the other hand, was unknown to the European continent until brought from North America by Columbus.[3]

The most important contribution of Hahnemann's explorations into the miasms is the concept that there exist *layers of predisposition* which underlie the waxing and waning of temporary ailments; these must be taken into account in treatment intending to be completely curative. In such cases, complete cure will take a relatively long time, while the prescriber systematically peels off layer upon layer of predisposing weaknesses by carefully prescribing each remedy based on the totality of symptoms in the moment (see Figure 9). Each layer is always the result of the underlying ones, and there is a definite sequence to the presenting layers. If a remedy is prescribed routinely, based merely on the past or family history and not on the presenting symptomatology of the patient, the remedy may actually disrupt any progress toward cure. Even worse, such a prescription may disorder the defense mechanism enough to make the image of the correct remedy much more difficult to discern.

The concept of predisposing layers had considerable practical value in chronic relapsing cases. For example, if a patient consults a homeopath for chronic headaches that began after exposure to cold, and the prescriber gives belladonna, he may find that the headaches disappear dramatically. If the patient has a quite strong constitution to begin with, the problem may remain cured for a long time. However, the vast majority of patients have been weakened through hereditary influence, drugs, or vaccinations, resulting in several layers of predisposition. At the time when the above patient first consults the homeopath, the totality of symptoms at that moment represents only the uppermost layer of predisposition. With time, the next layer will likely assert itself, and the patient may display symptoms such as great sensitivity to cold, excessive desire for sweets and soft-boiled eggs, vertigo from high places, and burning of the soles of the feet while in bed. The homeopath now perceives that the new complex of symptoms, while not as crippling to the patient as the headaches, still represents a limitation to the patient's freedom. Calcarea carbonica is

3. Folke Henschen, *The History of Diseases* (London: Longmans, Green, 1966).

prescribed on the basis of this new totality of symptoms, and the patient's health improves even further without relapse of the headaches. In this example, Hahnemann would have said that this second layer was due to the Psoric Miasm.

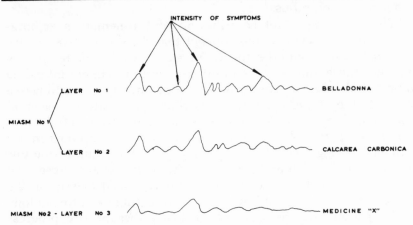

Figure 9: A schematic diagram representing the layers of miasms. Each miasm is manifest as a particular symptom picture, each symptom having a unique degree of intensity. In order to remove a particular layer, the specific remedy which resonates with that level of vibration must be prescribed. Then, with time, the next layer will manifest itself by a new symptom picture which may be similar but subtly different. A new remedy is prescribed for this layer, and the process continues. In this way, the patient eventually reaches a state of lasting cure after all of the major miasmatic predispositions have been systematically removed.

It is always necessary to remove the uppermost layer first. If a remedy is given which corresponds to a deeper layer, it will not cure. Moreover, it may change the symptom pictures of overlying layers enough so that the correct prescriptions may become obscured.

In this way, we can see the wisdom in Hahnemann's statement that homeopathic treatment must be continued until all the layers of predisposition have been removed. If the patient and homeopath were to be satisfied before all the layers were removed, the remaining untreated condition would be likely to slowly degenerate over time into an irreversible pathological process, particularly if further exciting causes occur. Each layer shows itself in the beginning as a few relatively minor symptoms which may be difficult to discern. Over a period of perhaps years the image becomes more clear, and the appropriate remedy can then be prescribed. In some cases, this process of complete cure can take as much as 20 years of careful, patient prescribing.

The predisposing weakness of the defense mechanism can be affected fundamentally by three major factors:

1. Hereditary influence.
2. Strong infectious diseases.
3. Previous treatments and vaccinations.

Despite Hahnemann's investigations, any homeopath who has studied the course of degeneration of patients over a long period of time can attest to the presence of a large number of "miasms." To be sure, Psora, Syphilis, and Sycosis are major influences which are seen in daily practice. In addition, cancer, tuberculosis, and other major illnesses transmit from one generation to another characteristic disease-images which may not necessarily be equated with the particular pathological condition itself; for example, the child of a parent with tuberculosis may not get tuberculosis *per se* but is likely to suffer from asthmatic bronchitis, hay fever, sinusitis, emaciation, night sweats, restlessness, and a fear of dogs—all of which manifest in the provings of Tuberculinum, which is the potentized "nosode" prepared from an actual tuberculos abscess. Just so, another asthma patient coming from a family with a lot of cancer in its history may respond very well to administration of the nosode Carcinosin, which is prepared from cancer tissue itself.

In the same manner, a patient may acquire a chronic disease predisposition after a bout with a severe infectious disease, and this predisposition may even be transmitted to subsequent generation. Thus we sometimes see cases in whom well-selected remedies do not seem to be acting satisfactorily, yet who later respond to influenzinum (the nosode prepared from a collection of influenza viruses), after the discovery has been made of a serious influenza episode in the history of the patient or a parent.

Finally, allopathic drugs or vaccinations may engraft upon the organism a predisposition to a particular syndrome of highly individualized homeopathic symptomatology. Smallpox vaccination, rabies vaccine, polio immunization, cortisone, penicillin, tranquilizers, etc., are all capable of weakening the defense mechanism severely enough to predispose to chronic diseases of many types. In these instances, few provings have been done on the potentized vaccines or drugs, so the prescription of the corresponding nosode

129

may have to be made blindly, but we do see cases responding very nicely to potentized Variolinum (smallpox vaccine nosode), Hydrophobinum (rabies nosode, which has been proven), Penicillin nosode, or Cortisone nosode, when the patient's history or the family history shows a major chronic disease predisposition following exposure to one of these morbific influences. Again, it must be strongly emphasized that *routine* prescribing of such nosodes should be deplored by all conscientious homeopaths, because such indiscriminate prescriptions can be greatly disruptive to a case whenever the corresponding layer has not yet produced a full image.

Based upon what has been said thus far, we can now present a definition of miasms: *A miasm is a predisposition toward chronic disease underlying the acute manifestations of illness, 1) which is transmissible from generation to generation, and 2) which may respond beneficially to the corresponding nosode prepared from either pathological tissue or from the appropriate drug or vaccine.* From this definition, it is clear that there are a large number of miasms, and that the total number is constantly increasing with the advent of suppressive therapies.

Let us consider an actual clinical example to help clarify the influence of inherited predispositions in a case and how this concept affects actual prescribing. We will take a young man who has suffered recurrent episodes of asthmatic bronchitis for many years. With each acute episode, a variety of remedies such as Bryonia, Gelsemium, Bryonia again, Eupatorium perfoliatum, and finally Kali carbonicum are prescribed; each time, the acute attack subsides quickly, but over a period of one or two years it becomes clear that the fundamental predisposition to the attacks has not been affected.

Reviewing the symptoms over the entire period of treatment, we see few indications corresponding to Tuberculinum, so we inquire as to whether anyone in the family ever had tuberculosis. Indeed, one of the parents did, but the child never manifested any symptoms of it. Because we see a family history *and* because the patient displays homeopathic symptoms corresponding to its provings, we give Tuberculinum in high potency, and the attacks of asthmatic bronchitis dramatically decrease in intensity and frequency, finally disappearing altogether.

After another few years, the patient experiences an attack of bursitis in the right shoulder, treated with Sanguinaria. Over a period of time, he has arthritis in the left shoulder and later in the right knee, treated with Rhus toxicodendron and Agaricus, respectively. Again, we realize that there is an underlying layer of predisposition which is less deep than the first one, but is nevertheless not being cured by the specific remedies given during the acute crises. The case is reviewed over the previous year, and some indications of Calcarea carbonica are found; it is given, and the patient is again well for several years. We can name the second layer of predisposition Psoric Miasm, but Psorinum (potentized material from an itch vesicle) is not given. Instead, the *symptoms* indicate Calcarea carbonica, and indeed the clinical improvement confirms its resonance with the vibration level of the second layer.

Such an example is very instructive because it illustrates nicely the basic principles involved. Each prescription is based on the best totality of symptoms of the moment, but during the acute crises the acute symptoms lead us to relatively superficially acting remedies. As will be seen in the practical section of this book, it very rarely occurs that a remedy can be found which covers *every* detailed symptom of the patient. Consequently, there are always a few relatively minor symptoms which are disregarded. Over a period of time, however, recognizing that the predisposing layer has not been dealt with, we review the entire case and discover a few of these somewhat "hidden" symptoms which lead us to the deeper acting remedy. This illustrates the value of having the patient continue to return for appointments even when not suffering an acute crisis; often it is during the relatively quiet times that subtler symptoms are most easily discerned.

One might ask whether Calcarea carbonica should have been given at the very beginning in this case example. First of all, it is very unlikely that it would have been possible to even see the image of Calcarea carbonica at the beginning, because the topmost layer had not been removed. If by chance, Calcarea carbonica had been given, it very likely would not have acted because the resonant frequency at that moment did not match. If it were close enough to produce some changes, it would not have produced a cure and very likely would have changed the symptom image sufficiently to make later prescribing very difficult. This kind of misunderstanding can create havoc in a case and seriously interfere with the possibility of eventual cure.

Some homeopaths begin a case by routinely giving the various nosodes which correspond to the patient's past history and family history, on the theory that the miasms must be "cleared" before the constitutional remedy is given. A typical such routine might be to give the nosodes once a week or once a month in sequence, and then to take the constitutional case after the sequence has been completed. These routines are utterly unthinking and very dangerous. Who is to say which of the diseases in the past history actually created a miasm? And who can determine the precise sequence of layers? Sometimes, of course, one of the nosodes may produce some degree of benefit, but if insufficient time is allowed to elapse after its action, whatever benefit has been created will be disrupted by subsequent prescriptions. It is *always* necessary to take the entire case and prescribe only after careful thought about the best choice of remedy, the best choice of potency, and the correct timing according to the basic laws and principles which have been enumerated.

Sometimes a clear knowledge of miasms can have tremendous predictive value, which confirms the theory convincingly. One twenty-year-old woman was brought to the office by her father because she had been suffering for many years from chronic, severe headaches. When the case was taken, the totality of symptoms indicated quite clearly Medorrhinum, which is a very well-proven nosode prepared from gonorrheal discharge. The father was an important government official, a man of great distinction, and I thought it unlikely that he had had gonorrhea. Nevertheless, I took him into another room and asked him confidentially if he had ever had gonorrhea, in his younger years perhaps? His answer was, "Who did not?" Medorrhinum was given and the patient was promptly relieved.

This case illustrates an important distinction which must be made. The daughter did not herself have gonorrhea; it is even possible that her defense mechanism was weak enough that she would not at that moment be susceptible to gonorrhea even if she were exposed (although, *after* treatment her defense mechanism might be strengthened enough to make her susceptible). Nevertheless, the miasmatic influence displayed itself by specific symptomatology not limited to the particular venereal pathology. If we possessed provings on all of the nosodes corresponding to known miasms, as happened in this case, prescribing would certainly be much easier.

In Figure 10 we see a schematic representation of several layers of predisposition. At the base of each layer, there is the broadest possible health for that layer. At the top of each layer, the defense mechanism is weakest for that particular layer of susceptibility. If the level of health of the mother and father are

132

located as shown, then the predisposition of the child will lie somewhere in between the parents'; the precise location depends upon the severity of the predispositions in each parent. This refers specifically to the state of the health of the parents *at the moment of conception* of the child.

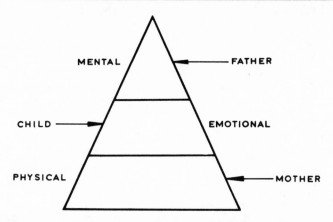

Figure 10: A diagram illustrating three miasmatic layers in triangular form. A child's miasmatic predisposition will fall within the range of the parents'. Precisely where the child's predisposition will fall depends upon typical factors which can be controlled by the parents—sleep, diet, exercise, consumption of alcohol, cigarettes, or drugs, etc.

The level of general health of the parents depends, of course, upon their own overall predispositions, but it also varies within a certain spectrum depending upon the amount of rest, the degree of emotional stress, the presence or absence of drugs and alcohol, etc. It is for this reason that it is very important for prospective parents to do everything possible to maximize their health—not only once the mother becomes pregnant, but even before conception. These transient changes in the state of health of parents explain the commonly observed phenomenon of children from the same parents showing great variation in health. In this way, conscientious attention on the part of parents to their own health during child-bearing years can save their children tremendous amounts of suffering throughout life.

Summary of Chapter 9

1. Disease is the result of an "exciting cause" and a "maintaining cause." The maintaining cause is the inherited chronic disease predisposition, "miasm."

2. Miasmatic predisposition is not merely a matter involving DNA, since diseases acquired during life can transmit their influences to subsequent generations.

3. Chronic disease predispositions are the primary reason why some cases continue to relapse despite good therapy.

4. Hahnemann's miasmatic theories have been largely misunderstood, ignored, or thoughtlessly transformed into routines for "clearing" a case of miasms.

5. Layers of predisposition are removed one layer at a time. A remedy given at an improper time either has no effect or creates actual damage of two types: it can interfere with progress toward cure, and it can disorder the defense mechanism enough to prevent a clear symptom picture from emerging.

6. Miasmatic predispositions are not merely the simple inheritance of a well-defined pathological condition, but rather the inheritance of a particular syndrome which corresponds to the influence of the miasm.

7. A miasm is characterized by transmission from generation to generation, and by relief from the corresponding nosode.

8. The predisposition of a child is a combination of the predispositions of the parents. The predisposition transmitted by the parents is a result both of the general state of health and of the specific state of health.

Annotated Bibliography for Chapter 9

1. International Agency for Research on Cancer and John E. Fogarty International Center of the National Institutes of Health, USA, *Host Environment Interactions in the Etiology of Cancer in Man* (Lyons: International Agency for Research on Cancer, 1973), p. 50. People in cancer families have a 300% increase in incidence of cancer compared to the general population. Children with leukemia have a 400% increased incidence in families compared with the general population. Cancer also correlates with diseases arising from chromosomal damage in families. Cancer incidence is the highest when familial tendencies to cancer or chromosome-

134

defect diseases occur at earlier ages. Childhood leukemia shows a 20% concordance rate in identical twins.

2. Jackson, Don, ed., *The Etiology of Schizophrenia* (New York: Publisher's Basic Books, 1960). First chapter is on the genetics of schizophrenia. The risk of schizophrenia if one parent is schizophrenic is 7-15%. If two parents have it, the risk is 40%. Twin studies show a concordance rate of 76-91% for monozygotic twins, and a 10-17% rate for dizygotic twins. P. 413: Studies show a higher incidence of various diseases in families of schizophrenics, including obesity, ulcerative colitis, peptic ulcer, asthma, rheumatoid arthritis, hypertension, prolonged convalescence from injury or surgery, acute leukemia, carcinoma, diabetes, scleroderma, and tuberculosis (the last doubtful).

3. Dubos, René and Jean, *The White Plague: Tuberculosis, Man, and Society* (Boston: Little, Brown, 1953), pp. 33-43, pp. 124-125. Tuberculosis families described; definitely higher incidence in twins, even when separated into foster homes.

Section II:

The Principles of Homeopathy in Practical Application

Introduction

As described in Section I, the processes involving health and disease are understandable through verifiable law and principles. Although these laws and principles have been known for centuries, it is only in recent times that the genius Samuel Hahnemann has enabled them to be formulated into the curative science of homeopathy. Just as physics moved from the Newtonian era into the concepts of modern physics, the field of medicine is slowly beginning to investigate the realms of energy fields in the human body.

The concepts presented in Section I are interesting and plausible in their own right, but they are merely sterile ideas until tested in the arena of actual clinical experience. It is in their application that the profound truths of homeopathy become alive with meaning and vivid in action. Having read this and other books on homeopathy, the reader may acquire an intellectually clear understanding of the Law of Similars, the laws of direction of cure, the fact of potentization, and the concepts underlying predispositions to disease. This intellectual understanding, however, is a long way from application. In specific terms, how is the totality of symptoms elicited from a patient so that the activities of the defense mechanism can be made visible? Likewise, how exactly do we arrive at the symptom picture elicited by homeopathic remedies? In actual practice, how do we match these two images when confronted with an individual patient? Once a remedy is given, pre-

139

cisely how do the theoretical principles manifest in response? Finally, everyone knows that human beings only very rarely fit into neat and simple patterns; how, then, can homeopathy be applied to complex cases involving various interfering factors?

Because homeopathy is a therapy based solely upon stimulating the energy level of the human being, the underlying laws and principles governing this realm must be understood very thoroughly by the homeopath prior to attempting to handle an actual case. Once the underlying principles have been understood, the next step is to plunge into the *art* of homeopathy. Each patient is an individual. The precise approach to each patient is therefore highly individualized. One can try to analyze, step-by-step, the precise manner in which basic principles are applied to the patient, but the actual process of prescribing a remedy is more akin to an art. Possessing an understanding of the principles, the homeopath learns the art of getting to know the patient, of drawing out of the patient the unique image of the pathological state, and finally of choosing precisely the remedy and potency needed by that particular patient. This begins a process which stimulates the defense mechanism, leading eventually to another decision as to whether the remedy has acted at all, and in what manner. Then the next remedy and potency must be chosen, and the process continues. Each decision demands a full understanding of the fundamental laws and principles, but in each instance this knowledge is fused in an artistic manner into a unique application for each patient.

The encounter between a patient and a homeopath is an intimate interaction for both. The patient, of course, has a responsibility to report as fully and accurately as possible every aspect of his or her own existence, even when describing the most private of symptoms. The prescriber, however, is not merely a passive observer, protected behind a wall of objectivity. Each patient engages the homeopath in a deep and meaningful way. Because of the very nature of homeopathy, the prescriber becomes an intimate participant in the life of the patient, involved in every aspect of it, and being at once sympathetic and sensitive as well as objective and accepting. For the homeopath, every day becomes a living process, and experience is gained very rapidly of the deepest regions of human existence. When homeopathy is practiced with this degree of involvement, it stimulates growth in the prescriber just as it does in the patient.

With each case, the homeopath faces a new variation on the

many ways in which the fundamental laws are applied to individuals. Each case is so unique that it is literally impossible to write a textbook which will apply with perfect precision to a specific individual. Even so, it is possible to describe patterns which are commonly seen in homeopathic practice; this is the purpose of Section II of the book. It is intended to provide guidelines by which homeopaths can learn to apply the principles enunciated in Section I.

It is very important to recognize that the art of practical application cannot be learned merely from books. Books can provide a general framework, but they are not enough to enable the prescriber to manage a specific case. Supervised instruction by an experienced homeopath is absolutely necessary. Such instruction teaches the beginner the case-by-case judgment needed to become consistently accurate in decision-making. In the beginning, mistakes are inevitably made quite frequently, but feedback from an experienced homeopath can enable the prescriber to learn from them. The very necessary quality of *circumspection* is learned—the ability to be decisive while simultaneously being willing to inwardly doubt all judgments. This takes a great deal of training in homeopathy as in all other professional endeavors.

Throughout this textbook, a moderate knowledge of standard medical information is assumed on the part of the reader. Such subjects as anatomy, physiology, physical and laboratory diagnosis, the many varieties of diagnostic disease categories, and standard medical treatments for such disease categories are important to any comprehensive view of what is occurring in a patient at any given moment. Even though standard disease labels utilized by medical science are never the basis for the selection of a homeopathic remedy, an accurate knowledge of the patient's pathological state does have importance for arriving at an accurate prognosis in any given case.

For this reason, medical doctors automatically have an advantage in learning homeopathy. They should presumably be ready to plunge directly into the purely homeopathic material presented herein. Experience shows, however, that for practical and doctrinal reasons, medical doctors are not likely to respond to homeopathy in sufficient numbers to satisfy the growing public demand. It can be expected, therefore, that many nonmedical students will endeavor to undertake the disciplined study of homeopathy. To these, it is important to emphasize that, although one need not be a true expert in standard medical subjects to become a good ho-

141

meopath, it is necessary to be *well*-acquainted with them in order to adequately fulfill one's responsibility to one's patients.

In this section, we will attempt to go into considerable detail regarding the various technical aspects of homeopathic prescribing. In every chapter, the principles described in Section I will be translated as much as possible into practical terms. For this reason these two sections are being combined into one volume: they are two ways of describing the same laws and principles.

Chapter 10

The Birth of
a Remedy

ONCE FUNDAMENTAL HOMEOPATHIC THEORY has been mastered, the next primary concern is the homeopathic remedy itself—the tool by which the process of cure is put in motion. To be effective, such tools must be highly refined in preparation and accurately tested. At the present time, there are literally hundreds of remedies derived from minerals, plants, and diseased tissues whose characteristics have been fully delineated through carefully conducted provings, and thousands more which have been at least partially proven. Nevertheless, as homeopathy continues to advance, it is necessary to perform provings on new remedies so that the therapeutic armamentarium can be further expanded. For this purpose, it is necessary to have clearly defined standards for the actual methods of performing an accurate and thorough proving.

The fundamental theoretical basis for the proving of drugs on healthy persons was enunciated originally by Samuel Hahnemann, as described in Chapter 6. In Aphorism 21, Hahnemann describes the basic principle:

Now, as it is undeniable that the curative principle in medicines is not in itself perceptible, and as in pure experiments with medicines conducted by the most accurate observers, nothing can be observed that can constitute them medicines or remedies except that power of causing distinct alterations in the state of health of the human body, and paricularly in that of the healthy individual, *and of exciting in him various definite morbid symptoms; so it follows that when medicines act as remedies, they can only bring their curative property into play by means of this their*

143

power of altering man's state of health by the production of peculiar symptoms; and that, therefore, we have only to rely on the morbid phenomena which the medicines produce in the healthy body as the sole possible revelation of their in-dwelling curative power, in order to learn what disease-producing power, and at the same time what disease-curing power, each individual medicine possesses.

Thus, we see that the purpose of conducting a proving of a remedy is to *record the totality of morbid symptoms produced by that substance on healthy individuals;* and that totality will then be the curative indications upon which is to be prescribed the curative remedy in the sick individual.

It is likely to be a new concept to many people that literally *any* substaance can have a wide and varied spectrum of highly individualized symptoms. Because we have the possibility of varying the dosage of the substance, this spectrum of symptoms can become evident by sufficiently careful testing. The fact that substances do indeed produce specific reactions is stated clearly by Hahnemann in Aphorism 30:

The human body appears to admit of being much more powerfully affected in its health by medicines (partly because we have the regulation of the dose in our own power) than by natural morbid stimuli—for natural diseases are cured and over-come by suitable medicines.

Indeed, it is possible to poison an organism with any substance whatsoever if given in sufficient quantity. This is true whether the substance is a poison or even a food. Something as ordinary as table salt, if given in large doses daily for a long time, can generate a variety of symptoms in relatively healthy people. *If we give a test substance in great enough quantity, it will disturb the vital force sufficiently to mobilize the defense mechanism, which in turn generates a group of symptoms which are entirely peculiar to the substance being tested.*

When a *substance* is administered and the resulting symptoms are noted down, we are recording the specific manifestations of the defense mechanism—which is the only way we have of identifying the resonant frequency of the action of the remedy. Similarly, when we note down the symptoms of the *patient*, we are recording the peculiar manifestations representing the resonant frequency of the defense mechanism. By matching the symptom-picture of the remedy to the symptom-picture of the patient, we match their resonant frequencies, thereby accomplishing cure by strengthening the defense mechanism at its weakest point.

If a substance is given in poisonous or toxic doses, virtually every organism will react to it, but the reaction will be too gross to be of value in homeopathy. Symptoms such as coma, convulsions, vomiting, or diarrhea will be recorded, but subtle, fine distinctions will not be evident. If small, even minute and potentized, doses are used, however, a wide variety of highly refined and specific symptoms will be produced, particularly on the mental and emotional planes. This is why homeopathy emphasizes testing upon healthy human beings who are capable of lucidly describing even very subtle changes. The allopathic method, by contrast, tests drugs first upon animals and then upon sick human beings. Animal testing, of course, is inadequate for any truly therapeutic purpose because the only symptoms which can be recorded are the crudest of physical symptoms. For homeopathic purposes, testing drugs on sick human beings is also inadequate, because disease symptoms can easily be mixed together with drug effects. In any case, it is obvious that allopathic drugs are tested merely for their ability to palliate specific symptoms or syndromes, and not for their effect upon the general health of the patient.

When a substance is administered to an organism, there are two phases of response. The *primary effect* occurs immediately, within a few hours, or within a few days; this represents the "excitation phase" of reaction and is usually somewhat dramatic. The organism, in its attempt to reestablish equilibrium, then compensates with a *secondary effect*. This usually occurs after a reaction time approximately twice that of the primary reaction. The symptoms generated in this secondary phase can be opposite to those of the primary phase. In any proving, it is important to record symptoms from both phases, even though they appear to be contradictory. Each phase represents a characteristic manifestation of the action of the defense mechanism and therefore must be accorded equal importance.

Homeopathic remedies are derived from plant, mineral, animal, and disease products (or from allopathic drugs which are potentized), and they are all highly standardized in their preparation. In countries most active in homeopathy, the strict quality of remedies is assured by conforming to very detailed homeopathic Pharmacopoeias which are used as universal standards.

In addition, the technique of the proving itself must be careful, thorough, precise, and standardized. Once a remedy has been gathered from a particular geographic location and then proven there, that specific preparation must be the one used by all homeopaths prescribing on the basis of that proving. The remedy

145

Pulsatilla, used by all homeopaths, must be the exact species used in the original provings; if a different species were to be used without being re-proven, it is probable that the specific symptom-picture would be enough different as to prevent the desired results. If a remedy is prepared and proven in India, then only that preparation must be used by the rest of the world. Only by adhering to these standards can our prescribing be sufficiently accurate to attain the reliable results possible in homeopathy.

In order for the defense mechanism to produce symptoms at all, the threshold of the vital force must be exceeded. This can occur in two ways: either the dosage of the substance must be strong enough to overpower the vital force, or the organism must have a relatively high degree of sensitivity to it. This is illustrated schematically in Figure 11. A wide spectrum of sensitivities, or resultant vibration rates, are shown for several provers. The vibration rate of the test substance is shown as indicated. In order to produce symptoms in provers whose vibration rates are very different from that of the remedy, high material doses (perhaps even toxic doses) must be used, and the resulting symptoms can be expected to be quite crude (involving mostly the physical body). On the other hand, if such a high material dose were to be used on provers very sensitive to the substance, strong and damaging symptoms could result. If, however, a minute or potentized dose is given to provers very near to the vibration rate of the substance, an array of highly specific and peculiar symptoms will be generated; in this case, the symptoms will be subtle, individualized, and characteristic, especially on the mental and emotional planes.

Finally, if by chance the vibration rate of one of the provers matches *exactly* that of the substance, the prover will experience a dramatic and lasting alleviation of any symptoms which might have existed prior to the experiment. Because of the principle of resonance, the best symptoms in a proving are elicited by the provers most sensitive to the substance being tested.

An important question which naturally arises is: Is it ethical to administer potentially toxic substances to essentially healthy individuals? First of all, it must be made clear that provings should *never* be done in toxic dosages; for toxic symptoms, we must rely solely on reports of accidental poisonings recorded in the toxicological literature. Always, the administration of the test substance is halted at the earliest indication of symptoms. Provers with little sensitivity to the substance experience little or no symptoms at all, and their health is not affected. Provers who are sensitive to the substance, however, experience a definite improvement in health during the course of the experiment and subsequently as well. The more sensitive a prover happens to be, the more marked will be the health benefit. Hahnemann himself observed this beneficial effect of provings and urged everyone to participate in them.

PROVERS

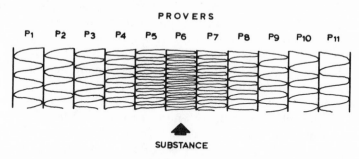

SUBSTANCE

Figure 11: Each prover represents a somewhat different resultant frequency of vibration. The vibration rate of the remedy will match very closely that of certain provers; these will be the most sensitive. If the remedy matches *exactly*, the provers will exhibit the most reliable symptoms and later will experience cure of the entire organism. If the remedy is close, but not exact, the prover will generate a variety of useful symptoms, even on mental and emotional levels. If the remedy is far from the vibration rate of the prover (for example, Prover 1 or Prover 11), then only toxic amounts of the remedy will produce symptoms, and those symptoms will tend to affect only the physical level in a gross manner.

Basically, there are three criteria for determining whether a remedy has been fully proven:

1. Symptoms must be recorded from provings on healthy individuals using toxic (as recorded from accidental poisonings), hypotoxic (i.e., low potency), and highly potentized doses.

2. The symptoms recorded must be drawn from all three levels of the organism—mental, emotional, and physical.

3. Symptoms must be included which have been cured in the process of treatment of the whole organism after administration of the remedy to a sick person.

Any remedy which has been proven by recording only physical symptoms is insufficient for homeopathic purposes. As mentioned, allopathic toxicology, even done by prestigious universities, is inadequate because it is based primarily on animal studies. In addition, such toxicological studies do not span the full range of potencies possible. Even the records of poisonings of human beings are inadequate, because symptoms are not described with sufficient individualization; for example, if a poisoning by a particular substance produces "mania," it is rare in the allopathic literature to describe the particular type of mania peculiar to each poisoning victim.

Finally, remedy descriptions which do not include cured symptoms present only a partial symptom picture. After all, cure is the object of the administration of the remedy, and symptoms eliminated during the process of a cure of the whole being are the most reliable of all because they indicate the highest degree of sensitivity to the remedy.[1]

Many times the question has been asked whether it is possible to find people who are healthy enough to be able to take part in such experiments. Indeed, it is nearly impossible nowadays to find perfectly healthy people. It is for this reason that provings must conform to a strict format designed to minimize recording any preexisting pathological symptoms. This must be done with great care and double-blind objectivity.

The following description of such a strict format will undoubtedly dismay some readers. It requires a relatively large number of people, it occupies approximately 2½ years of time, and it is of necessity rather expensive to complete. Nevertheless, these difficulties must be weighed against the fact that the information generated by such a procedure will be a solid foundation for prescribing for many generations. In our modern universities and medical centers, vast amounts of time, effort, and money are being spent to acquire data which are usually considered outdated within ten or fifteen years. The experiments described herein, on the other hand, represent only a fraction of such expense, yet the data remain reliable for all generations to come.

Preparation for a Proving

Today, in order to participate in a valid proving, a subject must comply with the following requirements:

1. The subject must be well-acquainted with homeopathic methodology, and above all, he or she must have a good knowl-

---

1. It should be made clear that a single cured symptom, *without* corresponding cure of the whole organism, is not to be considered as reliable.

edge of the symptomatology found in homeopathic materia medica. This requirement is necessary for the subject to fully appreciate the particular deviations that may manifest during the experiment.

2. The subject must be between 18 and 45 years old, so that the natural bodily degeneration that comes with age will not be a serious factor. The person should be reasonably healthy by orthodox medical standards.

3. The subject should not be a hysterical or anxious person. This is necessary because such individuals display a high incidence of "placebo-effect"; in other words, they generate symptoms simply because of the act of taking a medicinal substance.

4. The subject must be capable of appreciating the seriousness of the experiment.

5. The subject must be able to lead a life which is as normal as possible during the course of the experiment. This means that the life circumstances of the subject must be such as to allow a definite time for sleep, for walking, for eating, and to permit food free of chemicals, refined products, and spices or stimulants. Finally, the person must be able to maintain a reasonable degree of stability in relationship to job, family, friends—in the mental and emotional plane in general. In short, the subject must be able to live a life of moderation during the experiment, avoiding excessive influences.

The time of preparation before initiating the experiment must be at least one month in duration. During this time the provers should meticulously note down whatever symptoms or slight discomforts they experience on all three levels—mental, emotional, or physical. Diary notations must be made at least three times daily, to prevent even minor memory lapses. These observations must be made with the prover's full conviction of the absolute importance of the experiment. Each notation should record even the slightest deviation from the subject's normal state. It should include a description of each symptom in graphic and poetic detail, the intensity of the symptom, its duration, and all influences which make it worse or better. In addition, any possible "exciting causes" should be noted, in order to put the true significance of the symptom in proper perspective. An example of such a notation might be: a moderate stitching pain behind the left eye, radiating toward the left temple, occurring at 9 A.M., after being criticized by wife for forgetting to pick up the milk, lasting 40 minutes, aggravated by sudden motion and noise, better from pressure and cold applications. Another might be: irritability from too many details and from noise, accompanied by hunger, occurring at 3:30 P.M., unrelieved by walking or fresh air, relieved by eating. Once all these details of the subject's "normal" state have been recorded for at least one month, his "baseline" has been recorded sufficiently to begin the experiment.

Before starting, the panel of researchers carrying out the experiment collect all the notes of prospective subjects and check them in order to decide who can participate. The following people should be excluded from the experiment from the outset:

1. Those who note down a lot of emotional or mental symptoms. Too many symptoms in these realms confuse the final results.

2. Those who obviously omitted to recall symptoms or who exhibited superficiality in reporting. These tendencies indicate either a lack of mental clarity or a lack of sincerity.

3. Those who suffer from hypersensitivity diseases—such as asthma, hay fever, allergies, food hypersensitivities, etc.

Location for the Experiment

Ideally, three experiments should be conducted, each in different locations and on subjects of different nationalities. Because reactions vary so much depending on environment, provings should be conducted in the mountains, on the low plains, and by the seashore.

For a proving to be absolutely reliable, these ideal conditions should be met. However, it is unlikely that such elaborate experiments will be practical for some time. As a compromise, therefore, it is recommended that the experiment should be conducted in a place in the country, preferably at an altitude of about 1500 feet, with clean air and water. It should be a quiet environment, free of hectic and anxious urban influences.

The purpose of such a natural environment is to raise the health of the subjects as high as possible before the actual experiment. As an approximation, fifteen days in the country should suffice. After approximately the fifteenth day, symptoms reported are likely to represent expressions belonging to the person's true constitution. Once proper stabilization has been accomplished in such a natural environment, the actual experiment can begin.

The Experiment

The experimental proving of a new drug must always be carried out with a double-blind format in which neither the experimenters nor the subjects know the drug being proven. (Figure 12) The director of the experiment decides upon the substance to be proven and insures that the methods used during the experiment conform to the highest standards. The director also decides, according to routine randomization techniques, which subjects will receive the experimental substance and which will receive placebos. Approximately 25% of the provers are to be given placebos while the rest receive the test substance. The substance to be tested and placebos must be packaged identically, and the code identifying test subjects from placebo subjects must be kept secret from both the experimenters and the subjects. Strict instructions must be given to all provers that they must not communicate with each other about their symptoms under any circumstances.

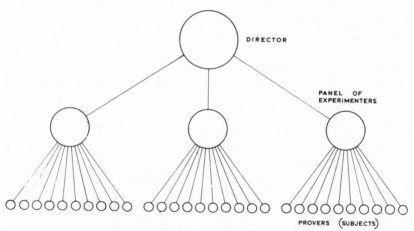

Figure 12: The director initiates the experiment; he or she is the only person knowing the actual remedy being tested as well as the code governing who receives the remedy and who receives a placebo. The panel of experimenters monitors the responses, inquiring in detail into each symptom recorded in the diaries of the provers. The provers maintain careful records and a stable lifestyle in order to maximize the possibility of obtaining meaningful symptoms.

The experiment begins with the administration of the test substance to the appropriate subjects in hypotoxic dosage. The potency should range from 1× to about 8×—1× being used for relatively nontoxic substances (e.g., edible plants) and from 8×— 12× for more toxic substances (e.g., hydrocyanic acid). Doses are given three times daily for a full month, or until symptoms appear. Careful instructions must be given that all doses should be discontinued whenever any definite symptoms out of the ordinary emerge. Nevertheless, detailed notations are continued three times daily, even after discontinuation of the remedy. Even after the month of administration of the remedy has been completed, observation should continue for another three months, or however long it takes to be certain that no more new symptoms are arising.

Assuming that 50-100 provers participate in such an experiment, only the very rare subject will experience cure of preexisting symptoms, some will develop new symptoms within the first few days, another larger group will show symptoms after the twentieth day, and the majority will display only few or no symptoms at all during the entire period of observation. This wide variation in response is perfectly expectable from the variation in sensitivity described in Figure 11. Those who produce symptoms immediately are the most sensitive to the remedy; these are the provers who will continue the experiment later with higher potencies.

After plenty of time has elapsed to be sure that no more new symptoms are emerging from the first phase, those subjects who reacted quickly to the hypotoxic doses are given the same remedy in the thirtieth potency, again with 25% receiving placebo in randomized fashion. This is repeated once daily for a period of two weeks. The subsequent observation period should be continued for at least another three months, or until it is obvious that no more new symptoms are emerging. As usual, if symptoms arise immediately, further doses are discontinued, and symptoms continue to be recorded under strict conditions until they are finished. When all symptoms have ceased, the prover may turn in the diary to the panel of experimenters and return home.

The final administration of a high potency should be delayed for a full year, during which time less formal observations can be made in the subject's normal environment. After this period of rest, the same subjects who received the thirtieth potency gather again in the rural experimental environment and spend another preparation period reestablishing "baseline" observations. They are then given one dose of a 10M or 50M potency (again with 25%

receiving placebos), and observed intensely for a further period of three months, or until symptoms have ceased.

At the conclusion of the experiment, the panel of experimenters collects all notebooks and, one by one, lists every symptom which represents a deviation from the subjects' normal state. The experimenters should meet with each subject and try to elaborate and clarify each symptom as carefully as possible—describing thoroughly the exciting causes, the timing, and the modalities. Finally, the experiment is "unblinded." Symptoms generated by placebo subjects are deleted from the records of the test subjects, unless there is a marked discrepancy in frequency or intensity. The experimenters then collate all the remaining symptoms and present them for publication.

Formulation of Materia Medicas

In the birth and emergence of a remedy, the above-described experiments are the first step. Such strict experiments, plus whatever information is available from toxicological literature, provide the raw data which form the basic foundations for the utilization of the remedy. As elaborate and detailed as the information is, however, it is as yet incomplete until tested clinically. The remedy is administered by reliable prescribers to sick people according to the symptoms generated in the provings. As clinical experience grows, careful records are made of symptoms which are cured during the process of a real cure of the entire patient on all three levels. It is very important to understand that only those symptoms cured during such a cure of the whole person are significant; occasional symptoms which randomly disappear without a corresponding curative change in the rest of the patient are disregarded.

Eventually, a complete picture of the remedy emerges from all sources: toxicological literature, provings, and clinical observations. Once such a complete image is available, the remedy can be included in a complete *materia medica*. It is finally possible for a homeopath sufficiently familiar with the remedy to create a gradation of symptoms according to their importance as expressions of the true personality of the remedy. Necessarily, such a gradation is highly subjective and may vary somewhat from homeopath to homeopath, but we can nevertheless offer a rough approximation of how symptoms are graded, from most reliable to least reliable.

The most important parameters in judging the reliability of symptoms are as follows:

1. Cured symptoms. Those symptoms cured as part of a total cure either during the experiment or in a clinical application.

2. Frequency. Those symptoms found most frequently among the provers.

3. Intensity. Those symptoms producing the most powerful effects on the provers.

4. Potency. Those symptoms occurring during the testing of the highest potencies are more reliable than those occurring from crude doses.

5. Timing. Those symptoms emerging in a prover immediately upon administration of the remedy, especially in a highly potency, are of greater significance than those occurring late.

Thus the symptoms given the highest grade are, of course, cured symptoms (as part of a total cure) which are also observed in a large number of provers with great intensity and speed and which are evident even upon administration of high potencies. The least reliable symptoms are those which occur weakly in just a few provers, which occur very late in a proving, which occur only in poisonings, or which were cured only incidentally without a corresponding general improvement in health.

As symptoms are graded and observed in actual patients, there gradually emerges an image of the *personality* of the substance being tested. Just as we do not view an individual as a collection of isolated characteristics such as hair color, body construction, mannerisms, attitude, etc., so we cannot view remedy expressions as being isolated entities. Once we have the totality of symptoms, we must spend time meditating on them as an integrated totality, especially in relationship to patients in whom we have seen the remedy act curatively. In this way, gradually we acquire a sense of the "essence" or "soul" of the remedy. This final integrated image of the remedy, in the last analysis, is beyond mere words; it is "known" in a living, experiential way—just as one gets to know a friend.

The symptom image of a remedy can be viewed diagramatically as in Figure 13. The totality of symptoms has an integrated "form" or "shape" as represented. Each bulge corresponds to a specific symptom. The shape of the illness in the patient, ideally, is similar to that of the appropriate remedy, but it is shown larger in size because of the intensity of its morbific influence in the patient. In this sense, the "shape" of the remedy and of the disease can be understood as having the same "resonant frequency," as we have discussed previously; the resonant frequency produces a particular pattern of symptoms in diseased individuals and in provers. It is this matching of symptom-pictures which is the primary task of the homeopath in prescribing a remedy.

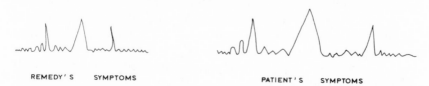

REMEDY'S   SYMPTOMS   PATIENT'S   SYMPTOMS

Figure 13: Each fluctuation in pattern can be viewed as a specific symptom manifested by either the prover or the patient. In the illustration, the patient's symptom picture is represented with greater amplitude because the intensity of symptoms can be expected to be greater. The goal in prescribing is to match the *pattern* of symptoms.

In the homeopathic literature, there are a variety of types of *materia medicas* offering descriptions at different levels in the process of emergence of a remedy. Perhaps the best way to illustrate this point is to follow the "growth" of the image of a remedy through several *materia medicas*. We will consider one of the most well-known medicines in homeopathy, Arsenicum album. To begin with, there are the highly detailed raw data of the original proving. This proving was quoted by Hahnemann in his *Chronic Diseases,* and it is one of the classic landmarks in homeopathic literature. Because this proving is so exemplary of the phenomenal detail and thoroughness which Hahnemann brought to all his work, it is quoted extensively at the conclusion of this chapter.

The results of such provings are then collected in voluminous *materia medicas* such as Allen's ten-volume *Encyclopedia of Pure Materia Medica* and Hering's ten-volume *Guiding Symptoms.* These are useful reference works for any homeopath to possess because, in addition to the detailed symptoms, they also used symbols to indicate the relative gradations of the most important symptoms.

Clarke's *Dictionary of Practical Materia Medica* is an example of a *materia medica* which has condensed the raw data into compact summaries of symptoms arranged by anatomical system. It is a valuable reference work because it is quite detailed, yet still convenient to use. In addition, each remedy is introduced by a section which lucidly describes the main clinical features of the remedy with illustrative cases which have been cured.

Finally, the "essence" or personality of a remedy is described in a *materia medica* best exemplified by Kent's *Lectures on Homeopathic Materia Medica with New Remedies.* This monumental contribution to homeopathy should be continually and meditatively studied throughout the career of any homeopath. Kent does not attempt to present a complete delineation of all the symptoms manifested by each remedy. Rather, he tries to describe the main "essence," the essential personality, of each remedy, as gleaned from his penetrating experience. Kent was a peerless clinician and observer, and it is the excellence of his knowledge and experience which make his *materia medica* so reliable.

A classic example of a carefully conducted proving is given in Appendix A. This is an extract from Hahnemann's original proving for Arsenicum album, one of the most commonly used remedies in the homeopathic *materia medica.*

Chapter 11

Preparation of Medicines

ANY THERAPEUTIC METHOD must master the technical aspects of the materials being used if there is ever to be any hope for achieving reproducible results. Standards of materials and methods must be carefully established and strictly followed. This is as true in homeopathy as it is in all other sciences.

Mostly, the burden of technical standardization has fallen on the shoulders of homeopathic pharmacists. Considering the smallness of the dose being administered to each patient, it is easy to imagine the problems facing these pharmacists in properly making a profit. Despite their difficulties, they have thus far done an admirable job in provdiing homeopaths the world over with excellent medicines of reliable standard. However, if these standards are to be maintained, every practitioner must take steps to support the pharmacists preparing and dispensing our precious remedies. It is not enough to simply gather remedies into our offices and blindly take for granted that the supply will always be there. On the contrary, we must make arrangements whereby the pharmacists are benefited by our prescriptions just as we and our patients are. If this is not done, the reliability, and eventually the availability, or remedies will disappear altogether; this can as surely bring about the death of homeopathy as can the opposition of governments of orthodox medical societies.

In considering technical standards for the actual production of homeopathic medicines, we must first put attention on the initial preparation of the plant, mineral, or nosode into a form amenable to potentization. Then, the specific standards for potentization must be considered. Finally, to be presented in Chapter 19, the storage, handling, and administration of remedies must be understood and followed.

Initial Preparation of Crude Substances

Materials of medicinal value occur in Nature in a variety of forms, some of which are chemically easily available for potentization and some of which require initial preparation.

A wide variety of plant species are used in homeopathy. Obviously, the first step involves selecting the correct species, grown under optimal conditions and collected at the optimal time. This requires the skills of a person highly knowledgeable in botany. Once a particular plant species has been used in a proving, all conditions of collection and preparation of the original plant must be duplicated in every detail in all later medical preparations.

In addition to careful attention to species, it is important to collect only plants found in a particular habitat, under conditions minimizing contamination from soil, water, and air pollutants. For example, a plant grown on a hilltop with plenty of access to sun and rain, free from run-off contamination by pesticides used in neighboring areas, is preferable to a plant grown next to a busy roadway, in a valley surrounded by crops which are frequently sprayed by chemicals.

The time of collection may be important. Some plants have much more vitality during certain seasons of the year, and others at different seasons. The season of collection, therefore, should duplicate the conditions of the original proving as much as possible; ideally it will occur at the time of greatest vitality of the plant. Usually, the best season would be spring, or secondarily summer, but individual species may peak at unique times of year. Ideally, the plant should be picked during a sunny day following a recent rain; this maximizes the likelihood that there is no contamination. Of course, the plant itself must be healthy, free of mold and free of infestation by bugs.

The provings of plant substances have in some instances included the entire plant and in other instances merely a portion of the plant. Again one must know clearly which was used in the original proving. If the original proving was done only on the

158

mature flower of a plant, rather than the entire plant, then one must use only the flower.

It would seem that the amount of technical information needed for each of the hundreds of medicines proven would be impossible for any practitioner to learn. Fortunately, this has all been compiled in standard pharmacopoeias. One of the most widely accepted is the *Homeopathic Pharmacopoeia of the United States.* At the time of this writing, it is currently being updated even further to conform to all modern standards of botany and chemistry, but we will refer herein to quotations from the Sixth Edition. To give an example of the detail involved in the selection of the proper plant for preparation into a medicine, the following is the description provided to Pulsatilla:

PULSATILLA. Wind Flower
Natural Order. *Ranunculaceae.*
Synonyms: Latin, *Anemone pratensis, Herba venti, Pulsatilla nigricans, P. pratensis, P. vulgaris;* English, *Meadow anemone, Pasque flower, Wind flower;* French, *Pulsatille;* German, *Küchenschelle.*

Description: *A deciduous, perennial herb, with a spindle-shaped, thick, ligneous, dark-brown, oblique, several-headed root. The stem, 3 to 5 inches high, is simple, erect, rounded. The leaves are radical, petiolate, bi-pinnatifid, with linear segments; at the base surrounded by several ovate, lanceolate sheaths. The flowers, varying in color from dark violet to light blue, appear from March to May, and are bell-shaped, pendulous, terminal, reflexed at the apex, surrounded by a distinct sessile involucre, composed of 3 palmately divided and cleft bracts with linear lobes. The plant, clothed with long, silky hairs, is inodorous, but when rubbed exhales an acrid vapor, and has a burning, acrid taste.*

Habitat: *Open fields and plains, in dry places in many parts of Europe, Russia, and Turkey in Asia. Fig., Flora Hom. II 102; Jahr and Cat. 254; Winkler, 109, 110.*

Part Used: *The fresh plant, when in flower.*[1]

Once a plant (or a portion of plant) has been collected in a correct manner, it is then prepared further to make it amenable to the standard process of potentization. Usually, this involves making a tincture of the plant. Preparation of tinctures is a standard

---

1. Committee on Pharmacopoeia of the American Institute of Homeopathy, *The Homeopathic Pharmacopoeia of the United States,* Sixth Edition, rev. (Boston: Clapp & Son, 1941), p. 475.

procedure known very well to botanists and herbalists, but for our purposes the standard description is given by Hahnemann in Aphorism 267 of the *Organon:*

> *We gain possession of the powers of indigenous plants and of such as may be had in a fresh state in the most complete and certain manner by mixing their freshly expressed juice immediately with equal parts of spirits of wine of a strength sufficient to burn in a lamp. After this has stood a day and a night in a close stoppered bottle and deposited the fibrinous and albuminous matters, the clear superincumbent fluid is then to be decanted off for medicinal use. All fermentation of the vegetable juice will be at once checked by the spirits of wine mixed with it and rendered impossible for the future, and the entire medicinal power of the vegetable juice is thus retained (perfect and uninjured) for ever by keeping the preparation in well-corked bottles further protected with wax to prevent evaporation and excluded from the sun's light.*[2]

Mineral substances and nosodes are also prepared to an equally strict standard. Nosodes are prepared from disease products such as gonorrheal discharge (Medorrhinum), syphilis chancre (Syphilinum), tuberculosis cavity (Tuberculinum), influenza virus (Influenzinum), rabies saliva (Hydrophobinum), etc., and also from drugs such as Valium, Penicillin, Cortisone, etc. Primary concern is for purity, simplicity, and chemical availability.

Many mineral substances, as well as some plants, are not chemically available for potentization. These must be prepared in some manner; the particular method in each instance varies according to the nature of the substance. Later preparations must conform to the exact method used in the original provings, even if modern techniques have been shown to be superior. For the best methods to use for particular substances, Hahnemann himself is one of the best resources. Hahnemann was a fully qualified chemist, and well-acquainted with alchemy as well, so his knowledge of how to prepare particular minerals was very specific and thorough. One example of the specific detail involved in preparing a specific metallic substance is given in the Annotated Bibliography to this chapter—Hahnemann's description of Causticum. This illustrates the incredible detail into which he investigated substances, both in their biological actions and their chemical characteristics.

The next step in preparation of medicines is the making of the millionth dilution ($6 \times$ or 3c potency). If the initial preparation or tincture is soluble in alcohol, then potentization to this level is

---

2. Hahnemann, *Organon of Medicine.*

carried out in the standard manner described below. If, however, the substance is not soluble in alcohol, a specific method of *trituration* is used to bring it to the millionth dilution in a form soluble in alcohol. This involves grinding the material with a specific amount of milk sugar in a mortar and pestle for a total of three hours. The method is highly specific and has not changed since Hahnemann's first description (see Annotated Bibliography).

As we know, such a first-level preparation enables the energetic potential of material substances to be liberated, but it also has purely chemical effects which are difficult to comprehend. Again Hahnemann describes this effect:

> Not only, as shown elsewhere, do these medicinal substances thereby develop their powers in a prodigious degree, but they also change their physico-chemical demeanor in such a way, that if no one before could ever perceive in their crude form any solubility in alcohol or water, after this peculiar transmutation they become wholly soluble in water as well as in alcohol—a discovery invaluable to the healing art . . .

> What can I say of the pure metals and of their sulphurets, but that all of them, without any exception become by this treatment equally soluble in water and in alcohol, and every one of them develops the medicinal virtue peculiar to it in the purest, simplest manner and in an incredibly high degree? [3]

Standard Preparation

Once the remedy has been prepared in a soluble form to the 6× potency the typical method of potentization described in Chapter 7 is used. One drop is diluted in a certain amount of solvent (either 9, 99, or 50,000 drops), and the resulting solution is shaken forcefully for a definite number of successions. One drop of this solution is then diluted and succussed similarly, and the process is continued indefinitely.

The dilution and succussion may be done either by hand or by machine. Nowadays, it is more efficient to use machines which can perform the process rapidly and tirelessly. Even with machines, however, a high potency remedy often takes as many as three months to make. A variety of machines have been devised to perform the successions. The important point is that the number of successions should be standardized; experiences shows that there should be between 40 and 100 successions at each potency level. Also, the force of each succussion should be equivalent to

---

3. Hahnemann, *Chronic Diseases*, p. 145.

or greater than the force that a man's arm can deliver when striking the hand-held vial forcefully against a firm surface (such as a leather-bound book, as described by Hahnemann). Machines must be monitored carefully as to the number and force of succussions, so that no mechanical errors can enter into the standardization of the preparations.

Of course, the practice of some unscrupulous pharmacies to succuss only after every 5 or 10 dilutions must be deplored and rejected. In addition, the modern tendency to develop machines which apply kinetic energy in unconventional ways (i.e., by ultrasound, by shooting a jet of solvent into a swirling vat, etc.) must be rejected. In a purely physical sense, such deviations might be effective, but the vast body of homeopathic experience has thus far been built upon medicines prepared by the standard method described above; therefore, major alterations introduce serious uncertainties into interpretation of results. Any changes in technique must be tested experimentally very thoroughly over a long period of time to confirm their validity. Conscientious practitioners must take the responsibility to determine the specific methods used in preparing their remedies and only purchase medicines from those pharmacies maintaining the highest of classical standards.

At present, there are two equally *valid* methods of preparing dilution. The Hahnemannian method takes one drop of the previous potency diluted into alcohol, succusses, and then discards the glass vial after preparing each potency. The Korsakoff method pours out the solvent from the previous potency, leaving a drop on the walls of the vial (which has been determined to be a consistent size each time), and then adds the new solvent for the next potency; thus by the Korsakoff method the same vial is used for each potency. Of course, even in the Korsakoff method, it is desirable from time to time to set aside intermediate potencies for storage, so the total number of vials used for, say, a 200 potency might be 6 or 8, whereas by the Hahnemannian method 200 vials would be required.

The difference between Hahnemannian and Korsakoff preparations has sparked considerable controversy among homeopaths. The argument against the Korsakoff method is that it might result in a mixture of potencies from one level to another. To me, this argument doesn't make sense. After all, when the dilution is made and the vial succussed, the entire solution and vial have been raised to a new amplitude of vibration. How can any one portion

162

of the solution avoid undergoing the same change as all other portions? Therefore, there cannot be "contamination" from one potency to another.

This is not a merely academic distinction. It has tremendous practical importance to homeopathic pharmacists. To perform the Hahnemannian method, a very large number of vials must be used, and old vials can be re-used only by heating in an oven to very high temperatures. Such a procedure is very expensive, of course, and unnecessary. In order to help preserve our pharmacies, and their standards, the Korsakoff method is preferable.

Hahnemann's original potencies were made in alcohol, but this again places a great burden upon pharmacies producing high potency remedies. Since alcohol cannot be re-used, tremendous volumes of alcohol would be required to make a high potency remedy. For example, consider the production of a 10,000 potency; to make such a potency would require approximately 50 liters of alcohol—an expensive proposition! It is unlikely that water or alcohol will make any difference in the actual process of potentization, as various mixtures of both have been used successfully in the past. It would therefore be preferable to use double-distilled water for all of the intermediary potencies. Any potency, however, which is to be stored for use as a remedy should be preserved in pure alcohol. Water is not a good medium for preservation because microorganisms tend to grow over time and might interfere with the action of the remedy. Alcohol, on the other hand, is an excellent preservative and can be relied upon to maintain potencies indefinitely.

In any case, careful attention should be paid to the standards of purity of all materials being used in this delicate process. As can be imagined, even small amounts of contamination can be exaggerated tremendously during potentization. Therefore, the environment in which potentizing machines are used must be as free as possible from dust, chemical odors, sunlight, etc. The vials used should be of high chemical standards. The water and alcohol used must be at least of high chemical standards and then at least double-distilled into even greater purity. The tops of the vials used, from experience, should be made of cork (or at least lined by cork), and the cork should be of high quality. The milk sugar used in trituration and for administration of remedies should be of high quality, and the mortar and pestle used should be heated to high temperatures before preparing each remedy.

Nomenclature

Terminology used in naming potencies on different scales has evolved over time. Unfortunately, it has led to conventions which are slightly confusing to the beginner.

The *decimal* scale is based on dilution of 1/10. The first 1× potency is a 1/10 dilution. The second dilution (1/10×1/10 = 1/100) is called a 2× potency. The eighth decimal dilution 1/10 × 1/10 × 1/10 × 1/10 × 1/10 × 1/10 × 1/10 × 1/10 × = 1/100,000,000) is called the 8× potency. Thus the potency on the decimal scale is equivalent to the number of zeros in the denominator of the final dilution.

The *centesimal* scale is the most commonly used in homeopathy. It is based upon serial dilutions of 1/100. Each centesimal potency, therefore, is equivalent *in dilution* to two decimal potencies. A 30c potency is the same as a 60×, considering only the amount of dilution.

Finally, some homeopaths are using potencies based on serial dilutions of 1/50,000 at each level. These are called *50-millesimal* potencies, but common parlance refers to them simply as *millesimals*. This unusual dilution factor was suggested by Hahnemann late in his life, based upon his preliminary experimentations with different degrees of dilution and succussion. For example, a 1m potency is a dilution of 1/50,000, and a 3m potency represents a dilution of 1/125,000,000,000,000 (1/50,000 × 1/50,000 × 1/50,000).

It is very important to understand that both *dilution* and *succussion* are important in producing a given level of clinically effective potency. For each potency level, a standard number of succussions are performed, as well as dilution according to the particular scale being used. Figure 14 shows a table in which potencies of equivalent number on different scales are compared as to their dilutions and the number of succussions received (assuming a standard 100 succussions at each level).

Since both factors are involved in potentization, it is incorrect to equate potencies according to mere succussion or mere dilution. For example, if we compare a 30c and a 30×, both have the same number of succussions (3000), but they have different dilutions ($1/10^{30}$ for the 30×, and $1/10^{60}$ for the 30c); so the 30c is a higher potency by some amount. Conversely, if we compare two remedies of equal dilution, a 30c to a 60×, we see that the 60× is of a higher potency because it has had 6000 succussions, compared to the 3000 given to the 30c.

Occasionally, the problem arises in clinical practice as to which potency on one scale corresponds in effectiveness to a potency on another scale. For example, suppose a patient has had a certain effect from a 30c, the same remedy is still indicated, but the homeopath wants to change to a millesimal scale. Which potency corresponds on the millesimal scale to the 30c? If a 9m is given, is it a higher potency because the dilution is greater? Or is it a lower potency because the succussions are much less? This question cannot be answered with precision as yet, but it should be a good subject for investigation in the future. Someday, it may be possible to devise a formula which would provide this comparison, but as yet there are too many unknown factors. For example, do succussion and dilution have equal importance, or is one more important than another? Or is one factor more important at lower potencies, and the other at higher potencies? Does a given number of succussions have a constant effect at different dilutions, or does the effect vary for different dilutions? Are there different effects below Avogadro's number, especially when appreciable amounts of the original substance are still present, or is the ratio of original substance to solvent irrelevant? Anyway, for the present, the only way of resolving this issue is by the clinical experience of the most astute observers in homeopathy; at the present time, the issue is still unresolved.

By convention and habit arising out of experience, there are certain potencies which are used routinely in homeopathy: 2×, 6×, 12×, 30c, 200c, 1000c, 10,000, 50,000c. For ease in communication, the "c" is deleted when describing potencies from 30c and above; thus we refer to a "200th potency" rather than saying "20-0c." Also, because some of the higher numbers are unwieldy, we adopt Roman numeral designations: 1000 becomes a 1M, a 10,000 potency becomes a 10M, a 50,000 potency is a 50M, 100,000 is called CM, and so on. The "M" is designated as a capital letter in this book to differentiate it from "m," which means "50-millesimal" scale of potentization. There do exist potencies called *ultra-high* potencies which go to MM (1,000,000c), 50MM (50,000,000c), CMM (100,000,000c), MMM (1,000,000,000c), etc. In addition, a homeopath may rarely give an unusual potency for certain reasons—such as a 17×, a 500c, etc.

As mentioned in Chapter 7, Avogadro's number corresponds in dilution to a 24×, which is a 12c or between a 5m and 6m. This means that beyond this point, there is no longer any molecule of the original substance remaining. Thus potencies of 10M or MMM are astronomically far beyond any possibility of maintaining any chemical effect of the original substance. The fact that the energy, or vibration rate, of the original substance is transferred to the solvent molecules was discussed in Chapter 7.

Centesimal			Decimal			50-Millesimal		
POTENCY	DILUTION	No. SUCCUSSIONS	POTENCY	DILUTION	No. SUCCUSSIONS	POTENCY	DILUTION	No. SUCCUSSIONS
1c	$\frac{1}{10^2}$	100	1x	$\frac{1}{10}$	100	1m	$\frac{1}{50 \times 10^4}$	100
2c	$\frac{1}{10^4}$	200	2x	$\frac{1}{10^2}$	200	2m	$\frac{1}{2.5 \times 10^9}$	200
3c	$\frac{1}{10^6}$	300	3x	$\frac{1}{10^3}$	300	3m	$\frac{1}{1.25 \times 10^{14}}$	300
6c	$\frac{1}{10^{12}}$	600	6x	$\frac{1}{10^6}$	600	6m	$\frac{1}{1.5 \times 10^{28}}$	600
30c	$\frac{1}{10^{60}}$	3000	30x	$\frac{1}{10^{30}}$	3000	30m	$\frac{1}{9 \times 10^{136}}$	3000
200c	$\frac{1}{10^{400}}$	20,000	200x	$\frac{1}{10^{200}}$	20,000	200m	$\frac{1}{9 \times 10^{919}}$	20,000

Figure 14: A comparison of dilutions and succussions at each potency level on each scale. This table can be studied in two ways. One can compare a certain number of succussions (say, 20,000) with the extreme differences in dilution found on different scales. Another way is to consider which potencies have approximately similar amounts of dilution yet have received quite different numbers of succussions.

Hahnemann, being a chemist, was well aware of Avogadro's number, but it is indicative of the openness of his mind and his emphasis or empirical observation that he went ahead anyway and used potencies that exceeded Avogadro's number—and he found them to be increasingly effective with fewer adverse effects than lower potencies. At this point, however, many of Hahnemann's followers could not follow him. Their belief was strongly grounded in the materialistic philosophy emerging at the time, so they found it inconceivable that medicines could act beyond the material level. This caused a major split in homeopathic circles, which eventually became called the split between *low potency* and *high potency* prescribers. (Generally, low potencies are remedies below Avogadro's number, and high potencies are considered those above it).

Describing this split as being based upon the potencies used by homeopaths does not adequately express the true nature of the schism. Those prescribers who broke from the leadership of Hahnemann tended to reject not only his use of high potencies, but many of his other principles as well. They favored mixing many remedies together, giving a variety of potencies at once, repeating remedies frequently throughout days or weeks, prescribing upon the organ affected or the diagnostic label, giving remedies to produce "drainage" of the system, etc. In short, the low potency prescribers by and large utilized homeopathic remedies in an almost purely allopathic manner. These practices are still in vogue in many areas of the world today and are seriously disrupting the possibilities of cure of many thousands of cases.

It is also misleading to describe classical Hahnemannian prescribers as high potency prescribers. A homeopath conforming to the strict laws of homeopathy is likely to use *any* potency, depending upon the individual needs of the patient. It is true that they most commonly rely upon potencies above Avogadro's number, but there are always circumstances when even a 6 X may be used. Thus the true schism has little to do with the potencies used but rather with the entire philosophy and method of prescribing.

Annotated Bibliography for Chapter 11

1. Hahnemann's description of Causticum:

Lime, in the state of marble, owes it insolubility in water and its mildness to an acid of the lowest order which is combined with it; when head to red heat the marble allows this acid to escape as a gas. During this process the marble, as burned lime, has received (besides the latent heat) another substance *into its composition, which substance, unknown to chemistry, gives to it its caustic property as well as its solubility in the water, whereby we obtain lime-water. This substance, though itself not an acid, gives to it its caustic virtue, and by adding a fluid acid (which will endure fire), which then combines with the lime by its closer affinity, the watery caustic (Hydras Caustici?) is separated by distillation.*

Take a piece of freshly burned lime of about two pounds, dip this piece into a vessel of distilled water for about one minute, then lay it in a dry dish, in which it will soon turn into powder with the development of much heat and is peculiar odor, called lime-vapor. Of this fine powder take two ounces and mix with it in a (warmed) porcelain triturating bowl a solution of two ounces of bisulphate of potash, which has been heated to red heat and melted, cooled again and then pulverized and dissolved in two ounces of boiling hot water. This thickish mixture is put into a small glass retort; to which the helm is attached with wet bladder; into the tube of the helm is inserted the receiver half submerged in water; the retort is warmed by the gradual approach of a charcoal fire below and all the fluid is then distilled over by applying the suitable heat. The distilled fluid will be about an ounce and a half of water clearness, containing in concentrated form the substance mentioned above, i.e., Causticum; *it smells like the lye of caustic potash. On the back part of the tongue the caustic tastes very astringent, and in the throat burning; it freezes only in a lower degree of cold than water, and it hastens the putrefaction of animal substances immersed in it. When Muriate of Baryta is added, the causticum shows no signs of sulphuric acid, and on adding oxalate of ammonia it shows no traces of lime.*[1]

2. Hahnemann's description of trituration:

In this preparation, peculiar to Homeopathy, we take one grain in powder of any of the substances treated of in the six volumes of Materia Medica Pura, and especially those of the antipsoric substances following below, i.e., of silica, carbonate of baryta, carbonate of lime, carbonate of soda and sal ammoniac, carbonate of magnesia, vegetable charcoal, animal charcoal, graphites, sulphur, crude antimony, metallic antimony, gold, platina, iron, zinc, copper, silver, tin. The lumps of the metals which have not yet been beaten out into foil, are rubbed off on a fine, hard whetstone under water, some of them, as iron, under alcohol; of mercury in the liquid form one grain is taken, of petroleum one drop instead of a grain, etc. This is first put on about one-third of 100 grains of pulverized sugar of milk, and placed in an unglazed porcelain mortar, or in one from which the glaze has been first rubbed off with wet sand; the medicine and the sugar of milk are then mixed for a moment with porcelain spatula, and the mixture is triturated with some force for six minutes, the triturated substance is then for four minutes scraped from the mortar and from the porcelain pestle, which is also unglazed, or has had its glazing rubbed off with wet sand, so that the trituration may be homogeniously mixed. After this has been thus scraped together, it is triturated again without any addition for another six minutes with equal force. After scraping together again from the bottom and the sides for four minutes this triturate (for which the first third of the 100 grains had been used), the second third of the sugar of milk is now added, both are mixed together with the spatula for a moment, triturated again with like force for six minutes; it is triturated a second time (without addition) for six minutes more, and after scraping it together for another four minutes it is mixed with the last third of the powdered sugar of milk by stirring it around with the spatula, and the whole mixture is again triturated for six minutes, scraped for four minutes, and a second and last time triturated for six minutes; then it is all scraped together and the powder is preserved in a well-stoppered bottle with the name of the substance and the signature 100 because it is potentized one hundred fold.[2] *[or labelled lc, as is done in modern times].*

---

[1] Hahnemann, *Chronic Diseases*, p. 558.

[2] Hahnemann, *Chronic Diseases*, p. 147.

Chapter 12

Taking the Case

THE HOMEOPATHIC SYSTEM is a scientific discipline based upon sound and verifiable laws, principles, and techniques. In its application to the individual patient, however, it is also an art. Nowhere is this artistic aspect of homeopathy seen so clearly as in the process of taking the homeopathic case. Although there are general guidelines for taking a case, each interview is a completely unique process demanding of the interviewer different kinds of sensitivity and different approaches to each patient. It is a living, fluid process which nevertheless leads to the information upon which scientific judgments are made.

Case-taking in chronic cases (acute case-taking will be discussed at the conclusion of this chapter) requires a great deal of experience and training which cannot be acquired from reading books. Books can provide the basic framework and a simple understanding of the goals of a well-taken case, but the drawback of book-learning in this setting is the tendency of the reader to conceptualize the process in terms of rules. In writing a book, the author of necessity must generalize his descriptions and examples, and the reader consequently gets an idea which is too pat, too simple, too black-and-white.

The only reliable way to learn the art of case-taking is to actually become involved in the process under the supervision of an experienced and effective homeopath. Initially, this may involve simply sitting in a corner and watching the homeopath take cases, and then comparing impressions after the conclusion of the interview. The ideal setting for this would be an office in which a one-way mirror has been installed; the interview can then be conducted in seeming privacy, while the students take notes on the other side of the mirror. Afterward, the instructor can look over the notes and offer suggestions regarding the subtleties and emphases involved in the case. Initially, his feedback in the very process of taking notes and interpreting the patient's responses is very valuable for the beginning student. It helps develop the necessary sensitivity to each patient, as well as the objectivity to accurately translate the expressions of the patient into information useable in the homeopathic framework.

Later, the student must become involved in taking cases personally. The homeopathic interviewer needs to become conscious of his or her own responses to the patient, and a certain discipline must be learned in the actual interview situation. A balance must be struck between the need for accurate objective information, sensitivity to what the patient is truly expressing, and the establishing of a rapport which enables the patient to feel comfortable enough to share the most intimate of feelings and experiences. This process as well should ideally be supervised by an experienced homeopath, so that the interviewer can further refine his or her interviewing skills. Every interviewer has a unique personality, and therefore a unique style of conducting an interview, and each patient requires an individualized approach. It is nevertheless necessary to refine the needed skills so that the information finally recorded on paper will be reliable enough for further study.

The information gathered during the homeopathic interview is fully half of the process leading to eventual cure. A well-taken case which provides living images of the patient and which is thorough can be fruitfully studied for hours on end, not only for the purpose of arriving at a remedy, but also from the standpoint of learning about fundamental interactions between health and disease. A well-taken case is a valuable experience for the patient as well, because it becomes an opportunity to consciously examine the most crucial and intimate regions of his or her life.

On the other hand, a poorly taken case can be a source of endless frustration. The more one studies such a case, the more one becomes confused about what is really happening with the patient, and any prescription based upon such information will be mere guesswork. If the information is not improved on subsequent visits, it is possible to follow such a case for years, continuing to disrupt the image by prescriptions based upon guesswork, until finally the case becomes incurable. Such is the experience of every homeopath in the early years while gaining experience, but the damage can at least be minimized by proper supervision and practical training.

The purpose of the homeopathic interview is to accurately arrive at the totality of symptoms which are meaningful to the patient on all three levels. It is this totality which expresses the pathological disturbances on the dynamic plane, and it is only by accurately and completely eliciting this totality of symptoms that the inner disturbance can be comprehended. In other words, it is this totality that expresses to our awareness the resonant frequency of the ailment. The interviewer is specifically *not* merely gathering a collection of data which can later be analyzed by a mechanical or computerized process to arrive at a conclusion. It is a living expression drawn out of the most intimate and meaningful regions of the patient's life, and so the interviewer must gently and sensitively encourage the externalized expression of this inner state.

It is in this sense that homeopathic case-taking is an art. The interviewer can be compared to a painter who slowly and painstakingly brings forth an image which represents in its essence a particular vision of reality. The artist begins a painting in a particular way, but as he proceeds the image changes its shape and becomes more distinct in ways not completely anticipated. The same is true of a homeopathic interview. In the beginning, the patient's description may seem to go toward a particular remedy, or a particular understanding of the evolution of the person's individual pathology, but with further description the concept may well change entirely. In this manner, then, the information acquired is as verifiable as any scientific data, but its acquisition is a true art.

The Setting

First, attention must be paid to the setting in which the interview is conducted. The environment should be quiet, with harmonious, simple, esthetic decor. Interruptions should be minimized, and the patient should not feel excessively rushed.

It is also important that the patient not be biased by too much preparation prior to the interview. A few simple instructions to clarify the fact that a homeopathic interview focuses upon the entire patient, and not merely on the immediate physical problem, are appropriate. But extensive descriptions of the precise kind of information needed in homeopathy and particularly the use of homeopathic questionnaires should be avoided. Such information is likely to cause the patient to focus too much on insignificant details rather than on the issues which are most meaningful to his or her life experience.

The prescriber's attitude is a very important factor which can make the difference between a successful and a poorly taken case. It is of utmost importance that *the interviewer be interested and concerned with the welfare of the patient.* This interest may be conveyed by a few unobtrusive questions posed from time to time during the patient's narrative and by listening with great care and attention. If the interviewer is sincerely interested, the patient will feel more motivated to provide the information needed.

There should be no implication of judgment on the part of the prescriber. Symptoms provided by the patient should be accepted with interest, but without judgment. Advice should not be offered, and moral injunctions should be avoided. If the patient feels judged, he will likely withdraw within himself and refuse to divulge the very information of most value.

An unprejudiced mind on the part of the prescriber is important not only for the comfort and freedom of expression of the patient, but also for the prescriber's own ability to perceive the truth of the case. All too often, the tendency is to try to catalogue symptoms into interpretations based upon previous experience or upon a knowledge of *materia medica.* This process is inevitable to some extent, but the interview must be very circumspect about it. One should be very suspicious about any habitual or unconscious attempt to pigeonhole the expression of the patient into preconceived categories.

This is the essence of the empirical approach to medicine; it is excellently described in Hahnemann's Aphorism 100:

> . . . it is quite immaterial whether or not something similar has ever appeared in the world before under the same or any other name. The novelty or peculiarity of a disease of that kind makes no difference either in the mode of examining or of treating it, as the physican must any way regard the pure picture of every prevailing disease as if it were something new and unknown, and investigate it thoroughly for itself, if he desire to practice medicine in a real and radical manner, never substituting conjecture for actual observation, never taking for granted that the case of

disease before him is already wholly or partially known, but always carefully examining it in all its phases.[1]

This point is then further elaborated by J.T. Kent, one of the greatest of homeopathic prescribers ever, who humbly admits how readily prejudices tend to creep into the process. In this paragraph, he comments on the above aphorism of Hahnemann:

Keep that in your mind, underscore it half a dozen times with red ink, paint it on the wall, put an index finger to it. One of the most important things is to keep out of the mind, in an examination of the case, some other case that has appeared to be similar. If this is not done the mind will be prejudiced in spite of your best endeavours. I have to fight that with every fresh case I come to. I have to labor to keep myself from thinking about thing I have cured like that before, because it would prejudice my mind.[2]

In listening actively to the patient, the homeopath's imagination and sensitivity must be highly involved. The homeopath must develop the capacity to *live* the experience of the patient. This is not merely a matter of putting *oneself* into the shoes of the patient, but rather one of perceiving the patient's experience in his or her *own context*. Since it is obviously impossible for anyone to actually experience the full range of expressions seen during even one day of homeopathic prescribing, it is necessary for the homeopath to suspend personal prejudices, and in imagination to crawl into the context of each patient in order to live that experience, if even for a moment.

The patient may describe a symptom foreign to the personal experience of the homeopath—for example, fear experienced in a crowd. The homeopath must actively wonder, What is this? Is it a feeling of oppression or suffocation because of the closeness of the atmosphere? Is it a fear that someone might cause bodily harm? Is it a fear of not being able to escape in case of some imagined disaster? Is it an emotional vulnerability to the sufferings sensed from those in the crowd? Is it a sensation of loss of personal identity while being merged with the identity of the crowd as a single entity? From such internal imaginings, the homeopath will be able to frame questions which will elucidate more precisely the exact meaning of this symptom to the patient. By living the symptom in this manner, the homeopath is also

---

1. S. Hahnemann, *Organon of Medicine.*
2. J. T. Kent, *Lectures on Homeopathic Philosophy*, p. 232.

conveying to the patient that he is truly interested and that he can actually understand even the most intimate of the patient's experiences or thoughts.

This process is identical with the process involved in studying *materia medica*. At first, when one approaches *materia medica*, one becomes frustrated over the overwhelming mass of seemingly unrelated data. But if each symptom is approached in the same way described above, gradually the remedy is experienced as an integrated, living entity. Each symptom should be read with great interest and solemnity; imagination must be brought into play so that the actual experience of the symptom and of the remedy can be lived. How does the experience of this symptom relate to the others? What must that be like? After meditating in this way on the meaning of symptoms and their interrelationship, the homeopath gradually gains a better understanding of the remedy, just as later he will gain a better understanding of the patient. If a patient feels cared for, understood, and not judged, he will finally yield up his inner state or essence. Just so, if a remedy is read with interest, understanding, and nonjudgmentally, it will finally yield up to the homeopath its inner essence. In the last analysis, it is the matching of these two living images or essences which is the fundamental process of homeopathy.

Eliciting the Symptoms

During the interview, the homeopath is relatively silent, merely asking a few discreet questions from time to time to clarify a point, to show active interest in what the patient is saying, or to direct the narration into more relevant areas. This is a gentle, catalytic process, and not merely a bored, mechanical, or routine process of gathering mere data. The homeopath is actively and intimately involved with what the patient is saying. It is not at all similar to the kind of interview conducted from a written questionnaire. The goal is not to acquire as much data as possible but rather to elicit a living image of the essence of the inner pathology of the patient.

Most interviews quite naturally begin by asking the patient to describe everything that is perceived to be a problem at the moment. Usually, patients then proceed to describe mostly physical complaints, and their descriptions are usually rather general. Quite likely, they will focus on information of an allopathic nature—laboratory tests, diagnoses from other doctors, etc. The interviewer merely allows the narration to continue until the patient has nothing more to say at the moment.

Initially, it is important for the homeopath to be satisfied about the allopathic nature of the complaint. Even though such knowledge is of little importance in prescribing the homeopathic remedy, it is quite important for judging the seriousness of the ailment at that moment, and it is particularly important for understanding the pathological prognosis for the future. Therefore, the homeopath may well wish to examine previous allopathic records and laboratory reports. If the pathological situation is still unclear, it may be important to gather more laboratory or radiological information, or even to acquire the diagnostic opinion of a specialist.

The homeopath may then ask the patient, "What else?" This question helps to convey to the patient that even nonallopathic or nonphysical symptoms are of importance. The homeopath may make a brief comment to assure the patient that the *totality* of the patient's problems is important.

Usually, the next step is to go back over what has been presented to clarify the meaning of each symptom, and to acquire the details so important to homeopathy. Inquiry is made into the exact location of each symptom, the precise sensation involved, the duration of it, its characteristic time of aggravation, over how many months or years is has lasted, and its modalities regarding such things as heat and cold, weather changes, activity or rest, position, rubbing or pressure, etc. Since these symptoms are the chief complaints of the patient, they should be elaborated in some detail, even though they may ultimately play only a minor role in choosing the remedy. Whatever physical examination is needed should also be performed to provide objective observation and to assure the patient that the problem is being investigated thoroughly.

It is natural to inquire next into the *evolution* of the present pathological state of the patient. This should not be a merely routine recording of the past medical history of the patient, but it should be an active questioning about the exact sequence of appearance of current symptoms. When did they occur? Were there any major events in the patient's life at about the time of appearance of the symptoms? What "exciting causes" can be considered factors in producing the symptoms? In particular, the evolution of the pathological state of the patient should focus on the following major influences:

1. Any mental or emotional shocks occurring in the patient's life. This might include such things as griefs, major financial losses, separation from loved ones, identity crises, and other life stress.

2. Any major illnesses which might have affected the overall health of the patient. Particularly, venereal diseases, prolonged infectious diseases, and mental breakdowns or imbalances should be noted.

3. Any treatments given throughout the life of the patient. Since therapies can frequently be suppressive, this factor can have major importance in the evolution of the pathology into deeper regions. For this purpose, one must consider such things as drug treatment, surgery, psychotherapy, natural therapies, and even meditative techniques. Particularly, cortisone, birth control pills, thyroid hormone, tranquilizers, and antibiotics must be inquired into. Often even merely inquiring into the these specific treatments will stimulate the patient's memory about an important episode in the past history.

4. Vaccinations which have been administered and the patient's reactions to them.

All of this information should be collected into a chronological sequence so that the homeopath can see the stages of development of the current pathology. Often, this inquiry will also prove to be very educational for the patient, who has probably not taken all of these factors into account in terms of his or her general health.

By this point in the case, the basic pathology and its evolution should be fairly well understood. The next logical step is to ask questions regarding the typical concerns of homeopathic symptomatology. These questions delve into areas of the patient's life which were probably not considered relevant to the picture, and thus it serves once again as an educational process in addition to the actual homeopathic information gained.

These questions should include as much information as is possible to obtain, of course, but they will tend to focus on particular areas of importance to the patient's daily experience:

176

1. Tolerance to temperature, humidity, weather changes, sun, foggy weather, wind, drafts, closed rooms, etc.

2. Changes which occur at particular times of day or night, and also during particular seasons.

3. The quality of sleep, the quietness or restlessness of sleep, position of sleep, times of waking and reasons for waking, need for covers over various parts of the body, whether the window must be open or closed, etc. Common dreams, somnambulism, peculiar sounds or gestures during sleep, etc.

4. Appetite, thirst, food cravings, food aversions, and food aggravations.

5. Sexual desire, sexual satisfaction, and particular inhibitions or obsessions regarding sexuality.

6. The functioning of the various systems of the body: endocrine, circulatory, gastrointestinal, eliminative, respiratory, skin, etc. In women, menstrual function and childbearing history should be elaborated.

7. Overall quality of energy available to function in daily life and under various circumstances.

8. Emotional limitations: specific anxieties, fears or phobias, depression, apathy, lack of self-confidence, irritability, etc.

9. The quality of the patient's life in relationship to loved ones, family, friends, and colleagues.

10. Mental symptoms such as poor memory, inability to concentrate or comprehend, delusionary or hallucinatory states, paranoia.

Such a list of symptoms should be viewed merely as examples; the actual questions in a given case will be guided by the nature of the illness itself. In inquiring about all of these things, great flexibility must be allowed, so that the patient can be as expressive as possible, once the breadth of symptoms of interest to the homeopath is understood by the patient.

Each symptom elicited should be further explored for accuracy and vividness. For example, if the patient reports "depression," it is important to inquire further into the patient's exact meaning. In these times of psychological fads, such a term has become generalized and vague, even though commonly used. To a particular patient, it might describe suicidal desire, mere suicidal thoughts, despair, discouragement, lack of self-esteem, anxiety, pessimism, apathy, mental lethargy, etc. The precise quality of the

177

symptom must be elucidated, and all the modifying factors should be included.

Most importantly, these symptoms must be elaborated into a *living image* of its meaning in the patient's life. When a generalized description is offered by the patient, the homeopath might ask, "Like what?" or "Can you give a concrete example?" In this way, the words being used come alive, and the homeopath can more accurately evaluate the importance and the individuality of the symptom. This principle of acquiring living images is of very crucial importance. If the homeopath gathers merely dry data, there will be no case whatsoever, and a curative prescription may well be impossible.

Once the detailed homeopathic symptomatology has been obtained on the physical plane, sufficient rapport should have been established to enable further inquiry into mental and emotional symptoms. These are of the utmost importance to the homeopath and should be elucidated with the greatest care. This is the realm in which patients are likely to harbor the most important secrets, so great tact and sensitivity must be used by the interviewer to bring them forward.

Chronic patients, in particular, harbor deep within themselves feelings, thoughts, or experiences which cause them great shame and embarrassment. They believe that these secrets are so shocking and so unacceptable that others would not be capable of handling them. In a Christian sense, they are viewed as deep, dark "sins" which must be repressed and hidden at all costs. These hidden images, feelings, or fears are of utmost importance to the homeopath, because they are the expression of the activity of the defense mechanism on the deepest levels of the organism. Once such symptoms are brought to the surface, particularly when accompanied with strong emotions, the homeopath can be assured that the deepest "essence" of the pathology is being revealed. Then and only then can a remedy be selected that will touch the deepest recesses of the defense mechanism and bring about a cure.

Bringing forth these deep symptoms is a very delicate matter indeed. The first clue of their presence may be revealed by a mere tension, or hesitation, or gesture, or cracking of the voice. Because walls have been erected around these sore spots, the patient will quickly attempt to skip over such symptoms and to move on to other less painful things. The interviewer must be quite sensitive to this dynamic. In our normal cultural context, there are innumerable subtle signals (nonverbal or verbal) which we use to warn others not to trespass into a "private" area. Much of this communication is done subliminally. The homeopathic interviewer, however, must become skilled in picking up these signals. Perhaps the best way is to be sensitive to one's own degree of emotional tension. If, during the course of an interview, the homeopath experiences discomfort about a particular topic (provided, of course, that this is not merely a tender spot for the homeopath himself), this area should be further explored, gently and sensitively, but resolutely.

Homeopaths are as human as everyone else; therefore, they want to be liked and respected by their patients. This motivation in itself can prevent the homeopath from probing into tender areas. If there is a sensitive area, the homeopath has a responsibility to the patient to nonjudgmentally and carefully encourage him or her to openly describe this symptom. Often even the gentlest probing into such realms will cause the patient to break down and weep, or to become agitated or angry. If symptoms are expressed with such emotional charge attached to them, their expression is beneficial to the patient and of great value to the homeopath. In these moments, the patient's guard is down, and whatever expression occurs is deep and essential to the case.

To some, this approach may be reminiscent of the cathartic method of a psychoanalytic interview. It is true that the skill involved in a homeopathic interview is superficially akin to that necessary in psychoanalysis, but the purpose of eliciting the symptoms is quite different. In homeopathy, these symptoms are brought out for the purpose of understanding deeply the true pathology, the precise way in which the defense mechanism is acting, and therefore of finding the most appropriate remedy that may lead to cure. A psychoanalyst, upon discovering such an important thought, feeling, or experience, will tend to pursue it further in an analytical manner. The homeopath, on the other hand, once satisfied that the symptom is elicited, will move on to other symptoms.

Recording of Symptoms

It would be preferable to be able to conduct a homeopathic interview without having to be distracted by the necessity of taking notes, but this is not possible. The homeopathic record is very important for the care of the patient. It provides a reliable method

179

of refreshing the prescriber's memory on future visits, and it provides a means by which the patient can be transferred from one prescriber to another without interrupting the continuity of the treatment. In recording the homeopathic case, the primary goal is to accurately and concisely describe all the important factors in the case, while eliminating irrelevant information. In addition, the record should communicate the relative intensity of emphasis of particular symptoms.

As much as possible, the patient's own words must be recorded in exact quotes. This is important because the entire homeopathic literature is based upon the graphic terminology of ordinary language. All provings record symptoms as closely as possible to the natural expressions of the provers. Of course, on occasion particular colloquialisms can be translated into more common homeopathic language. A vivid example of this is given by Hahnemann: it is permissible to translate words such as "show," "monthlies," or "period" into the terminology familiar to homeopaths—"menses." Such translations are quite safe to make when dealing with physical symptoms, but one must be very cautious when translating mental and emotional symptoms. Great care must be taken to encourage the patient to be very specific about such symptoms, so that they can be accurately interpreted in homeopathic language. Still, whenever possible, the best policy is to stick as closely as possible to the original phraseology of the patient.

It is also important to refrain from *putting words into the patient's mouth*. Questions should be phrased in a nondirective manner, so that the patient is not allowed to give the answer he or she thinks you are seeking. For example, the interviewer might ask, "How do you tolerate changes of weather?" The patient, faced with such a question, has a variety of possible responses and is therefore encouraged to examine the question in the light of true personal experience. Or the question might be asked, "Do you have any particularly strong cravings or aversions?" rather than a directive question such as, "Do you crave sweets?"

Direct questions, such as Yes/No questions on questionnaires, should be avoided at all costs. For example, if a patient answers affirmatively to the question, "Do you crave sweets?" the answer should not be recorded at all. To determine whether this is truly a pathological expression of the patient's individuality, further questions must be asked to determine its validity: "How strong is this craving?" "How often do you experience it?" "How difficult would it be for you to give them up?" "Can you give an example of circumstances when you most notice this craving?"

Hypothetical questions should also be avoided. For example, no useful information would come from a question of the following type: "Would you be irritable if you were late for an appointment, your car stalled while waiting for an unexpectedly long train at a train crossing, and the kids in the back seat were screaming and hitting each other?" Such a question would not provide any information truly expressive of the defense mechanism of the patient.

Sometimes the patient has no particular answer to give to the initial purposely nondirective question. Suppose the interviewer asks, "Do you have any fears or phobias?" The patient responds, "Not that I can recall." Because of the totality of the rest of the symptoms, suppose the interviewer specifically wants to know if the patient has a fear of heights. It would be improper to ask directly, "Do you have a fear of heights?" because the patient may infer that the interviewer is seeking an affirmative answer. Instead, the interviewer might give a variety of possibilities just to aid the patient's memory, such as, "Well, for example, do you have a fear of the dark, of being alone, of heights, of thunderstorms, of dogs, or any others?" Suppose the patient then responds, "Oh yes! I have always had a strong fear of heights! I just always avoid them." Such a response can be trusted because it was elicited among a variety of other possibilities presented with equal emphasis.

Important symptoms should not be left at simple face value. They should be probed further to be certain that the true picture is presented. For example, a patient may be asked, "Do you tend to be unusually fastidious or sloppy?" The patient replies, "Oh, I am quite sloppy." But if the question is further asked, "How do others see you in this regard?" the patient may well reply, "Very neat!" The fastidious patient is never quite satisfied and therefore sees himself as sloppy.

When a patient presents a particular symptom, it is advisable to write it down and then leave a space below it. One must not interrupt the patient merely to fill in the clarifications and modifications. Instead, a space is left, and this information is filled in later after the patient has run out of things to say. With certain patients, of course, particularly those who seem to enjoy rambling on about anything coming to mind, it may be necessary to interrupt from time to time in order to return to relevant topics. But even in such a situation, interruptions should be made only reluctantly, because there is always a chance that such ramblings may bring out clues to an important symptom.

A very important technique which should be used in all homeopathic cases is that of underlining. For any given homeopathic symptom, there are three factors which determine its emphasis: *clarity, intensity,* and *spontaneity*. A symptom of very great meaning to the patient which is given with great descriptive clarity, great intensity causing interference in the life of the patient, and spontaneity (i.e., volunteered by the patient rather than elicited after questioning) carries the most weight in a case. These three factors are combined in the process of underlining:

1. *No underlining:* Symptoms which are hazy, not given spontaneously, not perceived as very intense by the patient.
2. *One underline:* symptoms of greater clarity and greater intensity, yet still elicited only upon questioning.
3. *Two underlines:* symptoms of great clarity, moderate intensity, and volunteered spontaneously.
4. *Three underlines:* symptoms with the highest clarity, great intensity, and given entirely spontaneously by the patient.

These underlines should be used with precision, and they should apply equally well to follow-up visits as to initial interviews. By this means, changes in the emphasis of a symptom in the overall picture can be evaluated along with its mere presence or absence. This can provide extremely important clues for the progress or prognosis of a given case over time.

Finally, the record should include purely objective information such as name, address, age, birthdate, height, weight, and date of interview. A brief physical description of the patient, including body habitus, general demeanor, and gestures or posture, may be helpful in developing an image of the patient as an individual. Any laboratory or radiological data, as well as findings upon physical examinations, should be included.

At the conclusion of the record of each visit, the recommendations made to the patient should be recorded; if dietary changes or other therapeutic alterations are recommended, they should be noted, and the remedy prescription with potency and number of doses should be recorded.

Difficult Cases

All cases are taken in an individual manner. There are no set routines which should be followed, even though there are basic pieces of information which must be acquired in order to make a proper prescription. Every patient must be approached in an individualized way, and each presents particular challenges for the homeopathic interviewer.

There are, however, types of patients who pose particularly difficult problems. These, for various reasons, prevent the acquiring of a clear totality of symptoms. Each must be dealt with in a particular way, and symptoms coming from such individuals must be viewed with great caution until carefully confirmed.

The first group of such patients are the *timid*, sensitive, reserved, or withdrawn. They withhold many of their symptoms or describe symptoms with much less intensity than is true in reality. These people usually feel the interviewer is not interested in their little discomforts and will become bored or fatigued by them. They may consider it shameful to express some of their mental, emotional, or sexual symptoms. By withholding or downplaying their symptoms, such people mislead the homeopath into recording an incorrect picture, and therefore into prescribing an incorrect remedy.

With these people, an entirely special approach is needed. Each must be handled with great ingenuity. Primarily, reassurance must be communicated, and the patient must be shown that the interviewer is really interested in every detail, no matter how "insignificant" or "shameful." After gentle and accepting questioning and probing, the patient gradually begins to feel comfortable and becomes willing to expose the needed symptoms.

In "closed" patients who provide very few symptoms, objective observations take on added importance. The interviewer must note down every gesture, every nervous action, etc.—restlessness of the fingers, restlessness of the body or of the feet, excessive irritability, loquacity, the time taken to answer questions (whether too quickly or too slowly), difficulty in finding the right words, easy blushing of the face, facial expressions, swellings around the eyes, color of skin, falling of hair, biting of nails, timidity of expression, perspiration of palms or body, odors, etc.

The second group of difficult cases are the *hypochondriacs*. This group includes not only those who are excessively anxious about

183

their health but also those who compulsively observe every detail related to health, until all perspective is lost. These people tend to relate a tremendous volume of minute symptoms which cannot possibly be valued highly by the homeopath because of these patients' tendency to exaggerate. In such an instance, the hypochondriacal nature itself is noted, and perhaps the anxiety about health that may be present. Any other symptoms should be underlined only with great caution, and perhaps only after confirmation by objective co-workers or relatives. Often, these patients are very intent upon impressing the homeopath with how very sick they believe themselves to be. No particular approach on the part of the interviwer can counteract such behavior, but it is best to present a demeanor of objective understanding without excessive display of sympathy or alarm. Meanwhile, the patient should be encouraged to take an overall view of his condition, to summarize and highlight symptoms, and to communicate only those which are most persistent.

A third group of problem patients are the *intellectuals*—those highly educated people relying upon their minds for success in life. One might think that intellectuals would make the best homeopathic patients because their observations should be more astute than other people's. As a matter of fact, the opposite is true. Intellectuals tend to relate to reality according to what is explainable to their minds; if something is peculiar or unexplainable, they tend to block it out of awareness altogether. Thus intellectuals tend to see commonality in things, rather than individuality, and are unlikely to be able to report their own unique symptoms. They evaluate or interpret their symptoms in terms of what they have read, what theories are current, what conjectures fit their philosophy of life; in this way, they "explain away" the very symptoms of most value to the homeopath. A simple, uneducated man—a villager—expresses his symptoms with much more clarity and exactness than an intellectual. For example, if the intellectual admits that he has some anxiety, he immediately hastens to explain that this is natural because of the hectic environment he is forced to live in. Or if he has a fear, he explains it as being due to a traumatic experience in childhood, and asserts, "I am almost certain that that fear has been 80% overcome by now." Because of such conjecturing and reasoning, it becomes impossible for the homeopath to be sure whether the fear is a significant symptom or not. The homeopath then asks, "How do you sleep?" The intellectual replies, "Oh, I do have quite a bit of sleeplessness, but that is certainly due to the irregular night life I must lead."

In the end, after a long and involved interview, the homeopath has a mass of symptoms all of which are qualified by the phrase, "Yes, but . . ." In such cases, there may be no symptoms whatsoever upon which to prescribe with any reliability. These are very difficult cases to evaluate. The homeopath must be skeptical of the explanations offered by the intellectual patient, and must always keep in mind whether the severity of the symptom is in reality proportional to the explanations offered. For example, many people have traumatic childhood experiences or lead demanding lives with irregular sleeping hours, but how many develop a life-long fear or chronic insomnia? It is important to keep in mind the difference between the "exciting cause," which intellectuals tend to focus upon, and *susceptibility* to that cause.

Highly educated patients create another distortion as well. They have read many theories on diet, vitamins, cleansing regimens, etc., and they have adopted some of these ideas themselves without any consideration for the uniqueness of their own organism. For example, a well-educated professor suffering from hay fever, duodenal ulcer, constipation, and other problems may have become convinced by a nutrition book that salt is bad for the human race. He therefore avoids salt, even though it has been a chronically habitual and craved food in his case. His chemistry may have required a higher amount of salt than that of other people, but for intellectual reasons he has altered that balance in his own body. Not only does this remove from observation a symptom which might be important to the homeopath, but the resulting chemical imbalance might result in depression, or irritability, or easy fatigue, etc. For this new state, then, the intellectual studies other nutrition books and decides to take megadoses of B-vitamins to correct what he surmises to be a vitamin deficiency. This in turn produces other symptoms, and the process continues.

By the time the intellectual comes to the homeopath, he has used his mind to interfere so profoundly with his organism's own natural expression that it becomes virtually impossible to discover what the defense mechanism was trying to do in the first place. The intellectual, of course, can explain the reason for each and every alteration that has been made, but it is impossible to discern which symptoms resulted from previous alterations and which are

185

true expressions of pathology. In such a situation, the only thing to do is to recommend that the patient discontinue all the vitamins, follow a diet based solely on whatever is craved or desired, and return in several months for the homeopathic interview.

Another very big problem posed by intellectuals is their insistence upon making all the decisions for themselves regarding therapy. They want to know the reason for everything, and they want to participate in every judgment. Of course, patients must have overall responsibility for their health, and they must be bold enough to request basic information regarding their progress, their prognosis, and the rationale behind the therapy being used. But this process should not go so far as to involve the patient in every minute decision for which the homeopath has been trained over many years. At some point, a person must sit back and acknowledge the value of expertise.

This issue becomes most apparent in those intellectual patients who purchase *materia medicas* and study the remedies being given to them. Not having any training or clinical experience, they easily become confused over the various subtleties involved in choosing one remedy over another. Even worse, once they have read a few remedies in the *materia medica*, they naturally tend to describe their own symptoms in terms of what they have read. If this process goes far enough, the homeopath may receive only information arising out of intellectual theorizing and no symptoms at all expressing the true pathological state of the patient.

A related group of problem patients confronting the homeopath are those with sufficient wealth to visit specialists all over the world. From one doctor, such a "doctor-hopping" patient may have acquired a diagnosis of "neurasthenia," with the recommendation to rest. From another, "adrenal exhaustion," and a particular combination of vitamins, minerals, and herbs is prescribed. Then another nutritionist diagnoses the problem as "carbohydrate intolerance," and the patient learns to avoid carbohydrates. Finally, a clinical ecologist discovers by skin tests and controlled pulse testing that the patient is allergic to twenty-five different substances present in foods and the environment. The patient strictly avoids the harmful foods, goes on a rotary diet which is not based upon individual requirements, and undertakes a series of allergy shots to diminish the allergy. By the time she arrives in the office of the homeopath, she is on a very abnormal diet, is taking boxes full of vitamins, is groggy from Valium, and has just rushed to the office after receiving an allergy shot. Besides that,

instead of describing symptoms, the patient lists as chief complaints "neurasthenia," "adrenal exhaustion," "carbohydrate intolerance," and "chemical hypersensitivities."

Such people tend to view their homeopath as just another
doctor among an entire network of people being paid to create a
relatively comfortable state of "health" for the patient. They feel
completely dependent on the drugs, the vitamins, the allergy
shots, etc., and the mere suggestion that they discontinue them
throws such patients into a panic. These people are in a most pitiable state. The image which might have arisen from their defense
mechanism has long ago been suppressed into deeper levels, they
have lost track of their abilities for self-observation, and they become addicts of the health industry. Such cases are virtually hopeless for a homeopath to treat successfully. Unless they are willing
to return to fundamental laws of Nature and of healing, they are
doomed to continue their pilgrimages to doctors' offices, their pill-
popping, and degeneration in their chronic conditions.

Each of these groups of difficult cases raises a question to
those familiar with Eastern mysticism: What are the karmic implications of homeopathic treatment? By giving a remedy, are we
curing a state of suffering which is designed to be a spur to spiritual growth? The answer to this question lies in the fact that great
intelligence and consciousness are necessary for a patient to initiate homeopathic therapy in the first place, to cooperate with the
process of self-observation and confession necessary to finding a
remedy, and then to be patient enough to allow the pace of the
cure to complete itself without interference. Homeopathy demands a great deal of its adherents. In their life habits, they must
conform to a relatively natural and spontaneous diet, they must
avoid substances which can interfere with the functioning of the
defense mechanism, they must observe their responses to various
stimuli with a high degree of simplicity and objectivity, and they
must be willing to express the true experience of their inner state
of disequilibrium. If a patient is willing to undertake this rather
demanding task, then the karmic influences of the illness are
taken care of in the process of cure.

Taking the Acute Case

An acute illness is one which is self-limited. It is characterized
by a latent period, a period of exacerbation, and then a period of
decline of symptoms which may result either in cure or in death.

Acute diseases are such that the defense mechanism is capable of handling the disturbance on its own. In a truly acute disease, chronic sequelae do not occur. Indeed, whatever pre-existing chronic conditions were present retire into the background during the acute ailment, only to return again afterward.

The goal of the homeopathic remedy in an acute ailment is simply to accelerate the natural processes which were set in motion by the defense mechanism. The homeopath need only prescribe upon the dramatic symptoms of the acute phase and ignore the underlying symptoms belonging to the chronic state. This is relatively easy because the acute symptoms are dramatic and fresh in the mind of the patient. The important thing is to discover the specific reactions being generated by the defense mechanism in response to the acute stimulus alone.

During an acute illness, the homeopath collects information from three sources. The first, ideally, is the physical *environment* of the patient. If at all possible, making a home visit during a serious acute disease is extremely valuable. The homeopath observes whether the room is darkened or exposed to the light of day, whether the window is opened or closed, whether the patient is bundled up or throwing clothes off, whether a hot water bottle is being used, whether the patient is propped up in bed, whether a pitcher full of ice-water or tea is by the bedside, whether a chair is present for visitors, etc. In addition, the patient is observed directly: Is the expression anxious, peaceful, unusually cheerful, or stuporous? Is the color pale or flushed? Are the eyes clear or glazed? Are the lips dry and cracked, or moist? Are there any particular odors? Does the patient relate symptoms easily and freely, or would he rather be left alone and unbothered? Is he anxious or irritable? To a homeopath with a good knowledge of acute remedies, a simple visit to the sickroom of the patient provides a wealth of information within just the first few minutes.

The second source of information is the *patient* himself. If the patient is in a position to give reliable symptoms, all of the symptoms are collected, and their homeopathic characteristics are noted: the exact location, the time of appearance and duration, the precise type of sensation, and the modalities which make it better or worse. In an acute case, such information, is usually very easy to elicit because the symptoms are quite dramatic and the modifiers are fresh in the patient's mind. A clinical examination is then performed to determine the precise diagnosis, seriousness, and prognosis of the ailment at that moment.

The third source of information is the *friends or relatives* who have been attending the patient. Often, the patient is too stuporous to provide precise information, so the best information is elicited from the attendants who have a more objective perspective. Let us consider an example of an acute symptom and the pertinent factors which must be determined in relation to it. As an example, we will take the symptom: *fever*.

Fever could appear only in the afternoon, or only during morning hours, or only between 9 and 11 A.M., or just between 6 and 8 in the evening. Perhaps the fever goes down after eating, or it may rise only after eating. Perhaps it improves only with sleep. Occasionally, it will be found to affect only certain parts of the body or only one side of the body. It may be preceded by chills, or followed by them. There may be perspiration which relieves the fever, or perspiration may not relieve. There may be thirst with fever, or thirstlessness. Each of these symptoms may lead the homeopath toward a different remedy.

Each symptom must be scrutinized in exactly this degree of detail, until a totality of acute symptoms is arrived at. From this totality, the remedy for that particular moment can be determined. Of course, the pace of symptoms changes rapidly during an acute ailment, and another remedy might be indicated after a few hours. But whatever remedy is given based upon the totality of acute symptoms in the moment is likely to accelerate progress toward cure and relieve the patient considerably.

Chapter 13

Evaluation of Symptoms

ONCE THE PATIENT'S CASE has been taken and recorded with great detail and thoroughness, it is possible to begin the process of study which will lead eventually to the first prescription. For beginners, it is probably best to explain to chronically suffering patients that further study is needed to arrive at a first prescription, and therefore to ask the patient to return after a day or two for the actual prescription. This procedure helps to prevent hasty prescriptions which are the bane of all prescribers suffering under tight schedules. Such a policy will not disappoint the patient but on the contrary will improve careful homeopathic prescribing; this is useful not only for the necessary cooperation of the patient, but it also helps to impress upon the patient the necessity of accurate and thoughtful reporting of symptoms.

In the very beginning of a homeopath's career, it may be necessary to have several interviews with the patient before arriving at the final prescription. The beginning homeopath knows few remedies, and those only partially, and the questions asked are likely to be rather incomplete. Inexperience may cause the beginner to merely skim lightly over issues which later turn out to be very important. For this reason, the best procedure is to have an initial interview, and then take the record home and study it thoughtfully and carefully. During this study, inevitably new questions will arise, or doubts about areas of the initial case-taking. Meanwhile, the patient also is reflecting upon the interview and wishes to clarify a few points. So, a second, usually more brief, interview is held in which more details are covered. The homeopath may again wish to study the case further. This process should continue for as many times as necessary before the prescriber finally arrives at a prescription which is felt to be the correct one; always, each prescription must be made only after careful thought, whether arrived at after a period of days by a beginning prescriber, or whether settled upon after a relatively short period of time by a more experienced homeopath. If such great care is taken with each and every case, experience and knowledge of remedies will be gained rapidly and reliably, until finally the entire process can take place in a matter of minutes for some cases without diminishing the homeopath's confidence in the prescription.

Once the entire case has been taken, then the next task is to grasp the *totality* of the patient's symptomatology. Bearing in mind that the defense mechanism makes itself known to us *only* through symptoms produced on mental, emotional, and physical levels, the prescriber must read and re-read the written case until the entire case is grasped as a whole. To the mind's eye, the case should take shape in such a way that the major expressions of the defense mechanism are properly highlighted, and yet all of the minor details are understood as well. Etiological factors, miasmatic predispositions, and the general (nonpathological) personality of the patient are all fully understood as well.

The next step is to note down the major symptom expressions, in order of their importance. In this listing, only the most significant symptoms should be included; many minor symptoms will be ignored. This listing should be done *very thoughtfully*, and not merely according to some mechanical procedure (such as listing only those symptoms underlined three times, or beginning always with the main complaints of the patient). The criteria for listing of symptoms are described in Figure 15. Basically, symptoms are ranked according to their *intensity*, how *deeply* they reach into the organism (mental and emotional symptoms being considered most important), and according to their degree of *peculiarity*.

Often, this listing of symptoms will totally ignore the complaints causing the patient to consult the prescriber in the first place; for example, a patient may come to the office concerned about a few warts, or about chronic headaches, or a tendency to constipation, but the homeopath discovers on taking the case that the patient has a large number of phobias and anxieties and very

191

low stamina which have been present throughout the patient's life. In such an instance, the original complaints are virtually ignored in the evaluation of symptoms, and the major limitations to the patient's freedom are listed instead.

In Figure 15 the symptoms of most importance are found at the apex of the diagram, and those of least significance are found at the bottom. A mental symptom of great intensity, which is also very peculiar, is given the most weight in the evaluation of symptoms; for example, such a symptom might be Irritability Only When Alone, or Irritability Only While Reading, or Anxiety Which Is Ameliorated by Cold Drinks.

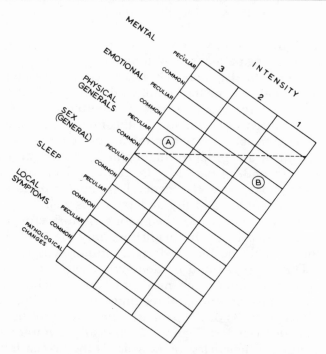

Figure 15: Three main factors are involved in grading symptoms: the location in the hierarchy of the organism, the degree of peculiarity, and the intensity of the symptom. Thus symptom A can be more important than symptom B because it is peculiar and highly intense, even though physical symptoms are *usually* considered less important than emotional ones.

On the other hand, a common symptom affecting only a local part of the body which interferes only occasionally with the patient's life is considered of least importance. An example of such a symptom might be a corn on the bottom of the foot, or a few warts on the fingers, or even a small blemish on the face which is only meaningful to the patient for cosmetic reasons.

For the purposes of homeopathic prescribing, a *peculiar* symptom is one which is not only unusual in human experience, but which is also listed in the Repertory as a rubric with only a small number of remedies. A patient, for example, may describe a constant paranoid delusion that everyone is trying to insult him. This is certainly an unusual symptom in human experience, but it is of no value to the homeopath because it is not described in provings of medicines. On the other hand, a patient may describe a powerful feeling of fear which arises only upon hearing music; in the homeopathic Repertory, such a symptom is found in only two remedies (digitalis and Natrum carbonicum), so it *may* be of great value to the prescriber. Of course, it must always be kept in mind that the provings, and the Repertory as well, may be incomplete. As valuable as peculiar symptoms can be, they must not be prescribed upon alone without confirmation from the rest of the case.

Common symptoms are those which are both common to human experience and have a very large number of remedies listed in the Repertory. For example, the symptom Aversion to Company, while not uncommon in human experience, is listed in the Repertory as having been produced by 100 remedies!

In evaluating symptoms, one must keep in mind which symptoms are truly representative of the defense mechanism of the patient, and which are merely common manifestations of the diagnostic category of the pathological entity. A patient suffering from the allopathic category "Rheumatoid Arthritis" is naturally expected to complain of pain in the joints. Such a symptom, although helpful for making an allopathic diagnosis, is of no help whatsoever to the homeopathic prescriber in finding the correct remedy. A joint can be very painful, red, swollen, and tender to the touch, and yet none of these symptoms assist the homeopath. On the other hand, a *painless* swelling of the joints of the upper limbs would be of great value to the homeopath, because it is a peculiar thing and only two remedies are listed under such a rubric.

General symptoms are those which describe the patient as a whole. Usually, such symptoms are described by phrases such as, "I feel . . ." or "I am . . ." Thus virtually all mental and emotional symptoms are general symptoms. A person tends to describe them in general terms: "I am anxious," "I am depressed," or "I fear . . ."

There are also *physical general* symptoms. These refer to physical states which apply to the person as a whole. The patient may say, "I feel very cold all the time," or "I cannot tolerate the sun," or "I am always tired." Even food cravings or aversions are considered physical general symptoms: "I crave sweets," "I hate meat," or "I am always thirsty for cold drinks." These symptoms represent manifestations of the entire organism, and not merely of the stomach.

Sex symptoms are considered next in importance to physical general symptoms. They include such things as the degree of sexual desire, the degree of sexual satisfaction, and aggravation or amelioration from menses. Such symptoms having to do with the particular genital organs, however, are listed as local symptoms: i.e., discharges, menstrual irregularities, or inability to develop or maintain an erection.

Of next importance are *sleep* symptoms, which, of course, are general symptoms. They arise out of mental and emotional states, certain hormonal and electromagnetic imbalances, physical restlessness, etc. Thus we list such symptoms as the position in which the patient sleeps, positions in which it is impossible to sleep or in which disturbing dreams occur, parts of the body which tend to become uncovered during sleep, times of waking, sleeplessness, sleepiness, etc.

Physical particular symptoms are given relatively minor significance. Even though such symptoms may be of great intensity, they affect only a part of the organism and are therefore a relatively insignificant manifestation of the defense mechanism.

Finally, of least significance are *pathological tissue changes*. These have tremendous importance for making an allopathic diagnosis, and also for determining a prognostic impression, but they are relatively unimportant for the actual selection of a remedy. For example, the common problem of delayed urination in an elderly man with an enlarged prostate gland cannot be used for homeopathic purposes. Constipation resulting from rectal cancer is equally useless, unless there are individualizing symptoms associated with it. Even such a serious symptom as dyspnea resulting from an enlarged thyroid gland cannot be used for the purpose of choosing a remedy without individualizing characteristics.

The process of arranging symptoms according to their relative importance is of crucial importance for later study of the case.

Other than the general guidelines listed in Figure 15, it is impossible to describe this evaluation more concisely. It is not a mathematical process, and it cannot be done by routine methods. It requires great thought, trained skill, and much experience. In the early years of prescribing, this process should be supervised by an experienced and skilled homeopath, for it can be as important to the ultimate prescription as the actual taking of the case.

The Homeopathic Repertory

Before proceeding further with the process of studying a case, it is necessary to take a little time to describe the contents and structure of the all-important tool: the Repertory.

Obviously, it would be entirely impractical for a prescriber to go thumbing through the many volumes of *materia medicas* trying to find the remedy which best fits the totality of symptoms of the patient. Consequently, cross references have been developed which compile lists of remedies in which a specific symptom has been found. During the history of homeopathy, several such Repertories have been developed.

From experience, the most thorough and useful Repertory is James Tyler Kent's *Repertory of the Homeopathic Materia Medica*.[1] This is a monumental work which has contributed immeasurably to the process of selecting a remedy. Kent's Repertory lists in great detail the many symptoms produced in provings of remedies known at the time (1877), but it goes even further. Kent was a vastly experienced and skillful prescriber, and he included in his Repertory a great deal of information gleaned from his personal experience. The reliability of his Repertory arises not merely from its thoroughness in recording the results of provings but also from the detail and depth of his own knowledge.

The purpose of the Repertory is to enable the homeopath to speedily review the many drugs known to have produced the symptoms being studied in a given case. Because of its grading of symptoms, it also helps the prescriber to interpret the intensity of symptoms as demonstrated in particular remedies. The Repertory is designed to serve as a reminder, as a hint. It leads the homeopath to think about certain remedies which otherwise might be forgotten.

It is very important that the Repertory not be exaggerated in

1. J.T. Kent, *Repertory of the Homeopathic Materia Medica* (Calcutta: Sett Dey, latest reprinting 1969, originally printed 1877).

importance. There is a natural tendency to use it as a kind of computer to be used mechanically, producing automatically and thoughtlessly the presumed remedy. Indeed, the contents of Kent's Repertory have actually been computerized. Of course, mere computerization of the data is not dangerous in itself; the true risk occurs when untrained people are taught to rely on the results of the repertorization as if they were sufficient for choosing a remedy. Repertorization can only be as helpful as the information which is gathered in the first place. Years of training are required to learn the proper skills involved in case-taking and the gradation and evaluation of symptoms.

In the last analysis, any prescription must be based on a careful study of *materia medica,* and the matching of the "essence" and totality of symptoms with that of the remedy. This matching requires great study and trained judgment. It must always be remembered that the Repertory is merely an aid to this matching process.

It also must be remembered that the Repertory, as admirable as it may be, is as yet incomplete. Kent's knowledge was vast, but could not have included everything. With further experience, the homeopathic profession will likely discover remedies which are incorrectly listed in the Repertory. There will be many additions made in order to include clinical observations of cured symptoms, and to include data from modern provings of both old and new remedies. Even the most thoroughly proven remedies, such as Sulphur, Calcarea carbonica, or Natrum muriaticum, can produce and cure symptoms not yet recorded in the Repertory. Therefore, it is important not to view the Repertory as an absolute, final reference, even though it is a work great inspiration. It is an indispensable tool but not the final word.

Simply described, the Repertory is a massive book containing a detailed listing of symptoms (called "rubrics") followed by the various remedies which have demonstrated such a symptom whether in provings or in cured clinical cases.

In Kent's Repertory, remedies are listed with three different gradations. Remedies in which the particular symptom is represented with the greatest intensity and frequency are printed in bold type, and are given three points. Remedies showing the symptom with moderate intensity are printed in italics, and given two points. Remedies with the least intensiy and frequency are listed in ordinary type, and are given one point.

The presence or absence of a remedy in a given rubric, as well as its grading, is subject to updating according to the experience of skilled homeopaths. As a routine practice, a prescriber should keep a record of symptoms found to be cured in the process of cure of the entire patient. When such a cure occurs, the homeopath should go over every cured symptom in minute detail, including all the modalities, sensations, and concomitants recalled by the patient—just as is done in a proving. Once a particular symptom has been observed to have been cured in this manner three times, the prescriber is justified to enter that remedy into the Repertory. Or, if the remedy was already listed, but in low degree, it can be upgraded according to the experience of the prescriber.

Kent's Repertory can be bewildering to the uninitiated beginner. It is not a merely alphabetical listing of symptoms; rather, it is arranged in a specific manner fitting the homeopathic method of case-taking.

The sections are arranged, first of all, from above downward and from general to particular. There are thirty-one chapter headings, arranged as follows:

Mind: including all mental and emotional symptoms, listed alphabetically according to major categories.

Vertigo: by which is meant all states of dizziness, not merely the specific allopathic definition of "vertigo."

Head: including all kinds of headaches, as well as eruptions, conditions of hair, swellings, etc. "Head" describes specifically the scalp region, excluding the face and neck.

Eye

Vision

Ear

Hearing

Nose

Face: including outer lips of mouth.

Mouth: including mucous membranes, gums, tongue, and palate, as well as speech as a function.

Teeth

Throat: including esophagus, pharynx, tonsils, and uvula.

External Throat: which is a separate chapter at the end of the section of Throat; this includes the anterior tissues of the neck.

Stomach: including all references to appetite, thirst, and food cravings and aversions (which are general symptoms, even though listed as part of a local region). Food Aggravations, however, are listed in Generalities.

Abdomen: including regions of "*Hypochondrium*" (below the ribs and above the umbilicus), *"Hypogastrium"* (literally, "below the stomach, but considered below the navel, *"Ileocecal,"* *"Crest of Ilium,"* *"Inguinal"* (groin), *"Sides,"* Liver, Spleen, and *Umbilicus.*

Rectum: including all references to its function. Diarrhea and constipation are listed under Rectum, while specific qualities of stool are listed separately.

Stool: qualities of the stool itself. Therefore, diarrhea would be found under Rectum, while "watery stool" is found under Stool.

Urinary Organs

Bladder: including Urination and Urging to Urination.

Kidneys

Prostate Gland

Urethra: both male and female.

Urine: specific qualities of the urine itself.

Genitalia

Male: (Note: Prostate Gland is listed separately under Urinary Organs)

Female: including menstrual symptoms. (Note: General symptoms having to do with sexual desire are listed under Genitalia.)

Larynx and Trachea: including Voice, which describes the specific quality of voice, such as hoarseness, etc. (Speech, describing functional qualities such as stammering, etc., is listed under Mouth.)

Respiration: including all functional aspects of breathing involving lungs, such as Difficult Respiration, Wheezing, etc.

Cough: a special section on cough alone.

Expectoration: describing solely the physical aspects of the expectoration.

Chest describing the chest wall, as distinct from respiration. Describes specific physical conditions of *Axilla, Clavicle, Diaphragm, Sternum, Ribs, Pectoral Muscles, Sides of the Chest, Lungs, Heart, and Mammae* (breasts).

Back: including entire length of it, beginning from *Cervical,* then *Dorsal* (thoracic), *Lumbar, Sacral,* and *Coccyx.*

Extremities: each symptom being broken down according to *Upper* and *Lower Limbs,* as well as specifics such as *Shoulder, Upper Arm, Elbow, Forearm, Wrist, Hands, Fingers,* and then *Hips, Thighs, Knees, Leg* (meaning below the knee), *Calves, Ankles, Foot,* and *Toes.* Also broken down in terms of *Bones, Joints, Muscles,* and *Tendons* in certain sections.

Sleep: including dreams and sleeplessness.

Chill
Fever
Perspiration
Skin: in general. Eruptions in specific locations should be looked up under Eruptions in the particular section.
Generalities: including all the physical generals, as well as most of the specific pathological descriptions in the book.

Each chapter is then broken down into major categories which describe various conditions, symptoms, pathological states, etc. Major headings under *Mind*, for example, include Anxiety, Fear, Dullness of mind, Delusion, Irritability, Restlessness (of mind as opposed to body), etc. In physical parts, such things are listed as Congestion, Eruptions, Heat, Numbness, Pain, Paralysis, Weakness, etc. These major headings are listed alphabetically within the chapter.

The next level of organization is most confusing to the beginner. From here on into more specific subdivisions, alphabetical order is not necessarily followed.

First of all, it must be understood that any given rubric describes either a particular sensation or condition, or it describes an Aggravation factor (unless Amelioration is *specified*). For each major category, specific subdescriptions are described according to a particular plan:

1. General heading
2. Time aggravations
3. Modalities which aggravate (or ameliorate, if specified)
4. Location
5. Extensions

This sequence is then repeated over again at each level of subdivision. Thus it can be seen that the entire plan of the Repertory is analogous to an inverted telescope; each level becomes more specific than previous ones, but always with the same sequence of presentation.

Let us take a specific example in order to elucidate the organization of the Repertory. Suppose a patient describes a headache, bursting in quality, located in the Forehead, worse in the morning at 10 A.M., and better while lying down. Such a symptom can be looked up in a variety of ways, becoming more and more specific at each level.

First, we open the Repertory to the Chapter *"Head."* Next, we

199

locate (alphabetically) the general heading *Pain* (which is 88 pages long!).

Immediately (on page 132) we encounter time aggravations having to do with headache in general, and there are several rubrics which might be helpful: Daytime, Morning, On Rising, On Waking, Until 10 A.M., Forenoon, and even 10 A.M. (which lists seven remedies). This is too vague for our purposes.

Next, we see modalities for headache *in general*, and note that lying, Amel. (p. 142), lists sixty-one remedies. Still too general.

We then move along to the location: Forehead. This is quite a large section, so we look further to *Head, Pain*, Forehead, 10 A.M., which lists only two remedies (p. 155). At this point, we have included the general pain, its location, one modality, and its time aggravation, so the chances that the remedy will be one of these two seem pretty good.

Finally, we recall the patient's description, "Bursting," and move further into the chapter to the section describing the specific sensations under *Pain*. "Bursting" begins on page 178, lists some time aggravations (of which we passingly note Morning), some modalities (of which we again passingly glance at Lying Down Amel.), and finally forehead. Under Forehead, there is only one remedy listed for 10 A.M., and also only one listed under Lying, While. Fortunately, they are the same remedy, which increases our confidence that it may be the remedy needed by this patient. So, the rubric which covers *all* the information given by the patient is found on page 179: *Head, Pain*, Bursting, Forehead, at 10 A.M. and also Lying, While. For this *particular* symptom, then, we would strongly consider Gelsemium.

Now, this sounds like a very cut-and-dried process, but in actual practice it is much more complex. It is quite unusual that a remedy will run through so many rubrics at all steps along the line. As we encounter smaller and smaller rubrics, we pay more attention to the remedies contained therein. But we must also be constantly aware of the vagaries of the entire process. Many questions are always kept in mind: How accurate is the patient's description of "Bursting"? Could this possibly be better described by "Pressing," "Lancinating," "Shooting," "Stitching," or "Tearing"? Is it really in the forehead, or might it be more in the temples, or even above the eyes, behind the eyes, or in the face? How reliable is the 10 A.M. aggravation? Should we use Morning, On Rising, or On Waking?

Also, we must always keep in mind the uncertainties about the

Repertory itself. When we get to the smaller rubrics, we must continually be wondering: Did Kent include *all* the possible remedies? Are there newer remedies whose provings might possibly include this symptom? Are there *old* remedies which might include this symptom, but which haven't yet been recorded?

It is because of all these uncertainties that we keep a careful eye open for all the rubrics along the way to the final one which includes all the characteristics given by the patient. In the above example, we would give strong consideration to Gelsemium because it was included in most of the rubrics along the way (although not *all*).

This painstaking process is continued for *every* symptom of importance given by the patient. It requires a great deal of study and reflection. Gelsemium may appear very strong for this symptom, but it may not show up at all for some other symptoms given by the same patient. It is at this point that skill, experience, judgment, and a very good knowledge of *materia medica* come into play.

It is all of these uncertainties which render routine computerized prescribing ineffective. The original case must be accurately and carefully taken; the totality of symptoms must then be listed correctly and with proper emphasis according to intensity, peculiarity, and mental/physical generality; and finally the actual selection of rubrics must be correctly made.

Once again, it must always be remembered that repertorization is merely a clue, a hint. It is designed merely to get us "in the ballpark." In the last analysis, the results of repertorization must be forgotten while the homeopath's full attention is placed upon a study of *materia medicas*. The goal, after all, is to match the "essence" and totality of the patient's symptoms with that of the remedy. The remedy is best described in the *materia medicas*, *not* in the Repertory, so we must study it meditatively and inquiringly, always trying to see whether our image of the patient matches our image of the remedy. When we finally are satisfied that the match is as perfect as it can be, we can then cautiously offer it as a prescription.

Chapter 14

Case Analysis and First Prescription

THUS FAR, we have discussed the process of case-taking and the general principles involved in grading symptoms and their listing according to homeopathic importance. We have also considered in a general way the organization of the Repertory and how an individual symptom can be studied in it. Now we are in a position to go into more depth about how a case is analyzed, and also how the first remedy is chosen.

Throughout this narrative, it will often seem that the analysis of a case and the choice of remedy are routine or mathematical judgments based upon concrete rules. This *seems* to be true because of the necessary difficulties of trying to translate a very complex process into language which is clear and understandable. The laws and principles involved in choosing a remedy, as described in Section 1, are definite and verifiable. However, their application to each individual case is a complex matter; the judgments involved result from a fusion between art and science. The reader should not get the idea that this process can be accomplished by thoughtless or computerized routines. Nor should the conclusion be drawn that prescriptions made by advanced prescribers are made somehow by psychic intuition or magical processes. There *is* a definite process involved which is soundly based upon solid laws and principles and yet which is also artistic in individual application. The homeopath uses a wide spectrum of

202

information from the patient, plus a broad knowledge of homeopathic principles and Materia Medica, and then fuses all of this into a "gestalt" understanding upon which the prescription is based.

This process requires a great deal of mental effort, a highly penetrating insight into the individual patient, and a massive amount of studying. Because of this, it can be expected that few will have the necessary motivation and patience to apply such a standard of homeopathy. There will always be a tendency on the part of prescribers to attempt shortcuts, to find "keynotes" which can be used in a routine manner, and to develop computer methods which can reduce the time and energy demanded of the homeopath in arriving at a correct prescription. Thus far, however, such attempts have in the long run yielded disappointing results which can only damage the public image of homeopathy. Very early in the career of any homeopath, a decision must be made as to whether strict and demanding standards are going to be applied—or not. Those who attempt shortcuts will obtain some results, but will be more and more frustrated by the confusion created by incomplete prescriptions. Those who, on the other hand, apply themselves to learning and applying the highest standards will discover a steadily increasing rate of success, and moreover they will find themselves truly *knowing* what is happening in each case. A career dedicated to such standards is indeed highly satisfying, not only for the patients but for the homeopath as well.

Practical questions frequently arise in the minds of beginning prescribers: "Can I make a living while applying such standards?" "Since it requires so much time with each patient, how can I possibly see enough patients to make a living?" It is true that each case takes a long time, and therefore the patient is charged a relatively high fee compared to what, say, an allopath might charge. However, it must be remembered that the results in homeopathy are far better than those in allopathy. Patients perceive this fact and are willing to pay for results. In the long run, homeopathic patients spend far less for their medical care than do allopathic patients, because as their health improves, the visits are spaced farther and farther apart, the medication is far less costly, and the need for laboratory tests and hospitalization is drastically reduced. Once a homeopath has mastered the highest standard of prescribing and is demonstrating reliable and consistent results, he or she can make an excellent living and be assured of a busy practice.

Initial Prognostic Evaluation

During the initial interview, one of the most crucial decisions which must be made regards the actual seriousness of the case. In the course of a day, a homeopath sees a variety of types of patients. Two patients may come to the office complaining of similar symptoms—say, stiffness of the knees. One patient with this complaint, after having the complete case taken, is found to be relatively unaffected on other levels in the totality. The patient is living a full and creative life, quite unencumbered by any problems except this occasional stiffness of the knees. The past history of the case is negligible, and all the parents lived to old age without difficulties and died quickly without prolonged illness. This person can readily be judged quite healthy, and the homeopath may be assured that such a case is likely to proceed smoothly and quickly to a complete recovery.

On the other hand, another patient may present exactly the same complaint, but the interview reveals an entirely different picture. Although the patient has learned to live with them, it turns out that there have been many anxieties, low self-esteem, periodic depressions, and a progressive process of introversion spanning a period of twenty years. As the patient talks, it becomes clear that his ability to express his inner emotions is greatly obstructed. He claims that he has enough energy to live his daily life, but further questioning reveals that he purposely limits his activities because of a lack of stamina and a need for an afternoon nap every day. In the past history it becomes clear that the patient was very sensitive as a child and then suffered a variety of severe disappointments. Over the years, everything became stressful: meeting new people, applying for a job, contemplating a move from one apartment to another—all have been felt as major stresses from which the patient requires days for full recovery. The family history reveals a strong history of cancer and diabetes, and a few relatives had been institutionalized for mental disorders. To a homeopath, such a case is very quickly recognized to have a poor prognosis. Even the best laboratory examinations might reveal merely "osteoarthritis." Yet the homeopath knows that within a matter of years, such a patient is likely to develop a serious pathological ailment; even good homeopathic treatment will be fraught with difficulties. In such a case, a partial prescription, or one which is timed incorrectly, may create such havoc that later prescriptions become almost impossible to discern.

The patient looks to the homeopath not only for a prescription, but also for information as to what to expect, whether the condition is curable, how long it will take, etc. If expectations are falsely raised so that the patient looks forward to dramatic relief within a few months, later stages of expectable problems experienced on the way toward cure may become profoundly disappointing. In such a circumstance, the patient may become discouraged enough to abandon homeopathy altogether.

Therefore, it is important to begin the study of a case with a judgment as to its seriousness. In the first example presented above, the homeopath may be confident that good prescribing will result in rapid and lasting relief of symptoms. In the second example, however, the prognosis is much more guarded; the patient must not be misled into believing that progress will be quick or easy. The patient should be taught to expect some difficulties, to learn patience, and to respect the necessity of conforming strictly to the laws of cure. Such a case will present many problems during the process of cure, and indeed the ultimate result may not be as complete as can be expected in the first example.

How exactly can a homeopath arrive at such a prognostic judgment? Basically, the following factors tend to signal an adverse prognosis:

1. *A limited degree of freedom of expression in life.* Even though a patient's original complaints are relatively minor, if the overall ability to live a happy and creative life are restricted, there are likely to be strong predispositions to chronic disease. Creative and selfless people, in general, can be expected to have good prognoses. People who have limited their horizons, who have purposely protected themselves from stress, or who isolate themselves from relationships with other people—such people carry a relatively less favorable prognosis.

Often, a homeopath can spot such tendencies from the earliest moments in the interview. Observation of the degree of openness of expression, the willingness to discuss sensitive subjects, the posture of the patient, the ability to make human contact with the interviewer—all of these are clues. In addition, simple clinical observations offer useful hints—color and texture of the skin, general muscle tone, clearness in the eyes, condition of the tongue, the sheen of the hair, etc.

2. *The center of gravity of symptoms.* If the center of gravity is mostly on the mental or emotional levels, a relatively poor prognosis can be expected; such patients commonly move toward cure

only slowly and with much difficulty. On the other hand, people with very few limitations on the mental or emotional spheres and with problems restricted to the physical plane can be expected to recover more quickly and more easily. The deeper the center of gravity, the worse the prognosis.

3. The degree of *hypersensitivity* to stimuli. People who are sensitive to every change in the environment, who are overly affected by suffering and violence, who react strongly to slight ridicule or rejection, who cannot tolerate confrontation, who must constantly watch the food they eat, who catch a cold very easily, etc.—such patients are more likely to have a poor prognosis. Their systems are unable to maintain a stable equilibrium, and the defense mechanism must be brought constantly into play in order to restore balance.

4. *The past history and the family history.* Patients with a history of deep and serious diseases, or who have had a great deal of suppressive therapy are more likely to encounter problems on the way to cure. Also, patients arising out of families with many deep miasmatic influences—i.e., deaths at early ages from serious pathological changes, relatives with chronic debilitating diseases, severe mental disturbances in the family, etc.—can be expected to have more difficulty during the course of treatment.

If any of the above factors are observed in a given patient, the index of suspicion should be raised immediately. Even one such factor should be taken as a clue to potential difficulty, and further questioning must be carefully directed to comprehend the depth of disease in the patient. Occasionally, a patient will exhibit only one of the above factors without carrying a strongly adverse prognosis. Usually, however, if one of these factors is present, the others tend to be there as well. Patients with all four aspects, no matter how minor the presenting complaint, should raise a "red flag" in the mind of the homeopath. In such cases, the minor complaint may be the "tip of the iceberg," and much time and energy will be required to bring such a patient to a reasonable degree of health.

Case Analysis for the Beginner

The next task in studying an initial case is to find the correct remedy, the *simillimum*. To the beginner with only a limited knowledge of *materia medica*, this decision can be very difficult, especially in chronic cases. Nevertheless, it must be emphasized that the choice of the initial remedy is the most crucial decision made in homeopathy. No shortcuts should be taken, and any judgments must be made with great circumspection. The first remedy is the one which opens up the case, which brings out the true healing potential of the defense mechanism, and which sets the case either in a direction toward greater order or toward confusion and disorder. Often, because the initial case has not yet been spoiled by previous incorrect prescribing, the choice of initial remedy is an *easier* decision than choosing later remedies; even so, it must be remembered that it is the most important prescription of all.

Occasionally (not often), the initial case is very obvious. The patient presents with a few simple complaints, the homeopathic image clearly fits a particular remedy, a few peculiar symptoms confirm that remedy, and no symptoms contraindicate it. Such a situation is obvious, and the prescriber can give the remedy with confidence. Even relatively inexperienced prescribers will see dramatic results when the initial image is clear and obvious. It is then very important to wait for a long time before either repeating the remedy or giving another one.

The more common circumstance, however, is a mixture of symptom pictures. A patient, for example, may present a highly characteristic mental symptom of Pulsatilla, and the prescriber naturally tends to believe that Pulsatilla will be the remedy. Upon further inquiry however, it turns out that virtually no other symptoms confirm Pulsatilla, and furthermore the patient is very chilly and desires fat (two symptoms which directly go against Pulsatilla). In such a circumstance, the homeopath must definitely not yield to the temptation to give Pulsatilla. More thought and study need be done to find a remedy that truly covers the totality of the symptoms. Every symptom may not be covered, but a remedy will hopefully be found which clearly covers the bulk of the most important symptoms.

In the beginning, it often happens that a seemingly confusing and unrelated collection of symptoms seems to fit no remedy at all simply because of the lack of knowledge of the prescriber. Someone with greater knowledge and experience may well see the correct remedy without difficulty. But what is the beginner to do in such a circumstance?

The best procedure is to "repertorize" the case. A careful list of the patient's symptoms is made according to procedures given in Chapter 13. Great thought should be applied to the choice of the symptoms to be used in repertorization, and then care should be taken to arrange them in their true order of importance.

To begin with, the very peculiar symptoms (those showing only a few remedies in the Repertory) should be excluded from the formal repertorization.

Then, beginning with the symptom at the top of the list, the homeopath writes on a sheet of paper every remedy listed in the corresponding rubric, including the correct grading of each remedy. This is done for each of the significant symptoms in the totality. *Every* remedy is included so as to reduce the chances of missing the true one (assuming that correct rubrics are chosen). Finally, notations are made of every remedy which "runs through" all of the rubrics.

In the ideal circumstance, such a repertorization will yield only one medicine running through all of the rubrics. This remedy is then carefully studied in the *materia medica*. If the "essence" of the remedy seems to fit the "essence" of the patient, and if the bulk of the symptoms are covered, then the remedy can be given with confidence.

This ideal is very rarely realized in actual practice, however. Usually, three or four drugs run through the rubrics, but only one must be chosen. Rubrics covering the peculiar symptoms are then consulted, and those remedies which have come through the full repertorization and are also seen in the peculiar rubrics are studied first. If the peculiar symptoms do not confirm any of the medicines from the repertorization, then all three or four drugs are carefully studied in the *materia medicas* to find the one most completely matching the totality of the patient.

Never should a remedy be given simply because it scores highest on repertorization. Even a remedy scoring much higher than the others should be rejected if its description in the *materia medicas* does not fit well with the patient. As mentioned before, repertorization is merely a clue; it is not a final answer.

Some homeopaths have developed "repertory sheets" which enable a numerical tabulation of remedies according to symptom. These sheets are handy to use, but they are not recommended for the beginner. Part of the purpose of studying a case in the early years is to gain a broader understanding of homeopathy and of medicines. The use of "repertory sheets" tends to prevent one from really thinking about each remedy in relation to the patient. The process of writing out each rubric with all drugs that can produce it, although tedious, can be a helpful way of learning the comparative value of remedies. As more and more medicines are learned, this method enables the prescriber to anticipate whether a particular symptom will be found in the proving of a particular drug. The process of actually writing out the rubric then provides feedback to the prescriber's "guess." This *is* a tedious process, but it nevertheless should not be given to assistants or secretaries, because a major part of its purpose is to add to the knowledge of the homeopath.

Attention should be paid to "small" remedies which run through a few rubrics in a repertorization, even though their grade was "1" all the way through. "Small" remedies are those whose provings are as yet incomplete, and therefore the number of symptoms listed for them is small. If such a medicine runs all the way through the repertorization, this can be an important sign. It should be carefully studied in as many *materia medicas* as possible. It may not cover the entire case, simply because the provings are incomplete, but enough of the image may be present to enable the prescriber to give it. Such a judgment is, of course, quite delicate and requires some experience, but it should be considered.

Very often, it will be found that a particular remedy runs through all rubrics except, say, the third and the fifth (as listed in order of importance); the first and most important symptoms are covered, as well as some lesser symptoms, but a few in the middle are not. If the rest of the repertorization has not produced an obvious solution, such a remedy should also be considered. It should be compared with any peculiar symptoms, and then carefully studied in the *materia medicas*. Since there are many uncertainties involved in case-taking, in the listing and grading of symptoms, and also in the recording of provings into the Repertory, it is frequently found that the *simillimum* will not cover all the important symptoms in a case. In such a circumstance, careful questioning about the missing symptoms should be made on follow-up visits to ascertain whether they are cured as part of a cure of the whole patient; if so, and if confirmed in other patients, that remedy may be added to the rubric as having produced a "cured symptom."

Using this tedious and painstaking procedure, the homeopath will steadily add to his or her knowledge of *materia medica*. After 10 years or so of practice, the homeopath will evolve to the point where the label "beginner" is no longer appropriate. As more and more experience is gained, the process of repertorization may be streamlined a bit by doing an "elimination" procedure. This modification should be undertaken only after the homeopath has gained an extensive knowledge of *materia medica*, because it distinctly reduces the opportunity to consider all possible remedies.

"Elimination" repertorization is done by first constructing a *very* carefully considered list of major symptoms. The most characteristic symptoms are pulled out and arranged according to their importance. This must be done with extreme care, taking into account a variety of factors: the severity of the symptom, its hierarchical level, how strongly it represents the essential pathology of the patient, its timing in relation to the evolution of the current pathology, etc.

The first symptom in such a list is then written down, and all remedies shown in that rubric are written on a sheet of paper, including the grading of each remedy. The second symptom is then written down, but this time only those medicines contained in the second rubric *as well as* in the first are written down. Drugs which are not present in the first rubric, but which are in the second, are eliminated. Next, the third symptom is noted down, and only those remedies included in it as well as in the previous rubrics are recorded. Finally, at the end of this process, only a small number of remedies should remain after the full elimination has been completed. These remedies are then thoughtfully studied in the *materia medicas*.

This method will appeal to everyone right from the beginning because it saves a lot of tedious labor. However, it is a risky procedure because the original listing of symptoms is very critical. For example, if a symptom is listed first but should be listed in third place, the chances are very good that the true *simillimum* will be eliminated from the analysis. The patient would consequently receive an incorrect remedy at the very outset of the case. Only a homeopath with a quite good knowledge of *materia medica* could spot such a mistake in time to prevent it.

Case Analysis for Advanced Prescribers

As experience is acquired, gradually less reliance is placed upon a formal repertorization. Possessing an extensive knowledge of remedies, the homeopath may have a very strong impression of the correct remedy by the end of the case-taking. Only a quick glance to certain rubrics in the Repertory will then suffice to confirm or deny this impression. In this instance, the homeopath may use a mere "finger" repertorization, which is my term for the process of inserting fingers into appropriate places in the Repertory, and then looking back and forth to perform the elimination procedure.

To a beginner observing an advanced prescriber, this process would seem easy indeed. Nevertheless, what seems so simple is in reality highly sophisticated. The same painstaking procedure occurs in the mind of the advanced prescriber as has been described for the beginner, but an advanced homeopath's grasp of the rubrics is so complete that remedies do not have to be physically written down. In the mind of the advanced prescriber, the pertinent rubrics are virtually memorized from long experience of writing them out time and again, so that repertorization is mostly done in the homeopath's head. Such prescribers can accurately quote, remedy for remedy, the contents of all of the most important rubrics.

An advanced prescriber has such a deep grasp of remedy "essences" that it is possible to match directly and immediately the essence of the patient to the essence of the remedy. If the essence is clearly and unequivocally seen, then only a few confirmatory symptoms are needed to select the remedy. Of course, the full case must be taken anyway, in order to be sure that no contra-indicating symptoms are present. Nevertheless, in a case which matches the "essence" of the remedy so closely, the process of case analysis will appear to be extremely rapid in the hands of an advanced prescriber.

If the essence of a remedy is perceived in the patient and a few other symptoms confirm it, then no further thought need be given to the prescription. The situation becomes more complex when there are one or two symptoms which strongly go against the remedy. Then the homeopath must go all the way back to the beginning and reconsider the entire case. In this circumstance, even the advanced homeopath will spend as much time and care selecting the remedy as the beginner. As a matter of fact, the procedure for selecting a remedy in such a case is essentially the same as would be true for the beginner. The entire totality is considered carefully, all uncertainties are taken into account, the appropriate rubrics in the Repertory are reviewed, and finally particular attention is paid to the peculiar symptoms. Great thought is put into the case; perhaps a somewhat compromise judgment is

211

made. Nevertheless, the final prescription will match as closely as possible the totality of symptoms of the patient with the totality of manifestations of the remedy.

In such complex cases, it may be necessary to "throw out" even important mental or general symptoms and to rely on seemingly less significant but more peculiar symptoms. Precisely how this is done cannot be described adequately in a book. Every case is so unique that it would be impossible to generalize about such judgments. They come from experience, and to a great extent they can only be learned in a supervised setting. Such judgments belong to the realm of art rather than science, even though there are always very cogent reasons for them.

Frequently, cases are encountered in which there are many common symptoms but only two peculiar symptoms. Acquiring a distinctive totality of symptoms is impossible. Repertorization is done, but because the symptoms are common, a large number of remedies come up which inevitably are those most widely proven—remedies which we call "polychrests." Such analysis and repertorization have little chance of producing the correct remedy. In this situation, it is permissible to focus solely on the peculiar symptoms—even disregarding the repertorization altogether. The remedy is selected from the rubrics describing the peculiar symptoms, and often the prescription will tend to be a rather unusual remedy. As always, careful study of the *materia medicas* must be made before deciding upon such a selection.

Occasionally, a case is encountered in which the chronic state arose very dramatically out of a powerful exciting cause. For example, a patient might be seen whose miasmatic background is quite insignificant but whose entire spectrum of, say, neurological complaints, dates from a severe head injury received in an auto accident. If, upon taking the case, one or two peculiar symptoms fitting Arnica or Natrum sulphuricum (noted for effects from head injuries) are found, then the prescription can be based solely upon the causative factor (confirmed by one or two peculiar symptoms). In this unusual circumstance, symptoms elicited during the rest of the case-taking are ignored for the moment, although they may become significant for later prescriptions.

As one can readily see, the selection of a remedy is a complex process. Many factors must be taken into account, balanced against each other, accepted in some instances, and rejected in others. The uncertainties involved underscore strongly the necessity for having a well-taken case in the first place. The principles

212

described, and particularly the exceptions to the "rules," are valid only if information derived from the original case is reliable. If the original case is sketchy, or misleading, or incorrect, then all of the delicate judgments later made while studying it are likely to be wrong. A correct homeopathic prescription depends upon a correctly taken case, correct information from provings, correct preparation of the Repertory, and finally correct analysis of the case.

It can also be readily understood that "keynote" prescribing can occasionally produce successful results. Sometimes the most careful and detailed study of a case by an experienced prescriber will arrive at the same remedy which a "keynote" prescriber would have chosen in a matter of minutes. In such an instance, the careful prescriber may seem foolish or even ignorant. However, "keynote" prescribing does not produce *reliable* and *consistent* results. Correct remedies may be selected here and there, but not in virtually every case—which *is* possible by strict application of deeply understood homeopathic principles.

Selection of Potency

Once a remedy is selected, the next decision facing the prescriber is the choice of potency. For this, there are no set rules, and experience and observation play a very large role. In this section, some general guidelines will be presented, but it must be fully understood that they are not designed to be adopted as "rules."

There is a tendency, particularly among beginning prescribers, to pay a lot of attention to potency selection. Strangely enough, it is more common for a homeopathic instructor to be asked why a particular potency is selected in a given case than why a particular remedy is selected. In actual fact, potency selection is secondary in importance to remedy selection. The Law of Similars is the primary law of cure, and the process of potentization is merely an accessory factor. If the correct remedy is selected, then it will act curatively in any potency, even though a correct potency will act more gently for the comfort of the patient; conversely, an *incorrect* remedy can be either inactive or disruptive to a case, regardless of what potency is given.

Proper guidelines for selection of potency are difficult to define, because in any given case it is impossible to say what would have happened if a different potency had been given. Suppose a patient is seen with arthritis, asthma, and anxiety about health;

Arsenicum is given in a 30th potency, and a lasting cure occurs over a period of six months. One might conjecture that a 10M potency would have produced a cure in three months. This, however, cannot be proven because one cannot go back and give the 10M in order to see! In addition, one cannot really compare two cases which *seem* similar and then give two different potencies; no two cases are ever exactly alike, so one case cannot legitimately be compared to another. The only circumstance where such comparisons have some validity is during a virulent epidemic in which many patients require the same medicine; indeed, it is in these circumstance that the effectiveness of higher potencies can be convincingly demonstrated, but this experience cannot necessarily be transferred to chronic cases. Chronic cases involve a wide variety of factors, so any guidelines for potency selection in chronic diseases can only be considered general impressions.

There are certain types of cases in which relatively low potencies should be used—at least initially. Patients who have weak constitutions, old people, or very hypersensitive people should initially be given potencies ranging, roughly, from 12× to 200. The reason for this is that higher potencies can overstimulate weakened defense mechanisms, resulting in unnecessarily powerful aggravations (aggravations will be discussed in the next chapter). This principle particularly applies to patients known to have specific pathology on the physical level—i.e., arteriosclerosis, cancer, coronary artery disease. When pathology has reached an advanced stage on the physical level, the constitution has likewise been relatively weakened, and administration of even the correct remedy in high potency can lead to severe sufferings. Thus in general it can be said that the more severe the state of physical pathology, the lower the potency that should be used for the initial prescription.

If a 12× potency is decided upon, it can be given frequently over a period of time, as long as careful instructions are given to discontinue it if any *dramatic* aggravation or amelioration of symptoms occurs. Amongst the patients weak enough to require a 12× potency, those with relatively greater vitality may repeat the doses three times daily for 30 days. If the patient's vitality is greatly weakened, however, this recommendation might be reduced to once daily for 20 days.

For example, suppose we have a patient who is an old man with a very enlarged prostate, which we suspect might involve cancer. If the patient has enough vitality to go about his daily activities to a reasonable degree, then a 12× might be prescribed three times daily for 30 days, with instructions to discontinue it if any dramatic change occurs for "better *or* for worse." On the other hand, an old man with an enlarged prostate who is so weakened that he spends most of his time in bed would be given a 12× (or sometimes even a 6×) potency only daily for about 20 days, along with the same instructions for discontinuation in the event of significant change.

Oversensitive patients present a unique problem for potency selection. These are patients who are excessively "nervous," reactive to all physical and emotional stimuli, usually lean and quick in their movements, restless, sensitive to odors and noise and light, and frequently suffering strongly from exposure to chemicals in the environment or in food. Such people are very reactive both to low potencies (on the physical level) and high potencies (on the electrodynamic level). Consequently, it is better to restrict initial prescriptions to 30 or 200 in such patients; depending upon their reaction, later potencies might go higher or lower. But, initially at least, 30 or 200 are the best elections for oversensitive patients.

Children who are suffering from *severe* problems should generally be given low potencies. An infant with a severe eczema or psoriasis is likely to have a severe aggravation if given a high potency. Consequently, such cases might be given just a few doses (say, daily) of a 12x, or just one dose of a 30 or 200.

Generally, cases with known malignancy should not initially be given potencies above 200. If a case is merely *suspected* to have a malignant or premalignant condition, the initial prescription should not be higher than 1M. Again, such potency restriction is in order to avoid unnecessarily powerful physical aggravations, which require considerable experience to manage.

If a case seems relatively curable and free of physical pathology, higher initial potencies may be tried, ranging from 30 to CM. The primary guiding principle here is the degree of *certainty* which the homeopath has about the remedy. If the medicine seems very obvious and covers the case very well, a very high potency may be given in a person with a curable system. If the remedy is not so clear, it is better to begin with a potency closer to 30.

For example, suppose a 30-year-old woman consults you complaining of a skin eruption on the hands of three-year duration. As you take the case, you discover that she has had very few other problems, and that she is quite free in her life-expression. She is quite creative, she enjoys her work, she has enjoyed traveling in various cultures, she has deep friendships, and she is not obstructed in the sexual sphere. The homeopathic information leads to a very clear picture of Pulsatilla, and your observation of the patient confirms this impression. In such a case, you could easily prescribe Pulsatilla 50M or even CM with confidence.

On the other hand, another young person comes to you with a similar complaint, but you cannot decide whether she needs Pulsatilla or Sulphur. You finally decide upon Pulsatilla after many hours of careful study; in this instance, you would tend to give only a 30 or a 200 for the initial prescription because of the lack of clarity.

In still another case with a skin eruption, you may see clearly that Pulsatilla is indicated. Yet the patient reports that she is able to keep her skin eruption under control by using cortisone ointment "only" twice a week. Further, you observe that there are other weaknesses of the organism—a weak vitality, the patient is easily tired, easily affected by chemicals in the environment. In this type of case, you would not give a potency higher than 200; otherwise, you may witness an unnecessarily prolonged aggravation.

It is sometimes said that high potencies are for cases in whom the center of gravity is on the mental level, whereas lower potencies are reserved for cases centered on the physical plane. This point of view is false. It is true that mental symptoms are the most important in selecting a medicine; if they give a clear and obvious indication for a remedy, even though the physical symptoms may not match so perfectly, then a high potency can be given—because there is a high degree of certainty about the remedy, and *not* because it is a mental case. Another case with many mental symptoms which do not fit clearly into any particular remedy will be given a lower potency because the remedy is not clear.

Another mistaken idea is that no harm can be done if a beginning prescriber restricts potencies to below 30. As previously mentioned, *any* potency can have profound actions depending upon the similarity of the medicine to the patient. If the remedy is the *simillimum*, even a crude dose or a very low potency can have profound effect; indeed, if it is originally a poisonous substance and it closely matches the resonant frequency of an oversensitive patient, a lower potency can produce a severe and dangerous aggravation.

216

There are a few remedies which one should be cautious about giving high potencies. Medicines such as Lachesis, Aurum, and deep-acting nosodes (especially Medorrhinum) have strong tendencies toward physical pathology. For this reason, they should usually be restricted to lower potencies (30 or 200) unless the individual case is demonstrated to be quite free of physical pathology.

Finally, a few guidelines should be given for prescribing in acute cases. In general, the same principles apply, but repetition may have to be more frequent if the remedy action is quickly exhausted. In children with acute ailments (because their defense mechanisms are quite strong), it is best not to give potencies lower than 200; thus 200 to CM potencies can be given, depending upon the certainty of the medicine for the acute ailment. If the patient is elderly, chronically weakened, or even if severely weakened by the acute ailment (for example, if it has developed into a severe pneumonia), a 200 potency would be preferable for the initial prescription, even if the remedy is quite obvious.

Even in acute ailments, one dose of the remedy should be given, and then the effect observed. If a lower potency has been given, it is possible that its effect will be exhausted in a matter of a few hours, in which case another dose should be given. This should not be done routinely, however; the case should be re-taken to be certain that a different remedy is not needed. It is common practice in some homeopathic circles to routinely prescribe an automatic program of repetitions in acute cases (say, one dose every hour for six doses). Although such a practice probably does little harm, it is also usually unnecessary. If the remedy is clear and a high potency can be given, one dose usually will suffice; even if a repetition is needed, the case should be re-taken to determine if a new prescription is necessary.

Single Remedy

One of the most fundamental principles of homeopathy is that of prescribing only one remedy at a time. This is such an obvious principle that it applies to every healing practice.

If more than one remedy (or therapeutic technique) is prescribed, any beneficial or adverse effects cannot possibly be evaluated with accuracy. There can be no way to decide which of the components of a combination has acted. In addition, no one can possibly predict the interactions which might occur between a combination of therapeutic influences. If a particular medicine acts in a particular manner when given singly, who can say what it might do after being altered in an unpredictable way by a combination?

Suppose a patient is given a combination of six different homeopathic remedies, and a definite deterioration ensues. What is going on? Is some kind of complex aggravation occurring? Has one remedy produced a healing crisis while another is antidoting any previous progress which might have been made? Is one remedy acting within a few days, while another is acting after a week? Is the patient unusually sensitive to one particular substance? And if so, which substance is it? If the aggravation is judged to be truly serious, how does one go about finding the next remedy that will save the patient?

Conversely, suppose a patient is given a combination of six remedies, and definite improvement occurs over a period of three months. Which medicine produced the improvement? If the improvement proves to be only temporary, how might a related follow-up remedy be chosen? Suppose the active remedy was given in a potency too low for permanent cure, how would one then decide which remedy to give in a higher potency?

There are even further questions. If remedies are proven in the context of separate, carefully-conducted provings, what would happen if they are combined? Would the resulting action be merely a mixture of the separate provings, a "sum of the parts"? Or would the result be a drastically different symptom picture? No provings have ever been conducted on combination remedies, so how can anyone predict what set of symptoms such combinations could cure?

The practice of giving combinations of remedies obviously violates all of the fundamental laws of homeopathy—and common sense as well. Nevertheless, it is common practice in some parts of the world. Some homeopaths take a case, cannot see a medicine covering the totality of symptoms, and so they create a combination of medicines, each of which (according to their estimation) covers a fragment of the case. To make matters worse, it is common practice in such circles to mix potency levels as well, and even to give certain remedies at one time of day and others at other times of day. As the reader of this book now knows very well, the process of homeopathy is to find the remedy with the vibrational frequency most closely matching the resonant frequency of the defense mechanism of the patient. Combination prescribing, in this context, would be analogous to trying to create harmony by tuning six different radios to separate stations simultaneously in the hopes of creating a symphony.

Such practice can only create complete chaos, and indeed some of the most pitiable cases in homeopathic practice are those who have undergone years of such chaotic treatment. The defense mechanism of such patients is so disturbed that it is often completely impossible to restore their health to even the level prior to such prescribing, let alone bring about a cure.

For a conscientious and knowledgeable homeopath, combination prescribing can only be forefully and vociferously deplored. Even the attitude, "Well, we have our way and they have theirs," is insufficient, because such chaotic prescribing can only contribute to the ruination of the reputation of homeopathy. If one is conscientiously attempting to utilize a therapy based on energies beyond ordinary perception, then one must necessarily conform very strictly to the specific and refined laws governing the use of such energies.

Chapter 15

The Follow-Up Interview

IT IS COMMON in homeopathic prescribing to focus attention almost solely on the original symptom complex and the finding of the first remedy. Although it is true that the most important prescription in any given case is the initial one, it must be understood that it is equally important to be able to *interpret* correctly the patient's response to the original remedy. It seems easier for the homeopath to approach the follow-up visit as a simple matter of deciding whether the patient has or has not responded to the initial prescription. If the patient expresses satisfaction, the prescriber breathes a sigh of relief and confidently recommends the most common of all homeopathic prescriptions—"Wait." If, on the other hand, the patient does not seem satisfied and little seems to have happened, then the homeopath settles down to the task of trying to decide upon a better prescription.

Actually, the true situation is much more complex than this, and decisions made during follow-up visits cannot be made so simplistically or casually. Although the first prescription is the most *important* decision made in homeopathy, the follow-up prescription is very likely the most *difficult* prescription. In the first interview the goal is relatively simple: to analyze the case in such a way as to arrive at the correct remedy. Follow-up interviews, however, involve much more complex judgments. Is the patient *truly* better? Is the remedy producing the desired response, or has it missed, or produced only a partial effect? Now that the response to the initial prescription is known, what is the true prognosis of the patient? Should a remedy be given at this point, or should the potency be changed? Or is this the time to wait for further developments? Perhaps it is clear that the patient has not responded properly to the original remedy; is the current remedy image clear enough to make another prescription? Or should more time pass to allow the true image to emerge?

These are but a few of the dilemmas confronting the homeopath during follow-up visits. Indeed, it can be said that the follow-up visit, even more than the initial interview, demands more knowledge, more sensitivity, and more judgment on the part of the homeopath. It is during the follow-up visits that the entire range of knowledge of homeopathy is brought to bear. The principles involved in the decisions made during these visits are verifiable and scientific in the truest sense, yet, again, their application demands such complexity in each individual case that it can only be considered an art.

It is a natural tendency for homeopathic prescribers to focus attention primarily upon finding the remedy. In conferences, study groups, and consultations with other homeopaths the primary topic is generally whether this remedy or that remedy should be prescribed. This is quite appropriate for the first prescription, of course, but a more important issue during follow-up visits is, "What is really happening?" A profound knowledge of homeopathic theory is required for this judgment, and it is a far from easy question to answer in many cases. It is only after an adequate answer is decided upon that the homeopath can then decide whether to wait or whether to give another remedy. If further treatment seems to be required it must be decided whether it should be the same remedy or another, and whether a change in potency is necessary.

The patient, as well, faces new challenges during the follow-up visit. Usually, during the initial interview, the patient has been impressed with the incredible amount of detail needed by the homeopath. This may lead to a tendency to focus upon details instead of the overall pattern of change. There is a strong desire to report the precise information needed, but there is also a powerful hope that the remedy is truly acting. Different patients respond to these pressures in different ways. An emotionally "closed" patient, one who takes a strongly rational view of events and reveals information only when it is dramatic and definite, will tend to be overly cautious and may mislead the homeopath into deciding that the remedy has not acted. An emotionally "open" patient may become carried away with the desire to bring good news and thereby communicate information which is overly optimistic. A hypochondriacal patient, always intent upon impressing the prescriber with the importance of his or her problems, may emphasize insignificant details, disregard symptoms which have been alleviated, and exaggerate the seriousness of new symptoms. Oversensitive patients may experience dramatic changes after taking the initial dose, only to pay inadequate attention to more long-term changes.

Thus it cannot be overemphasized that patients must provide reports which are as accurate and objective as possible. Notes may be kept by patients who are liable to forget the pattern of changes, but they should *not* be kept by detail-oriented patients who are likely to lose track of the general picture. At the same time, the homeopath must be much more cautious about responses given during follow-up interviews. As mentioned earlier, there are particular problems associated with case-taking during the initial interview; this is even more true during follow-up interviews, but the problems are quite different. The patient's responses should always be inquired into in great detail in order to determine the true pattern of changes occurring. This must be done with great care, always keeping in mind the serious disruption which can occur from an incorrect remedy, or from one which is improperly timed. Many homeopathic prescribers are quite able to select the proper remedy at the first visit, but a considerable percentage of these later ruin the initial success by interfering at the wrong time or with incorrect remedies.

Take, for example, a patient of a relatively "closed" nature who has received the correct constitutional remedy, but during the follow-up visit is as yet uncertain whether the remedy has acted. He does not want to be overly optimistic, so he reports that he has not noticed any definite change. The homeopath then re-takes the case, notes only a few changes which are readily explained by environmental factors, and decides that a new remedy must be given because no significant change has occurred. Upon re-studying the case, the original remedy still looks very good, but because it didn't seem to work, a second-choice remedy is given. On the next visit, it still appears that very little progress has been made, so still another remedy is tried. After five months of prescribing, the patient finally comments. *"You know, of all the remedies that you gave me, that first one seemed to do the most good; I remember some definite changes back then."* This is the most exasperating situation for a homeopath, because after so many medicines it may not be possible simply to repeat the original remedy; the case may have become so disrupted that the original medicine is no longer indicated, but it also may have become so confused that even the current image is difficult to discern.

The danger of misjudging the response during the second interview can be so serious that I will sometimes resort to somewhat drastic measures. If I suspect that such a "closed" patient is withholding the true story, I may say, "OK. Since there appears to have been no progress at all, I am *forced* to make another prescription. Let us hope that it will not disrupt any beneficial effect which might be occurring from the first remedy." Once the patient realizes by such a threat that later prescriptions can seriously interfere with the action of the first remedy, he or she is much more likely to try harder to describe the true situation. It is in such moments that the real picture comes out.

There are numerous examples which could be cited to demonstrate the traps into which homeopaths and patients can fall. In this chapter, I shall attempt to describe the most common ones in my own experience. To thoroughly delineate every possible response to remedies in every conceivable situation would be impossible. Such knowledge can only come from experience. Nevertheless, the examples given in this chapter are an attempt to describe the most characteristic responses, their interpretations, and the appropriate therapeutic actions.

To begin with, we must offer a clear definition of the second prescription. *The "second prescription" is the one which follows a remedy which has acted.* It is not necessarily merely the second prescription given. If no remedies have acted at all until the third prescription, then the fourth remedy is the "second prescription." An incorrect remedy which is far removed from the resonant frequency of the organism has no effect whatsoever; thus it is not taken into account in considering follow-up prescriptions. If, however, a prescription has had even a minimal effect on the patient, it is considered a "first prescription," and its follow-up must be very carefully evaluated.

This point becomes an important factor in regard to so-called *inimical* remedies. For example, it has been found in homeopathic experience that Phosphorus and Causticum can create adverse reactions if prescribed one after another. This observation, however, applies only to those cases in which the patient has *responded* to one of the two medicines. If Causticum is given and absolutely no change occurred as a result, then one need not fear to give Phos-

223

phorus as the next prescription. If, on the other hand, Causticum did seem to have some effect, the homeopath should avoid following with Phosphorus.

Time Interval for Scheduling Follow-Ups

Once the first remedy has been given, the next issue is how much time to allow before seeing the patient again. Of course, this is largely an individual matter determined by the nature of the particular case. Acute cases, and severely suffering chronic cases, are seen sooner than average patients. After the initial interview, the precise course of events can never be predicted with perfect accuracy, so whatever decision is made, it must be explained to the patient that the next appointment can be altered if there are any dramatic changes needing attention in the meantime.

In acute cases, the appropriate time for follow-up depends upon the intensity of the illness. In severely ill patients, six hours would be an appropriate time to evaluate the action of the remedy. In more routine acute cases, the best time would be 24 hours. These are the best time intervals for evaluating whether the remedy has acted at all, as well as for choosing a new remedy if the picture has changed significantly. Of course, if the remedy has produced a dramatic amelioration followed by a definite relapse, the interval may be even shorter than planned.

In chronic cases, the *ideal* interval would be two months. In this period of time, the response could be reliably evaluated in virtually every case. For most patients, however, this is too long a period to wait in case there is no response.

For practical reasons, therefore, a compromise of one month can be recommended. If there is any change, whether positive or negative, it can be detected within one month in approximately 95% of cases. If the original remedy is the correct one, a very large percentage can be expected to show an interpretable result within one month. Often, for example, a patient will report no change (or perhaps an aggravation) until 20 days after the remedy, but then a definite amelioration occurs within the last week or so. On the other hand, only a small percentage of patients are likely to show a curative response which is not visible within one month.

Of course, it sometimes happens that some change has definitely occurred after one month, but the precise meaning of the change is as yet uninterpretable. In such a case, it may be necessary to wait another 15 days or even another month in order to be very sure of the nature of the response. Nevertheless, the one month follow-up visit is never wasted, because many valuable details are gathered which can be of great help in later interpretations.

An important principle to remember always is that it is not absolutely necessary to give a remedy at every visit. Such practice is a prevalent assumption deriving from the predominant allopathic philosophy of prescribing, but it can be seriously disruptive in a homeopathic case. If the course of events or the remedy image are not sufficiently clear, then the best prescription is always "tincture of time." The defense mechanism can always be relied upon to produce the necessary image if given enough time (assuming, as well, enough knowledge on the part of the homeopath to interpret the image it is trying to produce).

There are, of course, always circumstances in which the patient must be seen sooner than one month. Particularly in patients with very serious pathological changes, the pace of the ailment may be more rapid, and the patient may even have to be seen within a few days after the initial remedy. This is the case with hospitalized patients, but for out-patients in general the tendency to evaluate cases on a day-by-day or week-by-week basis should be discouraged. Although such frequent visits may be reassuring to the patient, they place undue pressure upon the prescriber to "do something." Such pressure easily leads to prescriptions which in the long run can be disruptive to the orderly process of cure.

Format for the Follow-Up Visit

Traditionally, follow-up visits are scheduled for shorter lengths of time than are first visits. This is natural and appropriate because it takes time to develop a full understanding of the patient at the first meeting, but this should not in any sense diminish the importance of the follow-up visit in the mind of the homeopath or the patient. The attitude of the prescriber must be as careful and thorough as possible, because the actual challenges are in some ways greater during follow-up visits. Notes must be taken with the same reliability and underlining of symptoms followed as painstakingly. The common practice of listing follow-ups in terms of simple notations of "better," "worse," or "unchanged" is inadequate, because far more is involved.

To the homeopath, a follow-up visit presents a series of decisions which must be made unerringly:

1. What was the response to the first remedy (independent of the patient's subjective interpretation)? Has the medicine pro-

duced a curative response? Was it only a partial remedy, producing only unimportant changes? Was it suppressive, causing ultimately a worsening of the overall health of the patient? Or was it merely an incorrect prescription, producing no significant response?

2. Is another medicine required, or is it best to wait?

3. If another prescription is required, what is the correct remedy and potency?

With these tasks in mind, a basic format can be described which highlights the important information. Of course, such a format cannot be rigidly followed. Each case is unique, and every interview is therefore different from every other one. Nevertheless, the information which is gained can be ordered into a basic sequence:

1. How does the patient feel *in general?* Has his or her health improved, declined, or been left unchanged by the remedy? Patients usually tend to focus on specifics, especially after experiencing the unexpected amount of detail involved in the inital interview, but it is important to discern the overall impression at the outset.

2. Has the degree of *energy* been affected? Is the patient experiencing greater energy and motivation during daily existence, has it declined, or has it remained unchanged? Has there been any change in the ability of the patient to cope with the various stresses of life?

3. Has there been any change in the physical *chief complaint—* the original problem for which the homeopath was consulted? What was the pattern of its change during the month, if any?

4. What changes have occurred on the *mental* and *emotional* planes? Since these symptoms represent the core of existence of the patient, even seemingly insignificant changes on this level can signal important effects of the remedy.

5. Next, the original case should be reviewed, symptom by symptom, to determine whether changes have occurred, for better or for worse. The usual tendency during follow-up visits is to stop once an impression has been gained of the overall effect. This tendency should be resisted. All of the symptoms elicited during the initial interview should be asked about, and the resulting condition appropriately noted down and underlined.

6. Any *new symptoms* should be inquired into. Sometimes these

will be symptoms from the past, in which case their previous timing should be noted carefully. If the symptoms are truly new, all appropriate modifiers and descriptions of them should be carefully recorded.

7. The patient should always be given a chance to *elaborate* further upon previously described symptoms. After the patient has had time to reflect upon questions raised in the initial interview and once a better rapport has been established, it becomes possible to penetrate further into the "essence" of the case. This, of course, can be vitally important, so the homeopath must not allow an insistence upon any specific format to interfere with expression of such information. As enumerated here, this aspect of the follow-up interview is listed last, but in reality it could and should be elicited at any point in the interview.

During a follow-up interview, by far the most important information is gathered from the first four areas of the above format. The overall state of health, the general energy of the patient, the chief complaint, and the mental/emotional changes all provide the most important clues to evaluating the response to the first prescription. These should be clearly identified in the follow-up record, and the reliability of these symptoms must be *very* carefully evaluated by the interviewer. An error made by too readily trusting a patient's answers in these categories can lead to serious mistakes in prescribing. The remaining symptoms are accessory clues for interpreting action of the initial remedy, but they eventually provide the basis upon which further prescriptions are based.

The Homeopathic Aggravation

The issue of the homeopathic aggravation is perhaps the most controversial and most misunderstood aspect of curative prescribing. It is in this respect, perhaps, that homeopaths depart most dramatically from other therapeutic systems, and misunderstandings over this issue have created serious schisms within the homeopathic profession as well.

Since the *simillimum* for a given patient produces similar symptoms in healthy individuals, it must be expected that it will produce the same symptoms in the sick individual as well. Thus it is logical to assume that a truly curative response will be preceded by some degree of *aggravation* of symptoms. As has been de-

227

scribed at great length in Section I, the defense mechanism of a patient can only manifest its activity by means of symptoms. Our purpose in giving a homeopathic remedy is to stimulate the defense mechanism of the patient in such a way that it can finally cure the illness against which it has been struggling. In order, therefore, to produce a truly curative response, it is not only expected but *desirable* that an aggravation of symptoms be produced after administration of the correct remedy.

The homeopathic aggravation can be considered as a way in which the organism is "encouraged" by the indicated medicine to "confess," to bring to light deep-seated troubles or evil tendencies that were oppressing it before. To be completely free, an organism must be fully expressive and creative in the context of its immediate reality. When its expression is inhibited, suppressed, rendered secret, or obstructed, then we have an ill individual. During the homeopathic interview, therefore, the prescriber must to some extent draw out this "inner" expression of the defense mechanism in order to discover the precise remedy for that patient. The remedy then produces a stimulation of the defense mechanism, which creates for a time a heightened exacerbation of the symptoms which are the only manifestation of its action visible to our perception.

In this way it can readily be understood that, especially in chronic cases, homeopathic aggravations are desirable. The common practice of some homeopaths, therefore, to try to suppress aggravations is actually a process which prevents cure. Attitudes and teachings based on prescribing remedies which are unlikely to produce aggravations come from people who have understood very little of the science of homeopathy.

Homeopathic patients many times are surprised when they call their homeopath to report an initial aggravation of their symptoms, and the homeopath replies, "That is a good sign. I am pleased." Of course, homeopaths are not callous. They do not wish to inflict unnecessary suffering. Insofar as it is possible, everything is done to reduce the severity and the length of homeopathic aggravations, but always the basic laws of healing must be observed. Even though it may *appear* cruel on the part of the prescriber, anything less is actually performing a disservice to the patient, because the patient's suffering will ultimately be prolonged because of lack of cure.

In the vast majority of patients, the homeopathic aggravation cannot be considered harmful. The defense mechanism always obeys the fundamental principle of cybernetics, which states that any highly organized system will react to any stress with the *best possible* response of which it is capable at any given moment. That is why if there is a pathological symptom which can cause damage to the system, such as very high blood pressure, this dangerous symptom will be immediately ameliorated while other symptoms may be aggravated during the therapeutic crisis. This is a very important principle to keep in mind while interpreting responses to medicines.

A major circumstance in which remedy aggravations *can* be harmful is repetition of a remedy which is not well indicated. If the prescriber misinterprets the response of the patient and continues to repeat the medicine, the defense mechanism can become *over*stimulated, and eventually damage can occur. Ordinarily, this requires a truly excessive repetition, and would be likely to occur only by the most thoughtless prescribing, but it is at least a theoretical possibility.

Another circumstance in which one must be cautious about homeopathic aggravations is in serious pathological cases with severely weakened constitutional power. In such cases, actual cure *is* possible, since there is enough strength to produce an aggravation, but this requires the utmost skill and experience on the part of the homeopath to manage. It is in this circumstance that good allopathic knowledge is important to homeopathic prescribers; in such serious cases, it is necessary that the homeopath be able to determine when a case is developing serious pathological change. One must then enter quickly with the correct new medicine at the appropriate moment, which may be within even a few days of the original prescription. Such aggravations are very difficult to manage, occurring usually in hospitalized patients; it is unlikely that a beginning prescriber would be confronted with such a situation. Nevertheless, every prescriber should be aware of the possibility.

The disease cholera offers a good analogy. Most infectious diseases create a reaction on the part of the defense mechanism which manifests as high fever, malaise, muscle aches, anorexia, and various other symptoms. In cholera, the defensive reaction itself becomes severe enough to actually kill the patient; it is not the microorganism which causes death, but rather the severe diarrhea (and resulting dehydration) designed to eliminate the bacteria from the system. This is why allopathic treatment for cholera saves lives—not by giving an antibiotic, but by providing intravenous feeding to counteract fluid loss. Once the defensive reaction is ended, intravenous fluids are stopped and the patient returns to normal. In this instance, it is the overactivity of the defensive mechanism which can lead to death. The same is true of a severe homeopathic aggravation in a constitutionally weak and deeply pathological patient. If such a reaction occurs, the correct remedy given at the precisely appropriate time can enable the defense mechanism to more efficiently bring about health, but a policy of waiting unnecessarily long in regard to the pace of the case could possibly lead to pathological damage.

Such severe aggravations, however, occur only in highly unusual circumstances which are unlikely to be tackled by beginning prescribers anyway. For routine cases seen daily in the office, the homeopathic aggravation cannot do significant damage. Such responses, therefore, should not be feared or avoided but rather welcomed. Whenever possible, choosing a more comfortable potency at the outset might reduce the severity of the reaction, but a particular remedy should never be selected merely in order to prevent a homeopathic aggravation. On the contrary, an aggravation is an encouraging sign that the medicine is acting and that the patient is on the road toward cure.

Evaluation at One Month

The first situation requiring great understanding by the homeopath occurs during the one-month follow-up visit. The first and most important task is to interpret correctly what effect the first prescription has really had. As has been discussed, this is no easy task. In the first place, the reliability of the information must be correctly established. There are many dynamics within the patient which can mislead the homeopath, in addition to the usual interviewing problems which can cause the prescriber to "lead" the patient into a misinterpretation.

The next variable is the homeopathic prescription itself. Was the remedy active in its original state? Was the prescription the true *simillimum*? Was it merely close to the exact *simillimum* and therefore only partially acting? Was it too far from the *simillimum* to be of any effect? Was the remedy close enough to create a suppressive or disruptive effect? Has the remedy been antidoted by some action of the patient? There are all issues which must be correctly evaluated if the second prescription is going to further help the patient. If the evaluation is incorrect, it may well disorder the action of the first prescription.

Another variable is the state of health of the patient. During the first interview, many clues are discovered which can help the prescriber decide upon a prognosis in the case. A *true* prognosis cannot be found, however, until there has been an opportunity to evaluate the patient's response to the medicine. It is at this point that the degree of incurability of a case can be truly determined.

Throughout the history of homeopathic prescribing, clinical experience has gradually evolved verifiable interpretations of the various responses patients demonstrate after taking a remedy. Usually, homeopathic literature has focused upon the issue of finding the correct remedy in each case. However, the most astute and careful homeopathic observers gradually began to discover patterns of response to remedies which have particular meanings. Finally, these observations culminated in the rule formulated by Constantine Hering as *Hering's Law: cure proceeds from above downward, from within outward, from the most important organs to least important organs, and in the reverse order of appearance of symptoms.* To this might be added an important corollary: cure proceeds by amelioration on internal planes coupled with the appearance of a discharge or eruption of skin or mucous membranes. This elaboration of the original law does not add any new concepts, but it does make more vivid the kind of changes which occur during the process of cure.

This rule of interpretation is a valuable guideline for determining whether a remedy is acting. It simply and correctly expresses the principles described in Section I of this book. During the process of cure, the defense mechanism generates changes in vibration rate which progressively move to more and more peripheral levels of the organism. If cure is in progress, symptoms will manifest at levels which are progressively of less crucial importance to the freedom of the individual to express fullness and creativity in life. This is the concept underlying Hering's Law. It is not that there are merely four specific directions of cure; there is in reality only one direction of cure which language can only describe clearly in terms of four specific observations.

In Appendix B we consider a variety of patient responses which can occur within one month after administration of the first remedy. Their interpretation is sometimes a difficult task; much training and experience is required before a homeopath acquires enough knowledge, judgment, and skill to arrive at a correct interpretation. Nevertheless, I attempt to describe the most common examples which are seen in daily practice. Of necessity, only

231

vague terms can be used to describe a phenomenon which is actually quite specific; it is hoped that even such generalities will provide the homeopathic student with a framework within which he or she can accurately interpret patients' responses to medicines.

Chapter 16

Principles Involved
in Long-Term Management

W HEN IT COMES TO INTERPRETING long-term changes during homeopathic prescribing, individual variations from patient to
patient become so complex that the only way they can be discussed is in terms of general principles and categories. It is impossible to consider every eventuality in a textbook, but in this
chapter I hope to provide the salient principles which guide the
management of cases over a long period of time. Perhaps the
actual case examples presented in Appendix B will illustrate in
more specific ways precisely how these principles can be applied
to individual cases.

Once again, when dealing with such difficult circumstances as
presented here, the reader must be cautioned that the art of long-
term management can only be gained from supervised instruction
under an experienced and knowledgeable homeopath. Such understanding cannot be gained merely from reading books.

In this section of the book, we are considering practical application, but it must always be remembered that everything we
are discussing arises from the general laws and principles described in Section I. The first step in learning to manage cases of
varying degrees of complexity is to become well-grounded in theory. A mere knowledge of *materia medica* alone is not enough.
Knowledge of theory must be combined with knowledge of *materia medica*, plus practical clinical experience, to determine how to
respond to any given situation. It is not so much a matter of

"finding the right remedy" as it is of *being able to determine specifically and precisely what is happening with the patient at any given moment during treatment.*

We have considered in some detail how to interpret the response of the patient one month after having received a remedy. To some extent, the same principles apply to long-term management of cases. In this chapter, I will first reiterate some of the most fundamental principles guiding the management of chronic cases over time. Next, I will consider three basic categories of chronic patients and how the fundamental principles apply to each category.

Fundamental Principles

The general principles apply to all cases at all times, although to varying degrees depending upon the severity of the case. Precisely how they manifest in a particular person depends upon the strength or weakness of the defense mechanism. In a patient with a strong defense mechanism, the basic principles of evaluating the direction of cure are highlighted very clearly. When the defense mechanism is very weak and tenuous, however, the principles are not so clearly manifest, and skilled judgment and experience on the part of the homeopath become of crucial importance.

Principle No. 1: If the patient within himself feels better, do not interfere. This should be considered the "Golden Rule" of homeopathy. It should be obeyed as fully and strictly as possible if the homeopath truly desires deep and permanent results. This principle, although not infrequently ignored by prescribers for a variety of reasons, necessarily underlies all other guidelines for interpretation. One must always strive to understand how a patient is doing in these terms first, despite whatever complaints or disappointments are initially offered.

Principle No. 2: Do not give another remedy unless the symptom picture is clear. This applies both to situations when the same remedy is indicated and when a new remedy is indicated. If the remedy image is unclear following the initial remedy, it is always best to wait for a clear image whenever possible. Of course, being able to perceive the "clarity" of a remedy image depends both on knowledge and experience; a beginning prescriber may well believe that the image is clear and correct when it is not. Conversely, the image may seem confused to a beginner when it would be obvious to a more knowledgeable prescriber. Nevertheless, when consultation with a more experienced prescriber is not available, the general principle is to wait whenever the image is not yet clear.

It frequently happens that a patient goes through a phase of suffering which "appears" to need a remedy. The suffering may be quite severe, and the patient may be telephoning the prescriber daily. Nevertheless, the first step is to determine whether the suffering is *really* as severe as before the original remedy. If so, the next step is to determine whether a clear image is emerging, and whether it has stabilized. One must not be in a hurry to prescribe *while symptoms are changing.* The situation may still be in a state of transition; the remedy image may have been present for only two or three days, in which case it is entirely possible that it will eventually move on to another image. Whenever possible, one must wait until the remedy image has stabilized for at least 15 days or so, in which case one can be reasonably sure that a remedy based upon the stable image will not be disruptive and may well be beneficial.

Of course, as we shall see, there are desperate circumstances when this principle cannot be strictly followed. Despite these exceptions, every effort must be made to let the patient push the limits of endurance in order to clearly perceive the next remedy image. In the long run, observance of this principle will shorten the period of suffering—even though in the moment it may seem to be a cruel course of action.

Principle No. 3: Do not be in a hurry to prescribe if an old symptom, or complex of old symptoms (especially), is returning. If a patient admits to having experienced the same symptoms within a few months or years prior to taking the remedy as are found within the first six months after taking the remedy—the best course of action is to wait. In this instance, it is very important to have taken a very complete case. In the confusion of the moment and the desire of the patient to have the homeopath "do something" in a situation which may seem a "degeneration" to a previous condition, the patient may be reluctant to report fully the fact that the new set of symptoms is indeed a manifestation of a previous state. The prescriber must inquire very carefully into this possibility in order to be perfectly sure of the real situation.

Principle No. 4: Do not prescribe a remedy if a skin eruption or discharge appears and is accompanied by a general amelioration. In chronic cases, it frequently happens that the correct remedy is followed by a reaction producing a skin eruption or discharge. In a patient with a strong defense mechanism, this eruption or discharge may be intense but brief. In someone with a weaker defense mechanism, the eruption or discharge may be severely disturbing and prolonged. This can become quite alarming to the patient (who thinks that his or her health is seriously deteriorating), and to the homeopath who is plagued by urgent telephone calls. Nevertheless, the prescriber must not be hurried into prescribing another remedy unless the situation is beyond endurance and the next remedy image is clear.

Principle No. 5: Do not prescribe another remedy if the remaining symptoms represent only a minor disturbance to the person. This is a corollary to the first principle. To anyone having a true understanding of the basic concept of cure proceeding from more central regions to more peripheral regions of the organism, this principle is obvious. Nevertheless, many mistakes are made by prescribers who are anxious to "complete the cure."

Principle No. 6: Do not prescribe another remedy if the symptoms are clearly moving from above downwards on the body. This is another principle clear to anyone familiar with Hering's Law. It applies most obviously to symptoms on the physical body, but it is also evident in terms of the conical-envelope diagrams presented in Section I.

Application in Particular Patient Categories

Once the above principles are understood, how do they manifest in individual patients? Specifically, how can these principles be used in patients of varying degrees of constitutional weakness?

To begin with, we must establish three basic categories of chronic patients. Necessarily, these are generalizations, but they serve as useful categories.

1. Patients with only *one or two layers* of disease predisposition. These patients, of course, have the best prognosis.
2. Patients with *more than two layers* of miasmatic predisposition. These patients represent considerably greater difficulty.
3. *Incurable* patients, in which cure is a practical impossibility, and palliation is the only goal.

This classification of chronic disease cases is very important because it clarifies many confusing ideas regarding the long-term effectiveness of homeopathic treatment in different situations. It is often asked, "How effective is homeopathy in treating cancer? Or myasthenia gravis? Or diabetes?" To a homeopath, of course, these questions are basically meaningless, since our prescriptions are based upon the totality of pathological symptoms, and not upon the specific disease entity. The true answer to such questions, however, is that it depends upon the miasmatic severity of the case in the first place. If the constitution is strong, the possibility of cure is great no matter what the disease category. On the other hand, even the supposedly least serious disease categories may be incurable in patients possessing defense mechanisms which have been weakened beyond the threshold of curability.

Within the first category, any type of chronic disease may be encountered—schizophrenia, cancer, multiple sclerosis, myasthenia gravis, myopathies, diabetes mellitus, tuberculosis, etc. Nevertheless, these diseases are all curable if the patient belongs to the first category; the defense mechanism was strong until the onset of the disease. In such cases, the most astonishing and miraculous results can be witnessed. These are the cases which are most satisfying and encouraging to any homeopath, and every homeopath can recall at least a few such dramatic cures. Upon careful inquiry, such cases will be found to have parents in relatively good health, no long-term allopathic treatment which might have engrafted miasmatic influences upon the system, and few vaccinations with adverse reactions; prior to the onset of the ailment, these patients will usually be found to have lived relatively healthy and emotionally balanced lives.

Patients belonging to the second category present many more problems for the homeopath. The same disease entities may be involved—schizophrenia, cancer, neurological ailments, diabetes, etc. Therefore, the perplexed homeopath may wonder, "Why could I cure this disease in other cases and not so easily in this one?" The answer, of course, is that the miasmatic influences are much stronger. The patient's hereditary history shows many more chronic diseases, there may be a long history of allopathic treatment with powerful drugs, vaccination may have had either no apparent effect or very severe reactions, and the patient's life may have always been full of anxieties, fears, and nervousness. Any case with all of these adverse influences will inevitably be fraught with more difficulties than a patient in the first category—even when the allopathic diagnosis is identical.

It is very important for the prescriber to learn to judge the depth of the miasmatic influence in a given case. In this way, problems in management can be foreseen, and both the patient and the doctor will not be misled into a false optimism.

The same disease entities may be found in the third category of patients, of course, but in these cases the defense mechanism is so weak that the usual allopathic prognosis is indeed accurate. Even so, careful prescribing can provide very effective palliation for such cases, and it is quite possible that their useful days and months may even be extended beyond expectations.

Now, how precisely can the fundamental principles of cure be applied to each category of patients? We will begin by considering patients in the first category—those with strong defense mechanisms.

The most ideal evidence that a given patient has a strong defense mechanism is a response described by Cases I-IV (see Appendix B). Provided that the remedy was correct and nothing was done to interfere with it, the patient feels unequivocably better "inside." Cases exhibiting this response have the best prognosis, despite the pathological diagnosis. They can be expected to remain in this dramatically improved state for six months to several years, provided no chemical interferences or overwhelming stresses intervene.

If such a patient acquires an acute ailment, it can be expected to be relatively mild and self-limited. There should be no need for homeopathic treatment. Indeed, it is preferable to allow the system to handle it itself. Of course, this principle does not always apply; the patient may encounter a very powerful morbific stimulus—say, a prolonged and severe exposure to the elements, resulting in pneumonia or severe bronchitis. In this unusual instance, homeopathic prescribing will be needed, but it should be relatively easy. A patient with a strong defense mechanism, even during an acute ailment, will tend to generate a symptom picture which points clearly to the needed remedy. Only one prescription, or at the most two, will be sufficient to cure the acute illness, and the chronic state will remain in a cured state.

Patients belonging to the first category tend to remain relatively well for two to five years after the original prescription. If they do return for more treatment, it is usually for minor problems. After the first consultation, the homeopath often hears nothing from such patients for several years, and it is easy to falsely assume that their response to the medicine must have been disappointing. It is only years later that the homeopath learns that the original prescription produced a "miraculous" cure.

Occasionally, even patients belonging to the first category undergo such a severe stress that the defense mechanism is overwhelmed, and a full relapse occurs. This could occur following a very severe grief, a profoundly damaging business reversal, or a very severe physical injury. In the case of such a relapse, the homeopath must carefully re-take the case in its entirety; very likely, it will be found that the original remedy is still indicated. It should then be given in a higher potency. It is also possible that a "complementary" remedy will be indicated.

In many homeopathic circles, it is common to refer to the "constitutional remedy," as if a particular individual requires only a single remedy. This terminology can properly be applied to patients possessing strong defense mechanisms who tend to require the same remedy over a period of years, whether for minor complaints or for relapses after severe stresses. As we shall see, however, this concept does not apply as readily to other categories of chronic patients.

It is not infrequent that a patient who has responded with a dramatic curative response to the first medicine later suffers a relapse because of an antidoting influence. This might occur because of taking allopathic drugs for some minor complaint, drinking coffee, or undergoing dental treatment. After such interferences, the patient's condition may appear to be returning to a relapsed state, but it is nevertheless important to wait 15 days or so (after discontinuing the antidoting influence). Usually, the defense mechanism is strong enough to handle the disturbance on its own without further homeopathic treatment. If, however, the relapse does seem to establish itself over a significant period of time, the case should be retaken. If the same remedy is still indicated, it should be given in the same potency and *not higher*. The reason for this is that the first remedy was antidoted. Therefore, one cannot know whether the original potency was truly optimal; for this reason, one must again try the same potency level.

Skin eruptions may well occur in such patients within the first 10 days or so. If such eruptions (or discharges) are accompanied by a general amelioration of the patient, one should not administer another prescription. This is a classic example of symptoms moving to the periphery on the way toward cure, and nothing should be done to interfere with the process.

If the eruption were to occur much later, say, after six months or one year, however, another remedy should be given. Usually, either the same remedy or a complementary one will be indicated, but one must not be in a hurry to prescribe. If the image is not yet clear, allow more time to pass to become perfectly sure of the next prescription. A hasty prescription at this stage could confuse the case and delay the cure of the eruption.

A similar eventuality might occur in a patient initially displaying severe mental problems—say, depression. After the first remedy, the mental state dramatically clears up, but the patient then experiences a severe gastritis. If this occurs within several days of the first prescription, then it is very probable that it is a curative response, and it should be allowed to run its course. This would be a typical example of cure proceeding from "within outward" in a very strong constitution. If, however, the gastritis were to occur a few months or a year after the original prescription, it will most likely require a new prescription—again, most probably a repeat of the original "constitution" remedy or a complementary.

It may occur that a patient belonging to this first category will demonstrate the Hering's Law principle of amelioration proceeding from above downward. This might involve a skin eruption clearing first upon the head, then the chest, and finally the palms or feet. Or, it might be observed in an arthritis case showing an improvement first in the cervical region, moving next to the lumbar region, then involving the sciatic nerves, and finally progressing to the feet or hands. During a curative response, these progressions are most likely to occur within a period of three to six months, and they should not be interrupted by further prescribing. If, by chance, the process should "stall" for a month or more at a particular level, then one would be justified in selecting a new remedy based upon the full totality of symptoms in the moment.

To conclude the discussion about members of the first category of patients, we can reiterate that they carry the best prognosis. Their defense mechanisms are quite strong, and, despite the original pathological diagnosis, they can be expected to be relieved on all levels for a long period of time. These patients demonstrate most clearly the workings of Hering's Law, and the interpretation of their responses should be relatively easy even for the beginning prescriber. They are like prisoners who have been suddenly and unexpectedly released from prison. Inevitably, every homeopath wishes that every case would go as smoothly as these; the fact that most cases do not is not a reflection upon the prescribing ability of the homeopath but rather upon the severe nature of the cases which end up consulting a homeopath in the first place.

Deep Miasmatic Cases

The first category of "constitutionally strong" cases generally are seen in cultures closely related to Nature. In Greece, these patients are commonly found among villagers living a simple life at high altitude. By contrast, patients belonging to the second category involving several miasms seem to come from cultural milieus which would be called "cultured" and "sophisticated" in modern terminology. This observation makes sense for a variety of reasons—the separation from earth cycles occurring in urban environments, chemical pollution from various sources, the hectic and artificial pace of life in urban environments, overeducation and intellectualization, dependency upon suppressive treatments of various kinds, and many other influences.

In any case, homeopathic practices in highly "sophisticated" environments see a predominance of patients with many predispositions toward disease. These cases require the highest degrees of homeopathic skill in order to accomplish cure. Such cases are the measure of truly accomplished homeopaths, as compared to mediocre prescribers. As mentioned previously, every homeopath can claim impressive successes in cases with strong constitutions, but the real test comes in cases belonging to this second category. These cases are still curable, but accomplishing cure demands great skill, training, judgment, experience, and time on the part of the homeopath. It demands even more of the patient.

As we consider the first principle in regard to such patients, we see at once that we face great difficulties. Such deeply ill patients generally do not show an easily discernible amelioration on the deepest levels. At even the initial interview, the past history and family history provide strong hints that the prognosis is guarded; with difficulty, an initial remedy is selected. Even then, the patient's response is not as clear as one would wish. Often, progress can be determined only by subtle indications or improvement in minor symptoms. If one is able to wait long enough, a slowly curative response may occur over a period of one or two years (requiring a few more remedies, carefully chosen).

The natural question arises, "Assuming the response is not very obvious and the patient is suffering, *how long can one wait?*" The answer to this question, of course, depends greatly upon the individual circumstances, and upon the experience of the homeopath. The most helpful clue is found in the regions of most central importance to the patient's ability to truly live creatively. If even

241

subtle changes for the better are occurring on the energy or mental/emotional levels, then the inclination will be to wait, even though the patient may be suffering severely on more peripheral levels. At each visit, progress must be evaluated very carefully, particularly in central areas.

Often, prescribers will encounter members of this category who complain that the original symptoms really are getting worse after the initial remedy. This aggravation of physical symptoms may become intolerable, say, between 20 days and three months after the remedy, in spite of the fact that the patient feels better in himself. The inclination, of course, should be to try to wait out the aggravation, but it sometimes happens that the local symptoms become unbearable. One can be justified to enter with another remedy in this situation, provided the image of the next remedy is definitely clear.

In patients of the second category, if a skin eruption occurs in response to the first prescription, it can be expected to occur with great violence—and it will not be the last problem the patient will encounter. In this situation, the defense mechanism is *trying* to bring about a cure even though its process is producing severe suffering on the surface of the body. One must wait to the very limit of the patient's endurance. This situation tries the souls of both the patient and the prescriber. If it gets to the point that a new prescription becomes absolutely necessary, then the prescriber must be completely certain that the new symptom image has fully emerged and achieved stability.

In such very difficult cases, it may be necessary to use a series of two or three different remedies in fairly quick succession, but they must always be prescribed only upon a full totality of symptoms. Any shortcuts or hasty prescriptions carry the very real risk of delaying the ultimate cure of the case by several months or more.

Deep miasmatic cases, in the process of treatment, may develop a variety of problems on the physical level on the way toward cure. Instead of skin eruptions or discharges, they may develop arthritic problems or headaches, or digestive disturbances. Again, the same principle applies. These sufferings should be prescribed for only if they become intolerable, and only then if the remedy image has matured and stabilized.

The principle of progress from a more important organ to a less important organ, in patients with deep miasmatic predispositions, presents great difficulty. In terms of location, the direction may be clearly favorable, but the intensity of suffering is likely to be very great. The patient, involved in his or her own present condition, may be inclined to complain that the new state of suffering is even greater than the one prior to taking the remedy. If the *direction* is beneficial, however, this statement should be vieved with suspicion. Ultimately, the homeopath may test this judgment on the part of the patient by threatening the possibility of antidoting the remedy by giving allopathic drugs. Usually, the patient will emphatically refuse such an option, realizing that in actual fact the present state of suffering is not as severe as the original one.

In patients belonging to the second category, it is unusual to see old symptoms return within the early months of treatment. Whenever they do return, they occur with a great deal of violence, and they do not ordinarily return in the original image. As usual in these unfortunate cases, one must exhaust the endurance of the patient while waiting for the emergence of a clear symptom picture. As soon as a stable image reveals itself, however, the new remedy must be given.

Deep miasmatic patients frequently arrive at a stage in which a nosode or a characteristic miasmatic remedy is clearly indicated by the symptomatology. Whenever this occurs, even if it is only a week after the last medicine, the remedy should be given, and progress can be expected to ensue. Further medicines will be needed as well, but one should keep an eye out for the miasmatic nosode or remedy.

In deep cases, a new set of symptoms usually means that a new drug is required. Therefore, one cannot say that there is a "constitutional" remedy in such instances. After a period of years of treatment, such cases may settle into a pattern of response which may require a repetition of the same remedy, but this emergence of a so-called constitutional remedy is relatively unusual. This is true because there are so many miasmatic layers to be penetrated that continually new symptom pictures keep coming to the surface.

Acute ailments in such patients can be expected to be very severe. They tend to be both deep and prolonged, and often three or more prescriptions are needed to deal with the situation. Under the impact of a severe acute ailment and several homeopathic prescriptions, a relapse to the previous level of progress is quite likely to occur. For example, suppose a deep miasmatic case has been treated with three medicines over a period of six months, each having a beneficial effect—but during the sixth month, the patient acquires a very severe bronchitis. Suppose it requires three prescriptions to control the bronchitis. In such a circumstance, it is likely that the patient's chronic state will relapse back to the state just prior to the third prescription. If the resulting symptom picture happens to be the same as the third remedy, then it should be repeated in higher potency. If it is a different symptom picture, however, the new remedy should be prescribed at whatever potency is indicated by the clarity of the image and the degree of pathological change.

In patients of this second category, there is constant pressure to prescribe at every visit, and during moments of crisis in between. The patient is undergoing a great deal of suffering, and the constant complaining always presents a powerful temptation to give another remedy. If one succumbs to this temptation merely in order to stop the complaining, eventually a confusion of the case will occur. Recovery from mistaken prescriptions in patients with very weak defense mechanisms takes a very long time—so such hasty prescriptions in the long run will only maximize the suffering of the patient and minimize the reputation of the prescriber. As a general principle, such patients should be allowed to suffer to the very limits of their endurance, and then they should be prescribed for only when the new image has become clear.

A solid knowledge of physical pathology is an important prerequisite for a homeopath attempting to manage such patients. It is all too easy to allow a patient to suffer while thinking that it is merely a phase in the direction of cure—when in fact pathological damage is occurring. Even for very knowledgeable and experienced clinicians this can be a very difficult judgment to make in many instances, but the possibility that there may be pathological damage must always be kept in mind.

It is in patients with deep miasmatic weaknesses that the most mistakes in prescribing are made. Sometimes the mistakes are made because of sheer lack of knowledge of *materia medica*; in such instances, simple referral to a more knowledgeable or experienced homeopath may clear up the case. Even more often, however, mistakes are made by incorrect *timing* of remedies, and the eventual result is a case which is so disordered that cure may have become nearly unattainable.

A common situation is encountered when the patient returns complaining of a relapse when not yet truly in a full relapse.

244

Because of the patient's complaining, the homeopath misinterprets the severity of the situation. No clear image of a remedy is visible, but the prescriber, feeling under pressure, gives a remedy based upon the best guess. There are two directions that such a case may take. The incorrect remedy may lead to further "relapses," which are further treated, until finally a truly full relapse occurs. If one is fortunate, the current image may have returned to the original remedy picture, and it can be given again with success (if further temptations to prescribe hastily are resisted).

If the final image is completely *unclear,* then the homeopath is faced with a very delicate judgment. It may be that one remedy has worked quite well in the recent past; in this circumstance, it can be repeated in the hope that it will bring enough order into the case to restore progress. Most likely, however, the best alternative is to attempt to antidote the effects of all of the remedies which have disordered the case. This can best be done by giving allopathic drugs to palliate the symptoms for two or three weeks; then the drugs should be discontinued, and the case given another one or two weeks to stabilize before choosing another remedy. Coffee or camphor can be given in a similar manner if allopathic drugs are either inappropriate or ineffective in palliating the symptoms. Homeopathic antidotes should be avoided, because they are more likely to add further confusion to the case.

Incurable Cases

The third category of patients requiring long-term management are those who have already crossed the threshold into incurability. These patients demonstrate the fundamental principles of cure the least of all. Their defense mechanisms are so weak that typical curative reactions are impossible.

For example, if such a patient has been given a correct homeopathic remedy after the initial visit, the patient may return with the report: "I feel definitely better." Among this group of patients, this report generally means that the acute suffering has been alleviated considerably, but in actual fact the general state of well-being has been unaffected. Because the previous suffering was so severe, these patients have the impression that their overall state is improved.

Incurable cases can never be expected to demonstrate a jump from one major level of health to another more peripheral one.

The only reasonable goal is palliation of immediate sufferings so that the remainder of the patient's life can be relatively comfortable.

In such cases, relapses occur very quickly and frequently. When relapses do occur, the remedy image has almost certainly changed, so the prescriber must be very astute and attentive to new remedy images.

If skin eruptions or discharges occur, they are unlikely to be accompanied by real amelioration on deeper levels of the patient although amelioration will definitely ensue in a small percentage of cases. The suffering from such eruptions or discharges can be expected to be very severe and obstinate. Frequently, some prescription rapidly becomes an absolute necessity in such cases, even though the new remedy image has not yet become clear. Nevertheless, the homeopath must settle on the remedy most close to the case in the moment. This, of course, requires great skill; therefore, such cases should generally not be undertaken by beginning prescribers.

In incurable cases, the return of old symptoms is usually not observed; the defense mechanism is too weak to return to an earlier level of vibration.

Assuming excellent prescribing, incurable cases have a chance to survive in relative comfort for many years, depending of course upon the original severity of the condition. Their manifestations rarely follow the traditional directions of curative response, so only the skill and experience of the homeopath can bring about effective palliation.

This chapter may seem to imply that under homeopathic treatment, patients suffering with severe chronic diseases suffer inexorably. This can be true, of course, in the severest of cases, but the fact remains that during the whole time of treatment they definitely suffer *less* than their original state would have produced in the absence of homeopathic treatment. Homeopathic treatment is always worthwhile in such cases, for it is their *only hope.*

Chapter 17

Complicated Cases

IN THIS CHAPTER, we will consider cases which come to the initial consultation already in a highly disordered or terminal state. These cases demand the utmost skill, experience, patience, and time on the part of the prescriber. As a general rule, most such cases should be flatly refused by beginning homeopaths, because the likelihood is that relatively unskilled prescribing will result in even further confusion of the case, and the patient will have suffered needlessly. It often seems that homeopathy is the *only* chance for the patient, since allopathic medicine and other therapies have been found to be unsuccessful. However, since both the beginning prescriber and the patient have no concept of the extreme suffering and chaos which can be encountered in severe cases, they undertake the treatment and quickly discover themselves in over their heads. The most compassionate course of action may be to simply refuse such cases or to refer them to a more experienced homeopath, in order to prevent the terrible suffering which may be required in order to have any chance for cure; if the homeopath is not capable of handling the confusions and complications, this suffering may in the end go for naught.

Of course, there is no comparison between the damage the "correct" allopathic treatment can cause to a chronically ill patient and that which can be caused by an "incorrect" homeopathic one. The side effects of allopathic treatment are dreadful in comparison with even poor homeopathic prescribing. Incorrect homeopathic prescribing does not do *direct* harm to a patient, but it can produce enough disruption to the defense mechanism that further prescriptions are made immeasurably more difficult.

In this chapter, we will consider three basic categories of cases which present themselves at the outset with highly complicated problems. We will discuss cases which have been disordered for a long time by inadequate homeopathic prescribing, cases which have been chronically taking strong allopathic drugs, and cases who comes to the homeopath already terminally ill.

Homeopathically Disordered Cases

Patients who have already had years of homeopathic treatment without significant benefit are those which cause any experienced homeopath to cringe inwardly. They are the most dreaded of cases because they are the most difficult to treat. In homeopathy, every prescription is based upon the totality of symptoms, which is the visible manifestation of the activity of the defense mechanism. When a patient has received numerous homeopathic remedies over a number of years, the defense mechanism's actions are altered, at first subtly and then profoundly. By the time the decision is made to refer the patient to a more experienced homeopath, the manifestations of the defense mechanism are so severely altered that finding the correct series of remedies, and interpreting their actions with precision, can be nearly impossible.

Basically, these disordered cases can be divided into two categories:

1. Curable
2. Incurable.

Curable cases are those in which the defense mechanism is still strong enough to be able to respond to well-selected prescriptions. Incurable cases, on the other hand, are those in whom the defense mechanism has been weakened beyond any hope of being able to respond curatively even to correct prescribing; in these cases, the goal can only be palliation, not cure.

How does one decide whether a case is curable or incurable? First of all, it is impossible to make such a judgment with absolute certainty. Truly hopeless cases are virtually nonexistent, but every experienced homeopath has encountered cases in which the best prescribing produces very limited results. Even in such cases, the prescriber does not "write off" the patient altogether, but prognostic judgments are necessarily made guardedly. Determinations as to curability or incurability in any given case are, as always, a highly individual matter, and the decision should never be considered final. Basically, the following factors are considered:

1. The pathological diagnosis. A severe pathological diagnosis does not in itself signify incurability, but it is one factor to be considered.

2. The strength of the patient's constitution, especially prior to the original homeopathic treatment. Younger patients with strong constitutions initially have a much better chance of recovery than elderly or weakened patients.

3. The nature of the response to previous remedies. To determine this, the entire history of the case must be reviewed. Perhaps the patient has had some response to, say, half of the remedies, and no response at all to the rest. The mere fact that there has been *some* response is not in itself an encouraging sign. If the responses were merely temporarily palliative, the prognosis is adverse. If there have been distinctive aggravation followed by lasting ameliorations, then the prognosis is more favorable.

4. The clarity of the image of the remedy in the moment. Often, a homeopath treating a case simply has never studied the remedy which is needed. In these cases, another homeopath may see the image very clearly. This prognosis would be more favorable.

5. The strength or weakness of the ancestors of the patient.

These factors must all be combined to form a judgment which, again, cannot be absolute or final. It is a difficult decision to arrive at, but it is of more than mere academic value. Depending on the curability or incurability of the case, the goals and approaches to treatment will differ.

Let us first consider the situation in which the case is judged to be relatively "incurable" after having many homeopathic remedies over a period of years. It is important to avoid routinely prescribing the remedy which last produced an amelioration. Incurable cases in general tend to change images very rapidly. It is quite unusual in such cases for a medicine to be needed twice in succession. Therefore, the case must be carefully re-taken at each visit, and whichever remedy is given must fit the image *in the moment.* For example, suppose an incurable case suffered a month ago from loss of urine upon straining or coughing; later, it turns out that the patient has a strong aversion to sweets. Causticum would naturally come to mind, but the chances are that the original stress incontinence has already disappeared and become replaced by another symptom which fits more precisely, say, Graphites. Each prescription must be based solely upon the *current* image.

In incurable cases, the goal is to find the remedy which will produce an immediate amelioration of symptoms. Of course, such an amelioration will quite likely be followed by relapse after a relatively short time, and the relapse will probably require a different remedy. For this reason, the homeopath must see such cases very frequently. The patient should be instructed to contact the homeopath at the first indication of a relapse. In these cases, one does not wait for a clear image to emerge, because the relapses can become very severe in a short period of time. One must enter right away with the correct remedy in order to maintain the state of palliation. This is the reason why I specify that only experienced homeopaths should undertake such cases; if even a single slip is made, the case can degenerate quickly into a severely relapsed condition and will show no clear signs or symptoms for a precise prescription. The prescriber does not have the luxury of being able to wait for a full symptom picture, and there is no margin for error. Only a very experienced and knowledgeable homeopath has any chance of being able to manage such a case, and even then mistakes will inevitably be made.

Incurable cases will often react to a remedy by producing symptoms which are pathognomonic of that remedy without a corresponding general amelioration. If this occurs, it is a bad sign, and a new prescription should be made quite soon. In a healthy individual, or one with a relatively strong constitution, such a "proving" can be a very positive sign, because there will eventually be an amelioration in the general health of the patient. However, incurable cases have a severe weakness in the defense mechanism. A remedy which is close, but not exact, can therefore stimulate the defense mechanism in a morbific way, rather than therapeutically. Therefore, the only thing to do in this instance is to take another look at symptoms which were present when the remedy was originally given; hopefully, a better medicine will be found which more precisely fits the image. This remedy will then return the system to order.

Now let us turn to the curable patients who have had their

cases disrupted by imprecise homeopathic prescribing. Even though the original diagnosis may be quite serious, there may be signs of a fairly strong constitution, the patient is relatively young, and there were some curative responses to one or two of the remedies given. However, for the past year or so, none of the prescriptions have seemed to have lasting effect. In such a case, the homeopath can reasonably judge that the case is still curable, and an attempt can be made to find a series of remedies which will bring about order and cure.

If the case is not very serious, the best procedure is to simply wait a long time for the defense mechanism to settle down into a recognizable pattern. This can take a period of 3-10 months, so it is not a very practical recommendation for the majority of patients. However, some patients *are* able to wait long periods of time, in which case this possibility should be remembered.

If it is possible to acquire the full case record of the initial visit—prior to any homeopathic prescriptions—one should study the initial symptom picture very carefully. Sometimes the original prescription was missed, and the case was disordered from the outset. In other instances, the original remedy was correct, but the homeopath impatiently followed with other remedies without allowing sufficient time for the first medicine to complete its action. By returning to the very first homeopathic consultation, it may be possible to discover a clear image upon which a prescription can be made which will return order to the case.

Such a maneuver can work even though the needed remedy does not appear to fit the *current* symptom picture at all. The reason for this is that, despite the years of prescribing, the first miasmatic layer was never successfully removed. Symptoms were changed around by a series of partial remedies, but a truly curative process was never completed. Therefore, the remedy which fit correctly the original symptom image can still reach deeply enough to bring about order.

An example of this maneuver can be offered by a case from my own experience. An M.D. with a few years' experience in homeopathy attempted to treat a child suffering from severe mental disorders. The patient had received approximately fifteen remedies, some of which had partial actions and others of which had no action. The case was sent to me, and the case taken during the initial interview showed clearly Veratrum album, which had been given only as the tenth prescription amidst a variety of others. Based upon this initial interview, Veratrum album 50M (it is best to go to high potencies if possible in such cases) was given again with instructions to wait after that for a full three months in order to fully evaluate the action of the remedy. After three months, the pathognomonic picture of nitric acid emerged, and it proceeded to produce a lasting curative response.

In this example, the initial miasmatic layer required Veratrum album, but by the time it was given later on, its action was too slow to be fully interpreted, so another remedy was soon given which interrupted the cure. When trying to correct a confused case, it is important to give the best prescription based upon the original case, and then to wait a long time for development of the next remedy—which will represent the next miasmatic layer.

If the original case records are *not* available for some reason, then the homeopath must work hard to help the patient recall all of the significant details of the original case. In order to accomplish this, the homeopath must first win the full confidence of the patient, explain clearly the importance of the needed information, and display a great deal of the patience with the attempts to recall symptoms. Every clue must be followed out, and perhaps even allopathic records must be studied for valuable hints.

If it turns out that the original case is totally unavailable and the case is very confused, the best procedure remaining is to try to antidote the effects of previous remedies and then to allow enough time to pass for the true image to emerge. Generally, the best way to accomplish this is to palliate the patient's symptoms with appropriate allopathic drugs for about three months. The drugs will relieve some of the symptoms of the patient, but they will also create a disruptive influence on the defense mechanism. The drugs should then be discontinued, and a period of about one month allowed to pass before attempting to choose the remedy. Exactly how long to wait before giving the remedy is a matter of clinical judgment, depending upon the seriousness of the ailment and the intensity of the suffering of the patient. Hopefully, the disordered defense mechanism will still have enough strength to settle down into a manifestation of the correct remedy.

Other methods of antidoting confused cases can be used, but they are usually less effective than allopathic drugs. Coffee can be taken several times a day. In my experience, this will antidote remedies within 3 days to 9 months, depending upon the constitutional weakness and sensitivity of the patient. A patient who happens to be very susceptible to coffee will react immediately, as will a patient with a very weak constitution. Since the length of time required to antidote prescriptions by coffee is difficult to predict in advance, this is a relatively impractical method. An attempt could also be made by covering the patient's body with a substance containing a large amount of camphor; usually, liniments and "vapo-rubs" are best for this purpose. Again, the amount of exposure required to successfully antidote remedies by this method is an individual matter. For this reason, if a disordered case *must* be antidoted, I would recommend allopathic drugs as the most reliable method.

Allopathically Disordered or Suppressed Cases

Every homeopath, without exception, is constantly faced with patients who are or have been taking allopathic drugs prior to the original homeopathic consultation. If the allopathic drugs are relatively weak, or only occasionally taken, then the obvious policy is to merely discontinue them and wait 15-30 days before taking the full homeopathic case. This should allow enough time for the image to become clarified in cases who, for example, take analgesics for migraine headaches, sedatives for sleep, or tranquilizers for "nerves."

The real problems occur, however, with patients who have been taking very strong allopathic drugs for many years or decades. This problem occurs most often in cases with chronic asthma, chronic rheumatoid arthritis, epilepsy, chronic heart disease, and severe mental disorders. If such cases have been treated with strong allopathic drugs for a long period of time, the main symptoms become suppressed powerfully into deeper regions of the organism, and the defense mechanism becomes severely hampered in its action.

Of all the powerful allopathic drugs, the ones which seem to be the most disturbing to the action of the defense mechanism are the systemic corticosteroids and ACTH. Corticosteroids, whether administered orally or by injection into muscle, fat, or joints, have a profoundly weakening effect upon the defense mechanism when administered over a period of a few months to many years. It is not clear exactly why this is true, but it is readily borne out by homeopathic experience. Patients who have been taking these drugs over a period of years are virtually impossible to cure. The problem is not merely the inevitable difficulty involved in finding the correct remedy while the patient is taking corticosteroids. It has also been found that even the correct remedy is prevented

253

from acting fully in the presence of such drugs. Therefore, the only possible procedure is to try to get the patient off the corticosteroids, which turns out to be virtually impossible for most severe cases. Corticosteroid withdrawal has its *own* characteristic withdrawal period of aggravation which can be life-threatening in some cases, and then it takes at least three months for a true remedy image to become clear after their discontinuation. For these reasons, the best recommendation is to avoid such cases altogether.

As a general rule, patients on strong allopathic drugs for long periods of time should be refused for homeopathic treatment. This should be the general policy for several reasons. The problems of perceiving the correct remedy in the midst of strong allopathic drugs are very difficult, and the severity of the illness after discontinuing allopathic medications may be extremely dangerous. The homeopath must have great allopathic skill to manage such cases, and must be unerring in the choice of medicines and their timing. Moreover, the prescriber's time can become totally monopolized by the hour-by-hour, day-and-night, care required by such patients. Often, these cases have to be hospitalized, and sometimes for considerable periods of time. Finally, the legal question must always be considered; such cases are so delicate that the risks of homeopathic treatment, coupled with the dangers of withdrawal from allopathic medicines, can place the prescriber in legal jeopardy. It is unfortunate to have to refuse these patients, because many of them are unwitting victims who might have been cured if treated homeopathically from the outset. However, until we have homeopathic schools and homeopathic hospitals, and until there are many highly skilled and experienced homeopathic physicians available for consultation, such cases should be refused.

Now, despite the above advice, there will occasionally be cases in which the patient is *very* motivated to get off allopathic drugs for purposes of being treated homeopathically, and the homeopath is moved to try to help the patient. For the sake of advanced prescribers, I will attempt to describe some principles from my own experience referring to this difficult situation. To begin with, such a project should be undertaken only after all of the consequences are perfectly clear *both to the patient and to the homeopath*. It is easy for a patient, in a moment of desperation and of hope, to agree to undergo the terrible suffering and risk which can occur. It is also possible for the homeopath, who may not yet realize the full implications of the situation, to agree to take on such a case—only later to regret the decision after weeks and months of crises and nights of lost sleep. For this reason, both the patient and the doctor should take time to think over such a decision, to discuss it with their families, and to enter into such an agreement only after careful consideration.

Such circumstances arise most commonly from patients who have been continuously on corticosteroids for many years. This can be presented as a general model for cases who are on allopathic drugs.

Every effort must be made to take the case fully and thoroughly throughout its *entire* history. If possible, the initial case should be acquired prior to the onset of the corticosteroids. This will be difficult for the patient to recall clearly, but whatever information can be gathered may be valuable. Then, one must search *throughout* the years of corticosteroid treatment for symptoms—particularly the most peculiar and individualizing characteristics—which have been present most consistently throughout the history. Finally, the current state must be recorded, again with emphasis on those characteristics which have constantly been present throughout the entire history.

This may sound simple, but it is actually a very difficult process. When a patient is on allopathic drugs, many of the modalities affecting particular symptoms are altered by the drug itself and its time of administration. For example, a severe asthmatic patient may take a corticosteroid dose in the morning, and then theophylline-adrenalin combinations throughout the day, finishing just prior to sleep. If this patient awakes at 4 A.M. with dyspnoea, is this 4 A.M. aggravation a homeopathic symptom suggesting Natrum sulphuricum or is it merely the time when the drugs are beginning to wear off? Because of these uncertainties, most of the symptoms being evaluated are not truly manifestations of the action of the defense mechanism at all but rather effects of the drugs.

After very careful gathering of *consistent* symptoms and thoughtful study, a remedy is selected. It should be given in a low potency with frequent repetition while the corticosteroids are continued at their customary dosage. For example, a 12× might be given 3 times daily for 10 consecutive days. If the remedy seems to have an effect, then the drugs are decreased as rapidly as possible. If the remedy is truly the *simillimum*, the allopathic drug may be decreased at a rate even more rapid than the usual allopathic

255

recommendation—but this procedure must be carefully monitored by the consulting physician.

The patient must not be allowed to become overly optimistic during this phase of treatment. For some patients, this may be the first time that the drug has been decreased to such a degree, and there is a natural tendency to look forward to a full and rapid cure. These hopes should be discouraged, because there is always a strong probability that a relapse might occur which would again require corticosteroids. This eventuality should not be viewed as a failure but merely as a phase in the process of slowly working toward cure over a period of several years.

If it *is* possible to discontinue the steroids, the next step is to try to handle the inevitable aggravation after the withdrawal of the drug. This can be the most critical phase in the case, because the symptoms and pathological changes can become severe indeed. It is the effects of this phase for which the patient and the doctor must be prepared in advance. It can be a horrendous period of time, but it may be possible to survive if both the patient and the doctor clearly understand both the goals and the risks. There should never be a sense of failure in using corticosteroids again if the symptoms become too severe, but it should also be understood that they will be withheld unless the situation becomes truly dangerous. This phase of treatment requires great allopathic *and* homeopathic skill on the part of the doctor, and great motivation and patience on the part of the patient and his or her family.

Once the corticosteroids have been successfully discontinued, the doctor should be careful not to prescribe one remedy after another, especially if the patient is doing tolerably well under the circumstances. The defense mechanism must be given time to return to a relatively normal state, and then a remedy image should become clear. From then on, the case is treated normally. During crises, corticosteroids are resorted to only during the most dangerous circumstances, and the case is managed as much as possible solely by homeopathic means.

Cases involving corticosteroids can be used as models for discontinuing other powerful allopathic drugs as well. During the remainder of this section, I will try to comment on specific situations which are commonly encountered in homeopathic practice.

Cardiac cases: Patients on heart medicines present special problems. These cases, especially, require special allopathic knowledge on the part of the homeopathic doctor. Each case must be judged individually. In general, elderly patients or people with demonstrable arteriosclerotic disease require a more conservative approach; drugs should be withdrawn only very reluctantly and cautiously. Younger patients have a better chance, but even these should be handled with caution. In general, one should not withdraw antihypertensive drugs from pheochromocytoma patients, coronary vasodilators from patients with demonstrable arteriosclerotic vascular disease, anti-arrhythmic drugs from patients with arrhythmias or cardiomegaly, etc. Common sense and clinical experience must guide these decisions. Do not be overly hopeful about the benefits of homeopathic treatment in any given case. One should always remember that even the best prescribers miss the remedy occasionally, and this could be a serious mistake while trying to withdraw a patient from a strong allopathic drug.

Schizophrenics: Deeply psychotic, violent, or suicidal schizophrenics on major tranquilizers should not be undertaken for treatment at all—under any circumstances. These cases are too volatile and too dangerous to attempt. Once a major tranquilizer has been successful in suppressing symptoms in such a case, the chances are very poor that the drug can safely be withdrawn long enough to find a curative remedy. In milder psychotic cases, and in neurotics taking minor tranquilizers such as Valium, the drug should simply be stopped—and then homeopathic prescriptions given according to whatever pace seems to be demanded by the individual case.

Diabetes: Juvenile diabetes is a particularly difficult problem to bring to cure. It does happen, of course, but the process is slow and difficult. The administration of insulin does not interfere with the action of homeopathic remedies, nor does it interfere with the remedy image when due consideration is given to common hyperglycemic and hypoglycemic symptoms. The patient should be warned that during the homeopathic treatment, the requirement for insulin may well change; the patient must not feel compelled to maintain the customary dosage while general improvement is occurring, because there would then be a danger of hypoglycemic reactions and coma. The goal in all diabetic cases is not only to help reduce or discontinue the insulin requirement; even more importantly, homeopathic treatment hopes to prevent or reduce the long-term sequelae—such as arteritis, retinitis and blindness, nephropathy, infections, etc.

Adult-onset diabetes is a different matter altogether. This is relatively easy to benefit and cure by homeopathy if complications have not become too serious. Oral hypoglycemic agents can simply be discontinued in most cases, diet controlled, and homeopathic treatment pursued as usual.

Epilepsy: Epileptics who have been on anti-convulsive drugs for years are extremely difficult to treat. Homeopaths are frequently sought out by such patients after the allopathic drugs no longer seem to be "holding" as well, and allopathic medicine has nothing else to offer. By this time, however, the case has been so severely suppressed that withdrawal or reduction of the drugs becomes excessively dangerous. When homeopathic hospitals become available, such cases will be undertaken in controlled hospital environments so that the patient need not risk harm. Drugs would be gradually withdrawn and the seizures observed until the proper remedy is found. At the moment, however, such hospitals are available only in certain areas of the world; therefore, severely suppressed epileptics must be refused for treatment at the present time.

Thyroid cases: Thyroxine is a drug which does not directly interfere with the action of the homeopathic medicine, but it does mask the symptomatology which would lead to the correct remedy. It can be very difficult to find the remedy in such cases. The procedure used in regard to corticosteroids should be followed here. Once the correct remedy is found, a time may come when the general health has improved sufficiently that thyroxine can be discontinued altogether.

Chronic febrile illnesses: There are some chronic febrile ailments, such as Brucellosis and others, which are commonly treated by chronic administration of antibiotics. Such cases cannot be treated homeopathically *during* the administration of the antibiotics. The procedure, then, is to simply discontinue the drugs and await the emergence of the symptom picture. In febrile illnesses, this should only take a few days, When the remedy is clear, give it, and do not return again to the antibiotic treatments.

A general principle that should be strictly followed without exception is that if the patient is feeling really well under *any* treatment, never undertake to replace his old treatment with a homeopathic remedy. If, in spite of taking the drugs, the patient does not feel well, then the above principles apply.

Terminal Cases

Not infrequently, the homeopath is confronted with a patient who is already in a terminal state—expected to die within a few days or weeks. If the patient is suffering from cancer, it is very common that cytotoxic drugs are already being administered; such cases cannot be helped. Other terminal cases are seen who have not taken any drugs, either because treatments are not known or because the patient mistrusts allopathic doctors. Such patients may be undertaken—with due regard to whatever legal limitations exist in the prescriber's local region—but one can only hope for palliation.

At first glance, it might seem that simple palliation would be relatively easy to accomplish in homeopathy. In actual fact, especially in terminal cases, palliation can be the most challenging task confronting any homeopathic physician. All of the difficulties discussed earlier in regard to incurable cases are present here. The patient must be seen daily, the remedy is likely to be constantly changing, and the timing of doses must be such as to prevent the severe relapses which can easily occur. Virtually every prescription must be exactly precise; otherwise the case may unravel to such an extent that even palliation becomes impossible.

For some reason that I do not yet understand, terminal cases tend to require predominantly *unusual* remedies—such as Aurum muriaticum, Euphorbium, Tellurium, and others. Of course, if Sulphur or another polychrest emerges, it must be given, but it has been my experience that deep, terminal cases tend to require small remedies, which beginning homeopaths are unlikely to know. For this reason, and because of the legal difficulties that can occur, beginning prescribers would be wise to avoid such cases.

While trying to palliate a terminal case, one should be content to accept relatively minor sufferings. It is often impossible to produce a completely pain-free state, even though the very intense suffering can be alleviated. If the homeopath tries *too* hard to attain perfect palliation, there is a very great danger that a prescription will be given which may result in a relapse. In this instance, the relapse could quickly become as intense as the disease *would* have been had it not been treated at all.

It is often said in homeopathic circles that giving palliative remedies in terminal cases may well mercifully shorten the final days of the patient. This point of view needs more investigation.

259

In my own experience, I have not observed such an effect. As an example, I can recall in my first years of practice a woman with cancer of the breast which had metastasized to the lumbosacral spine, the pelvic bones, and the ribs. She was in such pain that she screamed all day long, and no one expected her to live more than a few days. Doctors refused to hospitalize her because there seemed to be no point; it was recommended that she be allowed to die at home. Therefore, the family called me to the house for treatment. I explained that, in my experience at that time, the remedies might produce relief from the suffering, but the remaining days might be shortened. This was agreed to, and homeopathic treatment was begun. To my surprise, the remedies not only succeeded in relieving the most intense suffering, but the patient lived for another 1 1/2 years! She remained weak, and had to restrict her activities mostly to watching television, but she at least was not suffering severely, and she remained mentally active.

This case also illustrates the principle of being satisfied with minor sufferings; she had some pains in her calves which were not controlled by the medicines. An allopathic doctor declared these to be merely "rheumatic" pains, which he said could be controlled by vitamins. She was given high doses of vitamins, and within three days there occurred full relapse which was beyond the control of homeopathic remedies. Quickly, she was hospitalized, given allopathic drugs, soon became a human "vegetable," and within ten days she died.

Another impressive case in which the principle of palliative remedies shortening life seemed to be violated: a man of 74 had advanced lung cancer which had metastasized to various regions. The allopathic prognosis was that he would die within a few weeks. Palliative homeopathic treatment was undertaken, and the results were again surprising. For the next *three years*, the man was essentially free of pain and active enough to maintain his garden, until he died from a severe, sudden hemorrhage from the lungs. This case cannot in any sense be said to have been "cured," but the palliation was lasting, and the patient was able to enjoy several more useful years than would have been expected otherwise.

Chapter 18

Handling of Remedies and Interfering Factors

T HROUGHOUT THIS BOOK, reference has been made to technical factors which can prevent the action of a remedy. In this chapter, the specifics of these factors will be enumerated. On the one hand, attention must be paid to the actual handling of the remedy itself so that its delicately potentized state is not destroyed prior to being administered to the patient. And on the other hand, factors must be considered which can cause the remedy's action to be disrupted even months or years after it has been administered.

Once the remedy has been acquired from a homeopathic pharmaceutical company, it must be handled correctly. Most homeopaths maintain a supply of remedies in the office which are administered directly to the patient. Sometimes, arrangements are made with local pharmacists to administer remedies on a prescription basis. Either procedure is acceptable as long as attention is given to the storage conditions of the medicines. The remedy is usually received in a glass vial with a cork top or a cork-lined plastic top. In its storage state, the vial should be colored in order to screen out the rays of the sun, but vials which are dispensed to the patient may be made of clear glass. The medicines must be kept in a location in which they are not exposed to direct sunlight, to excessive heat or cold, to moisture, or to strong odors. Any of these physical exposures can destroy the potency of a remedy.

Individual homeopaths have their own method of administering the medicine, but I believe that the strict professional standards maintained by good pharmacies are the only guarantee of quality. Unless such standards are observed, it may frequently happen that a medicine becomes inactivated before even reaching the patient.

The problem is that an inactivated remedy is unlikely to be discovered for quite some time. If a patient returns with no result, the homeopath is likely to decide that the wrong remedy was chosen rather than to suspect the activity of the remedy. There are already too many variables in homeopathic prescribing; it is therefore recommended that the remedies be maintained in as carefully controlled conditions as possible.

For those who keep remedies in their own office, it is absolutely necessary to re-order the medicine from a homeopathic pharmaceutical company every time it runs out. A major advantage of this procedure is that it provides a continuing source of profit to pharmaceutical companies, which is the only way that we can be assured of a continuing supply of reliable medicines. Even if our remedies are continually re-ordered in this way, the expense will be almost negligible.

Despite this consideration, many homeopaths strongly desire to maintain a continuous supply in their own offices. A useful compromise plan, then, is to maintain two sets of remedies. One set contains the remedies in "dry" form (on lactose granules), ready for direct administration to the patient. A second set of "stock" remedies is maintained in liquid form. Whenever a vial of granules is used up, it is refilled with unmedicated granules, and these are then wetted with a few drops of liquid from the alcohol "stock" solution. In this way, any inactivated remedies become reactivated from the liquid "stock" solutions, which are stored in colored glass vials and are only rarely opened. Finally, when a liquid "stock" remedy runs out, it should be re-ordered from a pharmaceutical company.

Generally, homeopathic remedies are administered by placing a few medicated lactose granules on the tongue of the patient. These are allowed to dissolve on the tongue, but they may be swallowed as well. The homeopath must train himself or herself to pause a moment prior to opening a remedy vial in order to be attentive to any odors in the environment. Also, it is important that the patient not be wearing any perfume at the time of its administration.

The best time to take a remedy is in the morning before breakfast and before the teeth are brushed with toothpaste. The reason for this is that there should be no strong odors (particularly aromatic odors such as from camphor, peppermint, onions, garlic, etc.) in the mouth when the remedy is administered; if there were such odors present, the remedy might become inactivated in the very act of putting it on the tongue. If a remedy is to be taken after eating, at least 1 1/2 hours must be allowed to pass in order to minimize the possibility of any strong odor remaining in the mouth. Once a remedy has already been taken, however, the patient may eat within 10 minutes or so.

When frequent repetition is desired, remedies are often given in water. The best procedure is to dissolve a few granules in a glass (made of actual glass, not plastic) of *distilled* water. The water is stirred until the granules are fully dissolved, and then the entire contents are taken according to the instructions of the prescriber. If another dose is to be taken the next day, the glass is filled with more distilled water, covered tightly, and then shaken very vigorously. It can then be stored until the next day in a place which is not exposed to direct sunlight, excessive heat, excessive cold, or strong odors. The next dose is taken, and the process repeated as many times as needed. This procedure is known in homeopathy as "plussing," and it is generally used in low potency prescriptions. For example, suppose a patient is given a $12\times$ potency and instructed to take it in its "plussed" form daily for ten days. As a very rough approximation, it can be said that the dose on the second day will be a $13\times$ potency, the third day a $14\times$, the fourth day $15\times$; by the tenth day, the patient is taking a $22\times$ potency.

Once the remedy has been successfully administered, our attention turns to the many factors which can *antidote* its effect after the organism has responded to it. This occurs by interferences with the action of the defense mechanism itself. As a general rule, it can be said that literally anything which has a medicinal effect on a particular individual can antidote a remedy. Anything which produces a hyperactive, nervous state, or a chemically induced calmed or sleepy state, can antidote the action of a remedy.

It is important to remember that it is not actually the remedy which is antidoted (although this expression is commonly used for the sake of convenience), but it is the defense mechanism itself which returns to disorder under the stimulation of an allopathic drug, coffee, etc. Therefore, patients have a responsibility to be very strict about the particular substances which are known to disrupt the defense mechanism and cause relapse.

The most important antidote is allopathic drugs. In our world, drugs such as painkillers, antibiotics, tranquilizers, sedatives, etc., are so commonplace that people tend to swallow them without a second thought. Nevertheless, they are artificial substances with powerful effects which can quickly antidote homeopathic remedies. Therefore, allopathic drugs should be strictly avoided unless specifically approved by the homeopathic prescriber.

The only exceptions to this rule are minor painkillers, such as aspirin, which are not compounded with other drugs. Used in moderate quantities for acute conditions, these are actually preferable to homeopathic treatment. When a patient is undergoing chronic homeopathic treatment, short, self-limited acute ailments should not be treated with homeopathic remedies; rather, slight pains or ailments should be treated with a few doses of aspirin.

Coffee is a very well-known "antidote" to remedies. Homeopathic patients should avoid coffee altogether. Because it is difficult to know in advance which patients are likely to be sensitive to coffee and which may be relatively resistant, it is best to set an absolute policy that no one drink coffee. This applies to those who drink one cup per day as well as to those who drink three cups per day. It is not necessary to be concerned about very small amounts of coffee which are added to coffee cake or coffee-flavored ice cream. The idea is that coffee is a medicinal substance which overstimulates the nervous system. In a given patient, any amount which produces even a minor degree of such stimulation is likely to cause a relapse. Common substitutes such as black tea (if taken in amounts which do not produce overstimulation), decaffeinated coffee, coffees made of cereals, etc., are acceptable.

The common practice of using herb teas as beverages requires special attention. The common herb teas are noninterfering, but it is best to vary their use from day to day; the routine use of one particular herb tea can lead to a strong enough dose to produce a medicinal effect. In a given patient, if a particular herb tea is *known* to have a medicinal effect—stimulation, sedation, settling of the stomach, regulation of the bowels, diuresis, etc.—then it should be avoided.

Camphor is a substance which can antidote homeopathic remedies. Common liniments and "vapo-rubs" used for "chest colds" usually contain large amounts of camphor. In addition, most chapsticks contain significant amounts of camphor and should be avoided. Even a strong exposure to camphor fumes is capable of antidoting remedies. However, it is not necessary to become overly cautious about minute amounts of camphor in unlabeled cosmetics. A common-sense practice of reading labels and avoiding substances with strong aromatic odors should be sufficient.

Dental treatment has frequently been observed to antidote the action of remedies. If a patient is just beginning homeopathic treatment and knows that dental treatment is going to be required in the near future, it is best to postpone homeopathic treatment until the dental procedures have been completed. If dental work does become necessary after having received a homeopathic remedy, the amount of anesthetic used should be minimized as much as possible. Also, the dentist should be instructed to avoid using substances with strong aromatic odors—especially oil of cloves or strong mint compounds—as much as possible.

There are instances in which even the mint in toothpaste has been found to antidote remedies. These cases are relatively uncommon, but they occur frequently enough that the homeopath needs to at least be aware of the possibility.

Various therapeutic measures have also been observed to antidote homeopathic treatment. Mineral baths, high doses of vitamins, acupuncture, polarity massage, and herbal therapy have all been observed to antidote homeopathic remedies in specific cases. For this reason, they should be avoided during homeopathic treatment.

As a general rule, food substances do not disorder the system enough to antidote remedies. Common foods do not seem to have medicinal effects in ordinary amounts, and therefore they do not interfere during homeopathic treatment. Interestingly, the same seems to be true of cigarettes and alcohol; neither of these has been observed to interfere with homeopathic remedies.

Chapter 19

Homeopathy for the Dying Patient

THE LAST TWO CHAPTERS of this section will focus on a few speculations about the role of homeopathy. These opinions do not involve information needed by the homeopathic prescriber in actual practice, but they touch upon issues which are brought up in more philosophical conversations about homeopathy. These views are completely personal speculations and should not be considered part of the accepted body of homeopathic knowledge.

The event of death is a crucial point of transition which can be as important to the conscious growth of an individual as any other crisis occurring during life. For this reason, homeopathy plays a very important role in assisting the patient to make this transition. Every person should be allowed to die with the *minimum possible suffering and the maximum state of awareness.*

Everyone will readily agree with the need to minimize suffering at the time of death, but little thought has been given to the necessity for simultaneously maximizing the awareness of the patient. All too often, modern hospitals keep patients in a drugged state, like "vegetables," separated from the love and support of family and friends. The excuse for such practice is that nothing more can be done, and since they must do something in order to minimize the patient's agony, they feel justified to stupefy the unfortunate patient.

Throughout this text, it has been repeatedly expressed that human existence is not merely a random or accidental process.

There is a purpose to life on this plane of existence—a purpose which is grounded in spiritual realities and not merely involving material issues. The primary purpose is to harmonize one's whole being consciously with the eternal laws of nature and to remain fully involved in the realm of life as an inseparable part of it.

Just as life consists of a series of changes and challenges which are transitory, so it is possible to view an entire lifetime as a transitory phase in a large and more purposeful process. Each day of existence, the human being is faced with a series of circumstances—some seemingly insignificant and some momentous—which offer opportunities for growth toward greater love and wisdom. Throughout life, major crises occur which offer even greater challenges and opportunities for growth. Ordinarily, most of us tend to be somewhat lazy and indolent about these opportunities, putting off the lessons until we are finally given no choice. As long as we feel we can "get away with it," we avoid having to face our weaknesses, our cruelties, our dishonesties, etc. Nevertheless, the very purpose of the challenges we confront in life is to provide us with motivation to learn ever greater degrees of love and wisdom. Even the miasmatic predispositions which we inherit serve this purpose.

The crucial moment of Truth for most people occurs at or just prior to the time of death. At this point of transition, the individual is faced with the fact of termination of this phase of existence. Inevitably, the individual reflects on the events and meaning of his or her lifetime. Faced with the imminent and inescapable fact of the termination of life, the person looks at it with a different attitude. The materialistic values which were so enslaving throughout life are cast aside; the pitiful and dishonest behavior of the past is seen in a new light. A sense of deep sorrow and regret may threaten to overwhelm the individual unless the person is able to finally face realities and accept release through confession and repentance. Once this release is experienced, the individual feels free to face death with serenity and satisfaction.

Such a process can occur in the midst of the major crises occurring during life, but in most instances it occurs in relationship to death. One can say that this moment is the most important in the life of a person; it is even more important than the moment of death itself. Yet in order to make use of this instant of spiritual transformation, the individual must be allowed awareness. Unfortunately, this opportunity is all too often denied the patient by the administration of powerful narcotics and tranquilizers. Suppressive therapies are applied with such force that patients end up degenerating into states of senility, imbecility, and finally even coma. This insensitive and inhuman management of the dying patient is excused as being the latest approach in modern science, and later the physicians wash their hands of the situation saying, "We have done all we could." Meanwhile, the patient has been robbed of being able to experience the most important event in life.

The purpose of homeopathy during life is to maximize as much as possible the health and freedom of the individual so that all opportunities for spiritual growth and transformation can be fully utilized. As the time of death approaches, homeopathy's role changes from the process of cure to the goal of offering the patient the maximum degree of awareness with the minimum amount of suffering. In this way the patient is enabled to experience the transition of death with dignity, serenity, satisfaction, and freedom.

Chapter 20

Socioeconomic and Political Implications of Homeopathy

IT IS NOT enough to merely introduce an idea into the world and then passively wait for its acceptance by society. New ideas always challenge conventional viewpoints and traditional structures. For that reason, they are accepted only slowly and with great difficulty. Nevertheless, if an idea is based on fundamental truth, it will eventually be accepted in spite of the many obstacles. This is the situation facing homeopathy.

In homeopathy, we have a therapy which has profound value for the future of our societies. Not only is it a therapy which can effectively cure chronic diseases, but it is a method of stimulating the defense mechanism and balancing the constitution of patients. It is capable of enhancing the degree of productivity, creativity, and serenity of people by removing the susceptibility to disturbing influences. This fact alone has startling implications for our societies. If we imagine a time in the future when homeopathy has become the major therapeutic method, and homeopaths of high standards are available to everyone in the society, we can see clearly the powerfully beneficial influence that homeopathy could have. As more and more people are successfully treated, there would be less inefficiency in work, there would be fewer tendencies for the socially disruptive acts which plague our societies today, there would be less need for artificial drugs which are used in order to experience momentary relief from suffering, and there would be greater tendencies for people to work together for common values and the attainment of greater wisdom. As homeopathy becomes a more widely accepted therapy, world leaders would have access to treatment which would reduce their personal reactions to stress, and thereby create a situation in which nations can decide to avoid conflict and create ways in which to harmonize their relations.

This vision of the implications of homeopathy seems grandiose, of course, because no one really believes that a mere therapy can have such profound effects. This assumption, however, arises out of the fragmented and materialistic views which are prevalent in standard therapies of today. In homeopathy, we take a total view of the person as an integrated spiritual, mental/emotional, and physical being. Homeopathy does not merely remove disease from an organism; it strengthens and harmonizes the very source of life and creativity in the individual. This is very evident in the daily experience of good homeopathic prescribers and their patients; to them, the grand vision presented in the previous paragraph is not at all far-fetched, but quite reasonable and practical given the assumption of the adoption of high standard homeopathy as a widely accepted practice.

Now, that is a large assumption, of course. The medical industry of today is one of the largest single industries in the world, if one considers the many practitioners, the hospitals, the pharmaceutical companies, and all of the ancillary industries. There is a great investment in the allopathic perspective toward health and disease. One cannot hope or even wish that such a structure will change overnight. The forces which allow this accumulated power are not easily going to accept a system as radically different as homeopathy. Any change toward adoption of homeopathy will necessarily be difficult and slow.

However, society itself is already undergoing changes which create hope that such progress is possible. More and more people are becoming disenchanted with the failures of modern allopathic medicine in the face of chronic disease; the underlying assumptions of medicine are being questioned and openly challenged. Alternative therapies of many varieties are being tried out. In this climate, if the public sees clearly the systematic science of homeopathy and its principles which are grounded in timeless natural laws, there will be a powerful wave of support which can provide homeopathy with the leverage it needs to become accepted and widely disseminated.

The dissemination of homeopathy throughout the world will

naturally have to be a step-by-step process. It is not the purpose of this book to describe a detailed strategy for bringing homeopathy into its own, but a general outline of the obvious steps in this process can be offered.

To begin with, the highest and strictest standard of homeopathy must be established and tested thoroughly in the arena of actual clinical results. To this end, teachers must be trained thoroughly to the highest standards. These teachers, with the help of the finances and talents of an interested public, can then establish *full-time schools* for the training of homeopathic prescribers. The very professionalism and clinical successes of these schools should be able to overcome the inevitable political and legal resistance to the emergence of a new profession, and eventually licensing procedures will be established so that the public can have a way of identifying a qualified prescriber from an unqualified one. As schools are established and homeopathic prescribers become known in their communities, formal clinical research can be conducted to prove conclusively the success of homeopathic treatment. The allopathic profession can be openly invited to participate in objective studies comparing the effectiveness of the two methods. Simultaneously, research should be conducted by physicists to investigate the electromagnetic processes involved in homeopathic remedies and their actions. As the successes of high quality prescribers become more widely known, books and articles can be written to improve the public's understanding of the true laws and principles governing health and disease.

The acceptance of homeopathy according to this general scenario will necessarily be gradual and time-consuming. The financial implictions alone, of such a change are staggering. Although homeopathic prescribers are paid very well for the great amount of time they spend with patients, the total cost of the entire medical care of each individual would be drastically reduced. Instead of constantly spending money on palliative drugs and increasingly frequent hospitalizations, the society would merely have to pay for a relatively inexpensive course of homeopathic treatment which in most cases would involve intensive treatment for only a matter of months—or at the most a few years. From then on, visits would be quite infrequent and very inexpensive compared to the chronic costs of today's allopathic medical care.

The pharmaceutical industry would necessarily undergo drastic changes. Most likely it would be forced to decline to a mere fraction of its present size. Hospitals would have drastically reduced burdens and would be able to *reduce* costs (in contrast to the presently uncontrolled rise in hospital costs). The entire context of training of medical doctors would eventually be changed to take into account the natural mechanism of healing, rather than merely focusing upon the end-products of disease. Of course, the value of allopathic methods will never be lost. Such fields as emergency medicine, surgery, orthopedics, and obstetrics will always be needed, as well as a measure of palliative allopathic treatment, but the context of allopathic medicine would be placed in a more appropriate perspective.

Even though the current growth of homeopathy is and must be gradual, there is every reason to believe that it will continue at a steadily increasing pace as public understanding and acceptance grow.

Appendix A

Hahnemann's Proving of Arsenicum Album

It is difficult to convey the extreme detail with which a carefully conducted proving is done. In order to provide the reader with a good example of proving, extensive portions of Hahnemann's original proving of Arsenicum album follows. Arsenicum is one of the most commonly used remedies in the homeopathic *materia medica*. The symptoms listed are a compilation of both accidental poisoning symptoms and symptoms produced by actual provers. If the entire proving were to be printed, it would occupy approximately fifty-one pages. However, it is unlikely that any reader would read such a proving in its entirely in this text and therefore, only a fraction of the complete proving is included here (for the entire record, see Hahnemann's *Chronic Diseases*).

Arsenicum

The abbreviations of the names of my fellow-provers are: Bhr., Baehr; Fr. H., Friedrich Hahnemann; Htb. u. Tr., Hartlaub u. Trinks; Hg., Hering; Hbg., Hornburg; Lgh., Langhammer; Mr., Meyer; Stf., Stapf.

Mind.
1. Sadness and gloominess.
    Melancholy, sad mood, after a meal, with headache (aft. 80 h.)

Sad, sorrowful ideas, in the evening in bed, as if some misfortune might have happened to one's relatives.

Religious melancholy and reserve. [EBERS, in Hufeland's Jour., 1813, Oct., p. 8.[1]]

5. He wept and howled, and spoke but little and briefly. [Stf.]

Piercing wailings, interrupted by fainting fits coming on. [FRIEDRICH, in Hufeland's Jour., V., p. 172 [2]]

Piteous wailings, that a most violent constriction of the chest was taking away his breath, attended with an extremely disagreeable sensation in the abdomen; this compelled him to double up, rolling here and there, then again rise up and walk about. [MORGAGNI, de sed. et caus. morb., LIX.[1]]

Fits of anguish for a long time. [TIM. A. GUELDENKLEE, Opp., p. 280.[2]]

Anxiety and restlessness in the whole body (aft. 1 h.). [RICHARD, in Schenk, lib., VII., obs. 211.[3]]

10. Anxious and trembling, he is afraid of himself, that he might not be able to restrain himself from killing someone with a knife. [MERCUS, Ephem. d. Heilkunst, Heft., 111.[4]]

Anxiety and heat, not allowing her to go to sleep before midnight for many days. Anxiety in the evening, after lying down and after midnight, at 3 o'clock, after awaking.

Severe anxiety, at night about 3 o'clock, she sometimes felt hot then again like vomiting.

Anxiety, anguish. [MYRRHEN, Misc. Nat. Cir.—Neuemed, chir., Wahrnehm, Vol. I., 1778.—QUELMALZ, Commerc, lit., 1737.[5]]

15. Excessive anguish. [KAISER, in Hb. u. Tr. Arzneimittellehre.[6]]

The most intolerable anguish. [FORESTUS lib., 17, obs., 13.[7]]

Great anguish with constriction of the chest and difficult respiration. [KAISER, 1.c.]

Internal anguish. [KAISER, 1.c.]

Mortal anguish. [HENNING in Hufeland's Journ. X., 2.[8]]

20. Continual anguish, like remorse of conscience, as if he had acted in violation of his duty, without knowing in what particular.

Anguish of heart, interrupted by fainting fits coming on. [FRIEDRICH. 1.c.]

Anguish and anxiety, so that he reapeatedly fell into a swoon. [BERNH. VERZASCH. Obs. med. obs. 66.[9]]

Anguish, trembling and quivering, with cold perspiration in the face. [ALBERTI, jurisprud, med. Tom. II., p. 257.[10]]

Great anguish, trembling and quivering with severe tearing in the abdomen. [ALBERTI, 1.c.]

25. With inexpressible anguish, he seemed on account of his increasing pains to lie at the point of death. [MORGAGNI, 1.c.]

With great anguish, he rolls and tosses about in the bed. [GUELDENKLEE, ibid. BUEITNER, Unterr. ueb. d. Toedl. d. Wund.[1]]

He can find no rest in any place, continually changes his position, wished to get from one bed into another and to lie, now here, now there.

Restlessness, he desires to get from one bed into another. [MYRRHEN, 1.c.]

Restlessness and tossing about in bed with sadness and unquenchable thirst (aft. 24 h.). [BUETTNER, 1.c.]

30. Restlessness with pains in the head, in the belly and in the knees. [RICHARD, 1.c.]

Full of restlessness, the child is cross and whimpers.

Restlessness, and hypochondriac anxiety as from constant sitting in a room, as if from the upper part of the chest, without palpitation (at once). Anguish and fear; he sees an acquaintance who is not present lie dead on the sofa, and is much afraid of him. [Whl.]

He sees nothing but worms and bugs crawling about on his bed, from which he desires to run away, and of which he throws out whole hands full. [Whl.]

35. He sees nothing but rogues in his room, and therefore always creeps under the bed. [Whl.]

His whole house, also under his bed, is full of rogues, which causes a cold sweat to break out, which runs down cold over his body. [Whl.]

In the night he runs all about the house, looking for thieves. [Whl.]

The greatest fear and anguish; night and day he sees ghosts.

He jumps out of bed for fear, and hides away in a wardrobe, from which he can only be gotten out with difficulty. [Whl.]

40. Lack of determination; he desires something, and when the endeavor is made to fulfill his desire, the merest trifle will change his determination, and then he is not willing to have it so.

Great seriousness.

When he is alone he falls into thoughts about disease and other things, from which he can easily tear himself away.

He despairs of his life. [RICHARD, 1.c.[2]]

Desponding and weeping, he thinks that nothing can help him, and he would have to die anyhow; at the same time he is cold and chilly with subsequent general weariness.

45. Super-sensitiveness and over-tenderness of mind; dejected, sad and lugubrious, she is troubled and solicitous about about the merest trifles.

Very sensitive to noise.

Inclines to be frightened.

Weak in body and soul, he cannot talk, without exhibiting peevishness.

Little talking, but complains of anguish. [ALBERTI, 1.c.]

50. Uncomfortable, he has no pleasure in anything.

Impatient and anxious.

Dissatisfied all day and extremely vexed at himself; he thought he had not worked enough and reproached himself most bitterly. [Lgh.]

Ill-humor alternating with gentle kindliness; in her ill-humor she will not look at anybody, nor listen to anything; at times also she weeps.

Ill-humor in the morning in bed; he pushes the pillows about in dissatisfaction, throws off the coverlet, uncovers himself, looks at no one, listens to nothing.

55. Vexed about trifles.

He is vexed at every trifle, and cannot stop talking about the faults of others.

Very peevish and dissatisfied with everything, she finds fault with everything; everything seems to her too strong and loud, all talk, every noise, all light.

Very peevish and sensitive; the least thing insults him and angers him. [Lgh.]

Very peevish and passionate, capricious, she takes every word ill and is cross when she has to answer.

60. Inclined to sarcastic mocking.

She became violently enraged when she was forced to eat something, while she had no appetite at all.

Her desires exceed her want; she eats and drinks more than what agrees with her; she walks farther than is necessary and is good for her.

Great indifference and lack of sympathy.

Indifference to life. [KAISER, 1.c.]

65. Life seems indifferent to him, he sees no value in it.

Calm equanimity; careless about their approaching death, then, neither hope nor wish to recover. (After-effects, with two suicides, who had taken Arsenic.)

Calmness of soul (in a despondent, melancholy woman). [LABORDE, journ., de Med., LXX., p. 89.[1]]

Of a calm, firm mind; he retained his equanimity in all events that happened. [Lgh.]

Cheerful disposition; he likes to converse with others. [Lgh.]

70. More inclined to cheerfulness, and disposed to occupy himself. [Lgh.]

During the first minutes great tranquility of soul and serenity; but after half an hour excessive restlessness and anxiety; he imagined that the effects of the poison would be dreadful and desires to remain alive (in a despondent suicide). [Stf.]

Diminution of memory.

Very faulty memory, for a long time. [MYREHEN, 1 c.]

Forgetfulness, his memory fails him.

75. Stupid and weak in the head, about noon.

Stupid and dizzy in the head, so that he could not think. [Mr.]

Stupid and confused feeling in the head, as from severe coryza and vexation; the head feels like a lantern.

Stupid feeling in the head, as if he had not slept enough; from 11 A.M. to 6 P.M.

Dullness in the head, without pain.

80. Weakness of the reason. [EBERS, 1.c.[1]]

Chronic weakness of mind. [EBERS, 1. c.[2]]

Delirium. [KAISER, 1.c.]

Fantastic delirium, returning from time to time. [GUILBERT, Med. chir. Wahrnehm, Vol. II., Attenb.[3]]

Crowding in of various ideas, which he is too weak to shake off so as to occupy himself with a single one.

85. The organs of sense are morbidly active. [KAISER, 1.c.]

Absense of reason and of the internal and external senses; he did not see, for many days he did not speak, he heard and understood nothing; when anyone cried very loudly into his ears, he would look at those present like a drunken person awakened from a deep sleep. [MYRRHEN, 1.c.]

She lay in her bed perfectly senseless, muttered unintelligible sounds, with her eyes staring, cold perspiration on her forehead; trembling in her whole body; small, hard and quick pulse. [EBERS, 1.c.]

Consciousness disappears or becomes indistinct. [KAISER, 1.c.]

Loss of sensation and consciousness, so that he knew not what happened to him. [PYL, Samml. VIII., p. 98 sq.[4]]

90. Loss of consciousness and speech. [Misc. N.C., Dec. III., an. 9, 10. p. 390.[5]]

Ideas straying, while the open eyes are without consciousness of phantasies, either before or afterwards.

Insanity; first headache, excessive anguish, noise before the ears, as of many large bells, and when he opened his eyes, he always saw a man who sometime before had hanged himself in the garret of the house, and who incessantly motioned to him entreatingly that he should cut him down; he ran there with a knife, but as he could not cut him down, he grew desperate and wished to hang himself; being hindered in this, he became so restless that he could hardly be kept in bed; he lost his speech, though with full understanding, and when he wished to express himself by writing, he could only make unintelligible marks, whereat he trembled, wept, and with the forehead covered with the sweat of anguish, knelt down and raised his hands entreatingly. [EBERS, 1. c.]

Frenzy; he had to be handuffed and seeks to escape. [AMATUS LUSITANUS, Curationes, Cent II., Cur. 65.[1]]

Inner Head.

Numb feeling of the head. [PEARSON, in Samml. br. Abhandl. f. prakt. Aerzte, XIII., 4.[2]]

95. The head is strongly muddled, in the evening (3d d.).

Weakness in the head, from much pain, with weakness and qualmishnesss in the scrobiculus cordis, so severe that she was really ill.

Dizzy in the head when walking in the open air, aggravated on reentering the room (aft. ½ h.).

Numb feeling in the head. [BUCHHOLZ, Beitr. z. ger. Arzneik, IV., 164 [3]]

Silly in the head, after sleeping.

100. Confused feeling in the head. [Hbg.]

Stupefaction in the head as from precipitate haste in performing an excessive amount of work, with internal restlessness (aft. 2 d.).

Stupefaction, with loss of sensation and vertigo. [EBERS, 1.c.[4]]

Sensation of reeling in the head. [ALBERTI, 1.c.]

Reeling, stupid and dizzy in the head, while taking a walk, most of all in the forehead, as if intoxicated, so as to stagger now to this side, now to that, and every moment was afraid of falling (aft. 9½ h.). [Lgh.]

105. Vertigo. [KAISER, 1.c.; THOMSON, Edinb. Vers., IV; SENNERT, Prat. med. lib., 6, p. 6.[5]]

Vertigo when sitting.

Vertigo only when walking, as if he would fall to the *right side*. [Lgh.]

Vertigo every evening; she has to hold on to something when she shuts her eyes.

Vertigo, with obscuration of vision. [MYRRHEN, 1.c.]

110. Vertigo, with loss of thoughts when rising. [Stf.]

Violent vertigo with nausea, when lying down; he has to sit up to diminish it. [Stf.]

Vertigo, with headache. [KAISER, 1.c.]

Pains in the head. [GRIMM, Misc. N.C., Dec. III, ann. 7, 8.[6]]

Pains in the head and vertigo for several days. [G. W. WEDEL, Diss. de Arsen Jen. 1719, p. 10.[7]]

115. Headache of excessive severity. [JOH. JACOBI and RAU, Acta N.C.; KNAPE, Annal der Staats-Arzneikunde, 1, 1.[8]]

Headache in the occiput.

Semilateral headache. [Knape, 1.c.]

Headache, for several days, immediately relieved by applying cold water, but on removing it is much worse than before.

Headache above the left eye, very severe in the evening and at night. [Hg.]

120. Periodic headache. [Th. Rau, 1.c.]

Stupefying, pressive headache, especially in the forehead, in every position. [Lgh.]

Stupefying, pressive headache, especially on the right side of the forehead, just above the right eyebrow, paining as if sore on wrinkling his forehead. [Lgh.]

Stupefying, pressive headache, chiefly on the forehead, with fine stitches on the left temporal region, near the outer canthus, when walking and standing, passing off when sitting (aft. 2 h.). [Lgh.]

Pain, as from a bruise, on one side of the head, in the morning immediately on rising from bed (aft. 12 h.).

125. Sensation as if beaten on the front of the head.

Pain in the forehead and above the nose, as from a bruise or sore, going off for short time by rubbing.

Heavy and confused sensation in the head, so that he cannot easily rise; he has to lie down.

Great heaviness in the head, especially when standing and sitting. [Buchholz, 1.c.[1]]

Great heaviness in the head, with roaring in the ears; it goes off in the open air, *but at once returns when coming again into the room* (aft. 16 h.).

130. Excessive heaviness of the head, as if the brain was pressed down by a load, with roaring in the ears, in the morning after rising from bed (aft. 24 h.).

Heaviness of the head with pressive pain, in the morning (aft. 72 h.).

Pressive pain in the right temporal region, in all positions (aft. 3 h.). [Lgh.]

Pressive, drawing pain in the right side of the forehead (aft. 2¾ h.). [Lgh.]

Pressive, stitch-like pain in the left temple, not passing off by touching (aft. 2½ h.). [Lgh.]

135. Tension in the head; headache, as if stretched.

Pinching headache above the eyes, soon passing away.

Drawing headache under the coronal suture, for several hours every afternoon.

Tearing pains in the occiput. [Bhr.]

Tearing in the head and at the same time in the right eye.

140. Headache, composed of tearing and heaviness, with drowsy weariness during the day (aft. 4 d.).

Tearing stitches in the left temple.

Stitch-like pain in the left temple, which ceased on touching the part. [Lgh.]

Throbbing headache in the forehead, just above the root of the nose.

Violently throbbing headache in the forehead, on motion. [Stf.]

145. Violently throbbing headache in the whole head, especially in the forehead, with nausea on raising himself in bed. [Stf.]

Sharp, hard throbbing, like chopping, in the whole head, as if it would

278

drive her skull apart, at night (about 2 a.m.), with an outbreak of perspiration.

Hammering, like blows of a hammer in the temples, very painful, at noon and at midnight for half hour, after which for a couple of hours she feels paralyzed in the body.

Dull throbbing headache in one half of the head, extending to above the eyes.

On motion, a sensation as if the brain was moving and beat against the skull.

150. On motion of the head, the brain feels as if shaking about, with pressure on it, in walking. [Whl.]

Clicking sensation in the head, over the ear, when walking.

Outer Head.

The skin of the head pains, when touched, as if festering.

Painfulness of the hair on being touched.

Falling out of the hair of the head. [Baylies in Samml. br. Abhandl. fuer pr. Aerzte, VII, w, p. 110.[1]]

155. Pains as from a bruise on the external head, aggravated when touched.

Contractive pain in the head.

Formication on the integument of the occiput, as if the roots of the hairs moved.

Burning pain on the hairy scalp. [Knape, 1.c.]

Swelling of the head. [Heimreich in Act. N.C. II, obs. 10.[2]]

160. Swelling of the whole head. [Quelmalz, 1.c.[2]]

Swelling of the head and face. [Siebold in Hufel, Journ., IV, part I, p. 3.[4]]

Extraordinary swelling of the head and face. [Knape, 1.c.]

Swelling of the skin of the head, the face, the eyes, the neck and the chest with natural color. [Knape, 1.c.]

Itching gnawing on the head. [Knape, 1.c.]

165. Gnawing itching on the whole head, inciting to scratch. [Lgh.]

Burning itching on the hairy scalp. [Knape, 1. c.]

Painful itching like ulceration, inciting to scratching on the whole hairy scalp, which pains all over, but chiefly on the occiput, as if from suffused blood (aft. 7 h.). [Lgh.]

A pimple covered with scurf on the left side of the hairy scalp, inciting to scratching, and painful when rubbing as if festering underneath. (aft. 2 h.). [Lgh.]

Eruptive pimples on the whole hairy scalp, which pain, on rubbing and touching, as if festering below, or as if suffused with blood (aft. 11 h.). [Lgh.]

170. Innumerable pimples, very red, upon the hairy scalp [Vigat, 1. c.[1]]

Eruption of pustules with burning pain, on the hairy scalp and in the face. [Heimreich, 1. c.]

Pimples on the left temple, inciting to scratching, and discharging bloody water, and, after rubbing, pain as if sore. [Lgh.]

Two large pimples on the forehead between the eyebrows, inciting to scratching, discharging bloody water, and filled next day with pus. [Lgh.]

Corrosive ulcers on the hairy scalp. [Knape, 1. c.]

175. Ulcerous scab, a finger's breadth in thickness, on the hairy scalp, falling off a few weeks later. [HEINREICH, 1.c.]
Ulcerous scab on the hairy scalp, to the middle of the forehead. [KNAPE, 1.c.]

Eyes.
The right eye pained deep internally, with violent stitches in turning it, so that she could hardly turn her eye.
Pressive pain above the left eyelid and in the upper half of the eyeball, aggravated on looking upward.
Pressive pain under the right eye, continuing for hours, at night, so that she could not stay in bed for distress.
180. Pressure in the left eye, as if sand had got into it (aft. 2 h.). [Lgh.]
Drawing pain in the eyes, and quivering in the lids.
Twitching in the left eye.
Constant quivering of the upper eyelids, with tears in the eyes.
The (oedematously swollen) eyelids close firmly and spasmodically and look as if they were bloated. [Whl.]
Tearing in the eye, at intervals. [SCHLEGEL, in Hb. u. Tr.[2]]
Throbbing, like pulsation, in the eyes, and at every throb a stitch, after midnight.
185. Itching about the eyes and the temple, as if pricked with innumerable red-hot needles.
Smarting, corrosive itching in both eyes, compelling to scratch (aft. 3. h.). [Lgh.]
Burning on the edge of the upper eyelids.
Burning in the eyes.
Burning in the eyes, the nose, and the mouth. [N. med. chir. Wahrnehm., 1.c.]
190. Red, inflamed eyes. [N. med. chir. Wahrn., 1.c.]
Inflammation of the conjunctiva. [KAISER, 1.c.]
Inflammation of the eyes. [HEUN, allgem. med. Annalen, 1805, Febr.[1]]
Violent inflammation of the eyes. [GUILBERT, 1.c.[2]]
Swelling of the eyes. [QUELMALZ, 1.c.[3]]
195. Swelling of the eyelids. [N. med. chir. W., 1.c.]
Oedematous swelling of the eyelids, without pains. [Whl.]
Swelling, first of the upper, then of the lower left eyelid, then of the forehead, the head and the neck, without pain or secretion of mucus; the swelling of the head and of the neck reached an enormous size. [Whl.]
Swollen eyes and lips. [KNAPE, 1.c.]
Painless swelling under the left eye, which partly closes the eye, and is very soft (aft. 5 d.). [Fr., H.]
200. Yellowness of the eyes, as in jaundice.
Yellow white of the eyes, as in a person having jaundice. [Whl.]
Tired look of the eyes. [KAISER, 1.c.]
Dryness of the eyelids, as if they rubbed on the eyes, in reading by candle-light.
The edges of the eylids pain on motion, as if they were dry, and rubbed upon the eyeballs, as well in the open air, as in the room.
205. Watering of the eyes. [GUILBERT, 1.c.]

Constant, severe lachrymation of the right eye, for eight days. [Fr. 4]

Acrid tears, making the cheeks sore. [GUILBERT 1.c.4]

Watering and itching *of the eyes*, some pus in them in the morning. [Fr. H.]

Eyelids glued together in the morning.

210. The outer canthi are glued together by eyegum, in the morning. [Whl.]

Contortion of the eyes. [J. MAT. MULLER, in Ephem. N.C., Cent. 1, C. 51.5]

Contortion of the eyes and of the muscles of the neck. [Eph. N., Cent. X, app., p. 463.6]

215. Protruding eyes. [GUILBERT, 1.c.]

Protruded eyes. [KAISER, 1.c.]

Rigid eyes, directed upward. [KAISER, 1. c.]

Frightfully staring eyes. [MYRRHEN, 1. c.1]

Wildly staring look. [GUILBERT, 1.c.]

220. Wildly staring look. [Whl.]

Wildly staring look, without dilatation of the pupils. [KAILSER, 1.c.]

Wild look. [MAJAULT, in Samml. br. Abhandl. f. pra. Aerzte. VII, 1, 59 and 2, 69.2]

His eyelids close themselves; he is weary. [Hbg.]

Contracted pupils (aft. 1½, 5 h.). [Lgh.]

225. Weakness of vision, for a long time. [MYRRHEN, 1. c.3]

Obscure vision, as through a white gauze.

He does not recognize the persons standing around him. [RICHARD, 1. c.]

Obscuration of sight. [BAYLIES, 1.c.]

Obscuration of sight; everything looks black before his eyes (at once). [RICHARD, 1.c.]

230. Darkness and flickering before his eyes. [KAISER, 1.c.]

Almost total blindness, in a weak-sighted woman, with loss of the hearing and with long-continued dullness of the senses. [EBERS, 1.c.4]

Everything becomes yellow before the eyes, during qualmishness. [ALBERTI, 1.c.]

White dots or points before the eyes.

Sparks before the eyes. [EBERS, 1.c.5]

235. Sensitiveness to light, photophobia. [EBERS, 1.c.6]

Snow blinds the eyes, so that they water.

Ears.

Otalgia. [Bhr.]

Cramp-like pain in the external ears.

Tearing in the interior of the ear.

240. Drawing tearing in the left lobule.

Drawing tearing behind the ear, down the nape of the neck and into the shoulder.

Stitching tearing outwardly through the left meatus auditorius, chiefly in the evening (1st d.).

Stitches in the ear, in the morning.

Agreeable titillation in both ears, deep within, for ten days. [Fr. H.]

245. Voluptuous tickling in the right meatus auditorius, compelling to rubbing. [Lgh.]

Burning in the external ear, in the evening (aft. 5 h.).

Sensation of obstruction in the left meatus auditorius, as if from without.

Hardness of hearing, as if the ears were stopped (aft. 16 h.).

When swallowing, something seems to obstruct the ear from within, as with deafness.

250. He does not understand what is said to him. [RICHARD, 1.c.]

Deafness. [Hg.]

Ringing in the right ear, when sitting (aft. 1½ h.). [Lgh.]

Like ringing in the ears and in the whole head.

Roaring in the ears with every paroxsym of pain.

255. Roaring in the ears. [THOMSON, 1. c. BAYLIES, 1.c.[1]]

Violent rushing sound before the ears as from a near water-weir.

Nose.

In the root of the nose, pain in the bones.

Stitches in the bones of the nose.

Violent flow of blood from the nose, owing to vexation (aft. 3 d.).

260. Violent bleeding from the nose, after severe vomiting. [HEIMREICH, Arsen, als Fiebermittel.]

A fetid ichor flows from the nose, which is ulcerated high up, and dropping into the mouth it causes a bitter taste. [Hgh.]

Face.

Alternately a smell of pitch and of sulphur in the nose.

The face is sunken. [Htb. u. Tr.[2]]

Pale face. [MAJAULT, 1.c.]

265. Paleness of the face with distorted features. [KAISER, 1. c.]

Paleness of the face with sunken eyes. [J.G. GREISELIUS in Misc. Nat. cur. Dec. I, Ann. 2. p. 149.[3]]

Pale, yellow, cachectic appearance. [SCHLEGEL, 1.c.[4]]

Deadly paleness. [HENNING, 1.c.[5]]

Deadly hue of the face. [ALBERTI, 1.c.[6]]

270. Yellow face with sunken eyes.

Bluish, discolored face. [MUELLER, 1. c. Eph. N.C., 1. c.[7]]

Earthly and leaden complexion, with green and blue spots and stripes. [KNAPE, 1.c.]

Distorted features, as if from discontent.

Altered and disfigured countenance. [KAISER, 1.c.]

275. Death-like appearance. [ALBERTI, 1.c.]

Twitches in the facial muscles. [GUILBERT, 1.c.]

Pressure in the left upper jaw.

Itching in the face, causing it to be scratch till it is sore.

Bloated red face, with swollen lips. [Stf.]

280. Bloated, red face. [KAISER, 1.c.]

Swelling of the whole face (from an external application). [Htb. u.Tr.]

Swelling of the face. [J.C. TENNER, in Simon's Samml. d. n. Beob. f.d. J. 1788.[1]]

Swelling of the face, of an elastic nature, especially in the eyelids, and chiefly in the morning, in three persons. [TH. FOWLER, Med. rep of the effect of arsen., Sect. VIII.[2]]

Swelling of the face with swoons and vertigo. [SENNERT, prax lib. 6., p. 237.[3]]

285. Hard swelling like a nut on the two protuberances of the forehead; the swelling increases in the evening. [Sr.]
Eruption on the forehead. [KNAPE, 1.c.]
Little knobs, bumps on the forehead. [N. Med. chir. Wahrn., 1.c.]
Ulcers all over the face. [N. med. chir. Wahrn., 1.c.]
The lips are bluish. [BAYLIES, 1.c.]
290. Bluish lips. [KAISER, 1.c.]
Black-spotted lips. [GUILBERT, 1.c.]
Blackish appearance about the mouth. [ALBERTI, 1.c.]
Pinching, quivering, or twitching on the one side of the upper lip, especially on going to sleep.
Itching, as if pricked with countless burning needles, in the upper lip, up to the nose, and the following day swelling of the upper lip above the red.
295. Swelling of the lips. [Stf.]
Bleeding of the lower lip after a meal (aft. 1½ h.). [Lgh.]
A brown strip of shrivelled epidermis, almost as if burnt, extends through the middle of the red of the lower lip.
Red, tettery skin around the mouth.
Eruption broken out on the lips at the edge of the red, painless (aft. 14 d.).
300. Eruption about the mouth, with burning pain.
Painful knots on the upper lips.
Eruption of ulcers around the lips. [ISENFLAMM STEINNING, Diss. de rem. susp. et ven., Erlangen, 1767, p. xxvii [4]]
Eruption on the lower lip, like noma, with thick crust and a base like a leaf-lard. [Sr.]
An ulcer eroding on the lip, with tearing pain and smarting as from salt, in the evening on lying down, in the day while moving; worst on being touched and in the open air; it prevents sleep and causes waking up at night (aft. 14 d.).
305. Swelling of the sub-maxillary glands, with pain as from pressure and contusion.
Swelling of the sub-maxillary glands, with painfulness on external pressure. [Hg.]
Hard swelling of the left sub-maxillary gland; the swelling is especially severe in the evening. [Sr.]

Teeth.
Toothache, more pressive than drawing.
Jerking, continuous toothache, extending into the temple, relieved or removed by sitting up in bed.
310. Tearing in the teeth and simultaneously in the head, at which she becomes so enraged as to beat her head with her fists; just before the setting in of the menses.
Pain in several teeth (in the gums), *as if they were loose and would fall out;* but the pain is not increased in chewing (aft. 1 h.).
Painful looseness of the teeth; and pain as if sore, per se, and more yet in chewing; so also the gums pain on being touched, and the cheek on that side swells up.
One tooth becomes loose and prominent, in the morning; its gum aches on being touched; still more in that case, the external part of the cheek, be-

hind which lies the loose tooth; the tooth is not painful on biting the teeth together.

Convulsive gnashing of the teeth. [VAN EGGERN, Diss de vacill. dent Duisb., 1787.[1]]

315. Gnashing of the teeth. [KAISER, 1.c.]

Falling out of all the teeth. [VAN EGGERN, 1.c.]

In the gums, stitches, in the morning.

Nocturnal tearing pains in the gums of the canine tooth, which is unbearable as long as he lies on the affected side, *but is removed by the warmth of the bed;* the following morning the nose is swollen and painful on being touched (aft. 3 d.).

The tongue is bluish. [BAYLIFS, 1.c.]

Mouth and Throat.

320. White tongue. [ALBERTI, 1.c.]

Insensibility of the tongue; it is as if it were burnt dead, without sense of taste.

Stitching pain, as from a fish-bone in the root of the tongue, when swallowing and when turning the head.

Boring pain in the right border of the tongue, while half asleep.

Pain on the tongue as if there were on it vesicles full of burning pain.

325. Erosion of the tongue at the side of the tip with smarting pain (aft. 14 d.).

On the roof of the palate, long-continued feeling of roughness. [Bhr.]

Scrapy, scratchy sensation, behind on the velum pendulum palati, when not swallowing.

Scraping and sensation of rancidity in the throat, as from rancid fat, after the first morsel she swallowed in the morning.

In the throat a sensation as if there was a hair in it.

330. Sensation in the throat as from a lump of mucus, with a taste of blood.

Tearing pain in the oesophagus and all up the throat, also when not swallowing.

Burning in the throat. [RICHARD, 1.c.; BUCHHOLZ, 1.c.]

Burning in the fauces. [KNAPE, 1.c. KOPP, Jahrb. der Staats-Arzneik, II. 6. 18 2.[1]]

Inflammation of the interior of the throat. [RAU, 1.c.]

335. Gangrenous sore throat. [FELDMANN, in Comm. lit. Nor. 1743, p. 50.[2]]

In the fauces and stomach a sensation of rolling together, as if a threat was rolled into a ball. [RICHARD, 1.c.]

Sensation of constriction in the throat. [PREUSSIUS, Ephem. N.C. Cent. III, obs. 15.[3]]

Constriction of the fauces (of the oesophagus). [N. m. ch Wahrn., 1. c.]

His throat feels as if pressed quite shut, as if nothing would go down his oesophagus. [ALBERTI, 1.c.]

340. Deglutition very painful. [N. m. ch. Wahrn., 1.c.]

Difficult swallowing. [RAU, 1.c.]

Sensation of paralysis of the fauces and oesophagus; the chewed roll could not be swallowed down, it went down with difficulty with a pinching pressure, as if the oesophagus had not sufficient strength for it; he heard it rattle down.

Feeling of dryness on the tongue. [BUCHHOLZ, 1. c.]

Sensation of great dryness in the mouth, with violent thirst; but he only drinks a little at a time. [Stf.]

345. Sensation of dryness in the throat; she had to drink constantly, as she felt that otherwise whe should perish of thirst.

Severe dryness in the mouth and violent thirst.

Severe dryness in the mouth. [THILENIUS in Richter's chir. bibl. V, p. 540.[4]]

Dryness of the tongue. [GUILBERT, 1.c.; MAJAULT, 1.c.]

Much saliva ejected he had to spit out frequently. [Hbg.]

350. The saliva ejected tastes bitter.

Bloody saliva [N. m. ch. Wahrn., 1.c.]

Slimey in the mouth and throat (aft. 2 h.).

Ejection of grey mucus by hawking.

Salty expectoration (by hawking?). [RICHARD, 1.c.]

355. Bitter expectoration. [RICHARD, 1.c.]

Green, bitter expectoration (by hawking) in the morning.

Bitterness in the mouth, with yellow diarrhoea. [MORGAGNI, 1.c.]

Bitter taste in the mouth, after a meal.

Bitter disgusting taste in the mouth, after eating and drinking.

360. Bitterness in the throat, after eating, while the food tastes normally on alternate days *(like a tertian fever).*

Bitter taste in the mouth, without having eaten anything.

Bitter taste in the mouth, in the morning. [Hg.]

Wooden, dry taste in the mouth.

Rotten fetid taste in the mouth.

365. Putrid taste in the morning, as of putrid meat.

Sour taste in the mouth, all the food tastes sour.

All the food tastes salty.

The food tastes as if it had too little salt.

The beer tastes flat.

370. The unhopped beer tastes bitter.

Stomach.

Adipsia, lack of thirst.

Thirst. [PREUSSIUS 1.c.; RAU, 1.c.; PET DE APPONO, de ven.[1]]

Great thirst. [ALBERTI, 1. c., TOM. II.]

Severe thirst, constant. [BUETTNER, 1.c.]

375. Violent thirst. [MAJAULT, 1.c.]

Choking thirst. [FORESTUS, 1.c.]

Burning thirst. [MAJAULT, 1.c.[2]]

Unquenchable thirst. [BUCHHOLZ, 1. c.; GUILBERT, 1. c.; CREUGER.]

Unquenchable thirst, with dryness of the tongue, the fauces and the gullet. [GUELDENKLEE, 1.c.]

380. Uncommon thirst, so that he has to drink much cold water every ten minutes, from morning till evening, but not at night. [Fr., H.]

Extremely violent thirst and drinking affords no refreshment and refection. [KAISER, 1.c.]

He drinks much and often. [Stf.]

With great thirst, he drinks often, but always little at a time. [RICHARD, 1.c.[3]]

Violent thirst, but he only drinks little at a time. [Whl.]

285

385. Violent thirst, not without appetite for eating. [KNAPE, 1.c.]
Lack of appetite, with violent thirst. [STOERK, med. Jahrg. I. p. 207.⁴]
Lack of appetite. [JACOBI, 1.c.]
Loss of appetite. [KAISER, 1.c.]
Total lack of appetite. [BUCHHOLZ, in Hufel. Journ., 1. c.]
390. No appetite, but when he eats he relishes food.
Lack of hunger and appetite for ten days. [Fr., H.]
Aversion to all food, she cannot eat anything.
Loathing of food. [GRIMM, 1. c.; GOERITZ, in Bresl. Samml., 1728.¹]
Loathing of all food. [ALBERTI, 1.c.]
395. Irresistible loathing of all food, so that he cannot think of eating without nausea. [EBERS, 1. c.]
It is impossible for him to get his food down. [RICHARD, 1. c.]
The smell of boiled meat is unbearable to him. [RICHARD, 1. c.]
Repugnance to butter.
Desire for brandy. [Hg.]
400. Desire for sour things. [Stf.]
Desire for vinegar and water.
Great desire for acids and acidulous fruit.
Great desire for coffee.
Great appetite for milk, to which before she was averse.
405. While eating, a compressive sensation on the chest.
Soon after breakfast and after dinner, pressure on the stomach with empty eructations for three hours, causing a lassitude of body which produced squeamishness.
Before eating, nausea, and after eating or drinking, distension or pressure and cutting in the abdomen.
Eructation, after taking food.
Much eructation, especially after drinking.
410. Ineffectual efforts to eructate.
Eructation, caused by flatus coming upward.
Constant eructation. [GOERITZ, 1.c.]
Frequent empty eructation (aft. ½ h.). [Lgh.]
Frequent empty eructation.
415. Constant, severe, empty eructation, with numb feeling of the head. (aft. 36 h.)
Sour eructation after dinner.
Bitter eructation after eating with belching up of greenish, bitter mucus.
An acrid liquid rises into the mouth.
Frequent hiccup after eating, every time followed by eructation. [Lgh.]
420. Frequent hiccup and eructation. [MORGAGNI, 1.c.]
Convulsive hiccup. [ALBERTI, 1.c.]
Hiccup, at night, when rising, with scratching, nauseous taste in the mouth.
Long-continued hiccup, in the hour when the fever should have come.
Qualmishness at 11 A.M. and at 3 P.M.
425. Nausea. [PFANN,¹ Samml, merkw. Falle, Nurnb., 1750, pp. 129, 130; N. Wahrn, 1 c.; KAISER, 1.c.]
Nausea in the fauces and stomach.
Nausea, with anguish. [ALBERTI, 1.c.]

Long-continued nausea, with faintness, trembling, heat all over, followed by a shiver. (aft. some h.)

Qualmishness and nausea *compelling the person to lie down* in the forenoon, at the same time tearing about the ankle and the dorsum of the foot.

430. Frequent nausea, with a sweetish taste in the mouth, not immediately after eating.

Nausea, more in the throat, with gathering of water in the mouth.

Nausea, with abortive waterbrash, shortly before and after dinner.

Nausea, when sitting; much water collected in the mouth, as in waterbrash; while walking, the nausea passed off, followed by a discharge of a copious pappy stool (aft. 7 h.). [Lgh.]

Heartburn, at 4 P.M.

435. Sickness at stomach. [MAJAULT, 1.c.[2]]

Inclination to vomit. [KAISER, 1.c.]

Nausea, in the open air.

Empty retching. [RAU, 1.c.]

Nausea and violent vomiting. [Htb. u. Tr.[3]]

440. Nausea, qualmishness on raising oneself up in bed, and frequently, sudden vomiting. [Stf]

Vomiting. [MAJAULT, *1. c.*; GRIMM, *and many others.*]

Vomiting immediately after every meal, without nausea. [Fr. H.]

The child vomits after eating and drinking, and then will neither eat nor drink, but sleeps well.

Vomiting of all the ingesta, for several weeks. [Salzb. m. chir. Zeit.]

445. Excessive vomiting produced with the greatest effort, of drinks, yellowish-green mucus and water, with very bitter taste in the mouth, which remained a long time afterward. [Stf.]

Vomiting of a thick, glassy mucus. [RICHARD, 1.c.]

Vomiting of mucus and green bile. [ALBERTI, 1.c.[4]]

Vomiting of a thin, bluish, smutty-yellow matter, followed by great prostration and exhaustion. [KAISER, 1.c.]

Vomiting of brownish, dark matter, sometimes thick, sometimes thin, with violent efforts and increased stomachache, without subsequent relief. [KAISER, 1. c.]

450. Vomiting of a brownish matter, often mixed with blood, with a violent bodily effort. [KAISER, 1. c.]

Vomiting of bloody mucus. [N. Wahrn., 1. c.]

Vomiting of blood. [KELLNER, in Bresl. Samml., 1727.[1]]

Discharged blood upward and downward. [GERBITZ, in Ephem. Nat. Cur. Dec. III, ann. 5, 6, obs. 137.[2]]

When vomiting ceases, frequent, very watery diarrhoeic stools set in. [Htb. u. Tr.[3]]

455. Excessive vomiting and purging. [PREUSSIUS, 1. c.]

Violent, continual vomiting, with diarrhoea. [MORGAGNI, 1. c.]

Vomiting, with diarrhoea, as soon as the swoon goes off. [FORRESTUS, 1. c.]

During the vomiting, which continues night and day, frightful cries. [HEIMREICH, 1. c.[4]]

During the vomiting, complains of severe internal heat and thirst. [ALBERTI, 1. c.]

460. During the violent vomiting, severe internal burning, thirst and heat. [ALBERTI, 1. c.]
Frequent vomiting, with *dread of death*. [ALBERTI, 1. c.]
Pains in the stomach. [QUELMAIZ, 1. c.; RICHARD, and several others.]
Great painfulness of the stomach. [N. Wahrn., 1. c.]
Pains in the stomach, causing nausea. [RICHARD, 1. c.]

465. Excessive pains in the region of the scrobiculus cordis. [S. PH. WOLFF, Act, Nat. c., V, obs. 29 [5]]
Heaviness in the stomach, as if it were being violently distended in its whole extent and were being torn. [KOPP, Jahrb. d. Staatsarzneik. II, p. 182.]
Trouble in the stomach, as if it were tormented with flatus; much aggravated after vomiting and diarrhoea. [MORGAGNI, 1.c.[6]]
Bloatedness and distension of the stomach and the hypochondriac region, before a stool ensues. [RICHARD, 1. c.]
Bloatedness of the region of the stomach. [KAISER, 1.c.]

470. The stomach begins to raise itself, and is warmer than the rest of the body. [KAISER, 1. c.]
Sensation of fullness in the stomach, with distaste for eating, and stomachache after it; in the evening.
Heaviness in the stomach, as from a stone, after eating. [Hbg.]
Pressive feeling of heaviness in the stomach. [MORGAGNI, 1.c.]
Pressure in the region of the stomach and the scrobiculus cordis; pressure on the heart. [KELLNER, 1. c.; GOERTZ and many others.[7]]

475. It felt as if it would break her heart.
It felt as if it would break his heart. [Stf.]
Pressure on the mouth of the stomach and in the oesophagus, after eating, as if the food remained on top; then empty eructation.
Pressure about the stomach, so that he cannot stand it, whenever he had eaten anything, not at once, but some time after eating.
Pressure in the anterior wall of the stomach, on speaking (aft. ½ h.).

480. Hard pressure above the scrobiculus cordis (at once).
Cramp-like pain of the stomach, two hours after midnight.
Periodic cramp-like pains in the stomach and the bowels. [KAISER, 1. c.]
Cramps of the stomach, of excessive violence, with thirst. [BUCHHOLZ, 1. c.]
Cramps of the stomach, with violent bellyache, diarrhoea and faintings. [LOEW, in SYDENHAM. Op. II, p. 324.[1]]

485. Cutting pain in the stomach. [THILENIUS, 1.c.]
Drawing pain, in the evening while sitting, from the scrobiculus cordis to the left ribs all around, as if something were violently torn off there.
Dull tearing, transversely across the region of the stomach, when walking, in the afternoon.
Tearing, pressive, spasmodic pain in the stomach. [KAISER, 1. c.]
Violent, tearing, boring pain and cramp in the stomach and bowels. [KAISER, 1. c.]

490. Gnawing and prickling (sharp and fine throbbing) pain in the scrobiculus cordis, with sensation of tension.
Eroding, gnawing pain in the stomach. [RICHARD, 1. c.]
Heat with pain and pressure in the scrobiculus cordis [KAISER, 1. c.]
Burning in the scrobiculus cordis. [BUCHHOLZ, 1. c.; KAISER, 1.c.]
Burning all around the scrobiculus cordis.

495. Burning pain in the stomach. [EBERS, 1. c.[2]]
Burning in the stomach like fire. [RICHARD, 1.c.]
Constant burning and severe constriction in the stomach and in the chest. [BORGES in Kopp's Jahrb., 1.c.]
Burning in the stomach, with pressure as from a load. [MORGAGNI, 1.c.]
Burning in the scrobiculus cordis, with pressive pain. [GOERITZ, 1. c.]
500. Constriction in the scrobiculus cordis. [Hbg.]
Great distress about the region of the scrobiculus cordis. [MORGAGNI, 1.c; JACOBI and others.]
Wails and lamentations about an indescribable distress in the region of the scrobiculus cordis, without distension or colic. [MORGAGNI, 1.c.[1]]
Distress in the scrobiculus cordis, rising up from it, at night.

Abdomen.
In the liver, a squeezing pressure, on taking a walk.
505. The spleen, indurated before, now swells. [Hg.]
Stitches in the side of the abdomen, under the short ribs, and he cannot lie on his side.
In the region of the kidneys, stitches, when respiring and when sneezing.
Pains in the abdomen of the most violent kind. [DAN CRUEGER, Misc., N.C. Dec. II. Ann. 4. O. 12.[2]]
Excessive bellyache and pains in the stomach. [WOLFF, 1.c.]
510. Exceedingly disagreeable sensation in the whole of the abdomen. [MORGAGNI, 1.c.]
Pains in the hypogastrium, with heat in the face.
Violent pain in the region of the right epigastrium. [MORGAGNI, 1.c.]
Pains in the right epigastrium and the neighboring inguinal regions, which extends thence at times through the hypogastrium, at times into the right side of the flanks and the scrotum, like a renal colic; but with unchanged urine. [MORGAGNI, 1.c.]
Roving pains in the abdomen, with diarrhoea and pains in the anus. [MORGAGNI, 1. c.]
515. The pain in the abdomen established itself in the left side of the belly.
Pain, as if the upper part of the body was altogether cut off from the abdomen, with great anguish and lamentation over it. [ALBERTI, 1.c., Tom. IV.[3]]
Violent pains in the abdomen, with so great anguish that he had no rest anywhere, rolled about on the ground, and gave up all hope of living. [PYL, 1.c.]
Fullness in the region of the epigastrium, with griping in the belly.
Distension and pains in the abdomen. [MUELLER, 1. c.]
520. Severe, painless distension of the abdomen after eating; he had to lean his back against something to ease himself.
Bloatedness every morning, with passage of flatus a few hours afterwards.
Swollen abdomen. [GUILBERT, 1. c.[2]]
The abdomen enormously swollen. [Ephen. N.C., 1.c.]
As if there were cramps and griping in the abdomen, in the nervous, in the evening, after lying down, with breaking out of perspiration; then passage of flatus and very thin stool.

525. Spasmodic jerk, frequently, from the scrobiculus cordis to the rectum, which makes him start.

Squeezing, cutting pains in the bowels, in the evening after lying down, and in the morning after rising; at times the pains shoot through the abdominal ring (as if they would force out a hernia) as far as the spermatic cord and the perinaeum; when this colic ceases a loud rumbling and grumbling ensues. Colics, returning from time to time. [MAJAULT, 1. c.[1]]

Pinching pain, aggravated even to cutting, deep in the hypogastrium, every morning, before and during the diarrhoeic stools, and continuing also after them.

Cutting pain in the abdomen. [BUCHHOLZ, 1. c.; KELLNER, 1. c.]

530. Cutting pain in the side of the abdomen, below the last ribs, very much aggravated by touching them.

Cutting (tearing) and gnawing pains in the bowels and the stomach. [QUELMALZ, 1.c.[2]]

Cutting and tearing in the abdomen, with icy-coldness of the hands and feet and cold perspiration of the face. [ALBERTI, 1.c.]

Tearing in the abdomen. [PEANN, 1. c.; ALBERTI, 1.c.]

Tearing stitches in the left side of the abdomen, under the short ribs, in the evening soon after lying down.

535. Drawing pains in the abdomen, in the umbilical region (aft. 2.h.).

Drawing and pressing in the abdomen, as far obstructed flatus, and yet none passed off. [Whl.]

Twisting together of the intestines, and cutting in the belly, after previous rumbling there; then three diarrhoeic stools.

Contortion of the intestines, and squeezing and rumbling in the abdomen, before and during the liquid stool. [Mr.]

Burrowing, with pressure, in the right side of the abdomen. [Hbg.]

540. Twisting colic. [RICHARD, 1.c.[3]]

Twisting and griping in the abdomen. [KAISER, 1.c.]

Dysenteric colic in the umbilical region. [GRIMM, 1.c.[4]]

Uneasiness in the abdomen, but only during rest.

Anxious feeling in the abdomen, with fever and thirst. [MORGAGNI, 1.c.]

545. *Constant chilliness, internally, in the epigastric region;* cannot keep himself warm enough; externally the place feels warm.

Burning pain in the abdomen, at noon and in the afternoon, passing off with the discharge of a stool.

Burning in the abdomen, with stitches and cutting. [BUCHHOLZ, Beitr., 1.c.]

Burning in the abdomen, with heat and thirst. [ALBERTI, 1.c.]

Burning in the flanks. [Hbg.]

550. In the groin and the inguinal region of the right side, pain in stooping, as from a sprain.

Burrowing, burning pain in the inguinal tumor, excited even by the lightest touch.

Single, severe, slow stitches in both flanks.

Weakness of the abdominal muscles.

Rumbling in the abdomen, as if from much flatus.

555. Growling in the stomach, in the morning on awaking.

Rumbling in the abdomen. [THINLENIUS, 1.c.]

Rumbling in the abdomen, without stool.

The flatus tends to pass upward and causes eructations.

Rectum and Anus.

Passage of much flatus, with previous loud growling in the abdomen. [Lgh.]

560. Putrid smelling flatus (aft. 11 h.). [Lgh.]

(Clotted, insufficient stool.).

Constipation [GOERITZ, 1. c.; RAU, 1. c.[1]]

Constipated abdomen.

Constipation, with pain in the abdomen. [Htb. u. Tr.[2]]

565. Retention of stool, despite of violent urging. [ALBERTI, 1. c.]

Fruitless urging to stool.

Tenesmus, with burning. [MORGAGNI, 1. c.]

Tenesmus, as in dysentery; a constant burning, with pain and straining in the rectum and anus.

Unperceived discharge of stool, as if it were flatus.

570. Stools pass without his knowledge. [BUETTNER, 1.c.[3]]

Copious stools. [KAISER, 1. c.]

Pappy faeces pass, now more, now less (aft. 6, 13 h.). [Lgh.]

Diarrhoea. [MAJAULT, 1.c.; KELLNER, 1. c.]

575. Diarrhoea, which frequently becomes very severe. [KAISER, 1. c.]

Diarrhoea, with violent burning in the anus. [THILENIUS, 1.c.]

Diarrhoea, alternating with constipation. [Stf.]

Yellow, watery, scanty diarrhoeic stools, with subsequent tenesmus, as if more stool would pass, and painful colic about the navel. [Stf.]

Yellow, diarrhoeic stool, with tenesmus and burning pains in the rectum and anus.

580. Small stools, with tenesmus, first with dark-green faeces then of dark-green mucus, with previous colic.

Evacuation of lungs of mucus, with cutting pains in the anus, as of blind piles.

Mucous, thin stools, as if hacked.

Mucous and green evacuations. [PHILENIUS, 1.c.]

Viscid, bilious matter is often discharged with the stool, for two days. [PHILENIUS, 1.c.[1]]

585. Greenish, dark-brown, diarrhoeic stool, with a smell as of fetid ulcers. [Hg.]

A black fluid, burning in the anus like fire, is discharged after much restlessness and pain in the abdomen. [RICHARD, 1. c.]

Black, acrid, putrid stools. [BAYLIES, 1.c.]

A spherical lump, which to seemed consist of undigested tallow with layers of tendinous matter, went off with the stool. [MORGAGNI, 1.c.[2]]

Watery blood is discharged with the faeces and envelops them.

590. Bloody discharge with the stool, almost every moment, with vomiting and excessive colicky pains. [GRIMM, 1.c.]

Dysentery. [CRUEGER, 1.c.]

Before the diarrhoeic stool, cutting and contortion in the bowels.

Before the diarrhoeic stool, sensation as if he would burst. [ALBERTI, 1. c.]

291

During the stool, painful contraction close above the anus, toward the small of the back.

595. After the stool, cessation of the colic. [RICHARD, 1.c.]

After the stool, burning in the rectum, with great weakness and trembling in all the limbs.

After the stool, distension of the abdomen.

After the stool, palpitation and tremulous weakness; he has to lie down.

The rectum is spasmodically protruded and pressed out, with great pains.

600. After a flow of blood from the anus, the rectum continues to protrude.

Itching of the anus.

Scraping or erosive pain in the anus, with itching.

Pain of the anus as of soreness, on being touched.

Burning in the anus.

605. Burning in the anus. [MORGAGNI, 1.c.]

Burning in the anus, for one hour, going off after the discharge of a hard, clotted stool.

Stinging itching, anteriorly on the prepuce.

Severe itching on the glans, without erection.

The hemorrhoidal veins are painfully swollen, with tenesmus. [MORGAGNI, 1. c.]

Blind piles, with pains like slow pricks with a hot needle.

Varices on the anus, with pricking pain, when walking and sitting, not during the stool.

610. *Hemorrhoidal lumps at the anus,* which especially at night. *pain and burn like fire* and permit no sleep; during the day the pain becomes aggravated and changes into violent stitches; worse when walking than when sitting or lying down.

On the perinaeum eroding itching, compelling him to scratch (aft. ½ h.). [Lgh.]

Urinary Organs.

Suppression of urine. [GUILBERT, 1.c.; N. Wahrn., 1. c.]

Retention of urine, as from paralysis of the bladder.

Retention of urine despite of internal urging to urinate. [ALBERTI, 1. c.]

615. *Frequent urging to urinate,* with copious flow of urine (aft. 2 to 17 h.). [Lgh.]

Urging to urinate every minute, with burning in the bladder.

He has to rise at night three or four times to urinate, and each time he passes a good deal, for several days in succession.

Involuntary micturition at night, when sleeping, wetting the bed. [Hg.]

Involuntary micturition. [KAISER, 1.c.]

620. Involuntary micturition; she could not get to the utensil before the urine ran from her, though it was but a little.

Diminished micturition. [FOWLER, 1. c.[1]]

But little water passes, and it scalds during the flow.

Increase of urine. [FOWLER, 1. c.[1]]

Very copious and burning hot urine. [Hg.]

625. Almost colorless urine.

Exceedingly turbid urine (aft. 5 d.).

Greenish, dark-brown urine, turbid already when passed, like cowdung stirred into water, without settling. [Hg.]

Bloody urine. [O. TACHENIUS, Hipp. chym. cap., 24.[2]]

When beginning to urinate, burning in the anterior part of the urethra; in the morning (aft. 24 h.).

630. *During micturition, burning in the urethra.* [MORGAGNI, 1. c; N. Wahrn., 1.c.]

During micturition, contractive pain in the left iliac region.

After micturition, sensation of great weakness in the epigastrium, so that she trembled.

In the urethra, a stinging pain.

Frequent pain, like tearing, deep in the urethra.

Male Sexual Organs.

635. In the genitals, itching.

Burning anteriorly on the prepuce, with erection.

Involuntary passage of faeces. [KAISER, 1. c.]

Eroding itching posteriorly on the penis, compelling him to scratch. [Lgh.]

640. *Inflammation and swelling of the genitals, even to mortification,* with excessive pains. [DEGNER, Act. Nat. C. VI, app., pp. 8,9.[1]]

Sudden mortification of the male genitals. [STAHL, Opusc. chym. phys. med., p. 454.[2]]

Exceedingly painful swelling of the genitals. [N. Wahrn, 1.c.]

The glans is bluish-red, swollen and cracked in chaps. [PFANN, 1. c.]

Swelling of the testicles. [ALBERTI, 1.c.[3]]

645. Erection in the morning without pollution. [Lgh.]

Pollution at night, with voluptuous dreams. [Lgh.]

Pollution, at night, without voluptuous dreams, followed by long continued erection. [Lgh.]

Emission of prostatic juice during a diarrhoeic stool.

Female Sexual Organs.

Sexual furor in a woman; she desires coitus twice a day, and when it is not accorded, a discharge takes place of itself.

650. *Menses too early.*

The menses set in twice too early, returning in twenty days.

Menstruation too profuse.

During the menses, pinching, lancinating cutting from the scrobiculus cordis down to the hypogastrium, also in the back and in the sides of the abdomen; she had to bend herself double, standing and covering down, with loud eructation and loud groaning, wailing and weeping.

During the menses, sharp stitches from the rectum into the anus and the pudenda.

655. Instead of the menses, which were suppressed, she had pains in the region of the anus and the shoulders. [Sr.]

After the menses, a flow of bloody mucus.

A discharge of leucorrhoea while standing, with discharge of flatus (aft. 24 h.).

Discharge from the vagina about a cupful in twenty-four hours of yellowish, thickish matter, with smarting erosion and excoriation of all the parts it touches; for ten days.

Stitches from the hypogastrium down into the vagina.

The other half of the proving concerns the following:

Respiratory Organs.
Chest.
Neck and Back.
Lower Extremities.
Nervous System.
Skin.
Sleep.
Fever.

Appendix B

Patient Evaluations at One Month

The following descriptions and diagrams are not designed to cover *every* eventuality. Nevertheless, if they are studied thoughtfully, the student will perceive the basic principles underlying the interpretation. They should not be learned by memory—to be applied in a routine manner. Rather, they should be studied meditatively in order to arrive at the inner principles underlying them. Only in this way will the reader gain a true understanding of the single direction in which cure proceeds. These descriptions and diagrams, although often oversimplistic in themselves, bring to bear all of the laws and principles which have been described thus far.

One word of caution in interpreting the diagrams: the figures included in this chapter describe on the vertical axis the *intensity of symptoms,* and on the horizontal axis, time. To be truly accurate from the point of view of homeopathy, I would have to present the diagrams in terms of the overall *health* of the patient; in this way, I would show an improvement as moving higher on the graph rather than lower (declining intensity of symptoms) as is shown. It is presented in this manner because the patient is most likely to describe symptoms in this way. Even though it is somewhat incorrect in terms of the activity of the defense mechanism, patients do measure health in terms of presence or absence of symptoms. For this reason, this convention will be followed in these diagrams.

Another point to emphasize in interpreting the diagrams is that the lines shown are purposely *not* shown as straight lines. All patients show some degree of variation in symptoms from day to day. If symptoms are observed over time intervals which are too short, i.e., hours or days, the overall progress of the patient can easily be misinterpreted. On any given day, it can appear that a significant aggravation or amelioration is occurring, whereas in reality the changes are merely due to random daily fluctuations.

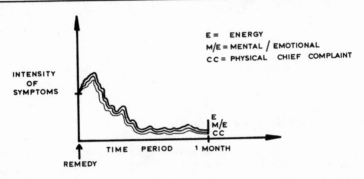

Figure 16:

CASE I:

Patient: "I feel much better—in every way."

Case: Definite aggravation, then definite improvement of all symptoms.

Interpretation: Remedy was precise. Strong defense mechanism. Good prognosis.

Prescription: Wait a long time—likely six months or more.

CASE I:

In this case the patient reports a dramatic improvement. Every major symptom—physical chief complaint, energy, mental/emotional symptoms—are reported to be definitely better compared to before administration of the first remedy. Even minor symptoms have undergone favorable change. The homeopath is encouraged by this report, but every detail is nevertheless checked for accuracy. Upon inquiry, it turns out that the patient did indeed experience an initial aggravation of some or all symptoms within a few days after taking the remedy. This was forgotten, however, in the face of the dramatic improvement which ensued during the rest of the month.

Of course, this is the best of all possible responses. This report is what every homeopath wishes for every patient. The initial aggravation signifies the stimulative effect of the remedy

296

upon the defense mechanism, and the definite and dramatic improvement confirms this action. In any practice, perhaps only 70% of such patients will actually recall the original aggravation. Another 30% may experience a response which is just as curative in the long run, but the initial aggravation is not clearly recalled. Sometimes this is because the symptoms were already so aggravated prior to taking the remedy that a further aggravation was difficult to distinguish. Often, the primary symptoms in such cases are mental or emotional, and quantitation is difficult. In any case, the key observation is that *all* symptoms on all levels have been improved within one month.

A distinct initial aggravation of short duration (from a few hours to three days) followed by a definite amelioration within one month signifies that the remedy was precisely the *simillimum*. It also means that the prognosis is very good for the patient, because the original disease was primarily focused upon functional levels and involved very little organic pathology. The patient's defense mechanism was already quite strong prior to administration of the remedy, and the well-selected medicine has further strengthened it in a curative direction.

After such a positive response, the equilibrium attained within the organism can be expected to last for a long time—say, from six months to many years. The patient will very likely not require further prescriptions for a very long time. Another follow-up visit should be held within another month, but there is every reason for expecting the amelioration to continue. If this turns out to be indeed true, later visits could be spaced out to every three months, every six months, and eventually every year. Of course, the patient should always be instructed that if any relapse occurs, or if intercurrent illnesses happen, earlier visits are encouraged. Nevertheless, it can be expected that any further ailments will be of a relatively minor nature.

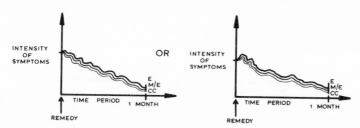

Figure 17:

CASE II:

Patient: "I feel very much better."

Case: Marked amelioration with little or no aggravation. Better in every respect—chief complaint, energy, mentally/emotionally.

Interpretation: 1) Precise *simillimum* and exact potency in a case with no pathological changes, or 2) case was already severely aggravated at the outset (severe chronic case, or an acute case). Good prognosis in both instances.

Prescription: Wait.

CASE II:

This circumstance is very similar to the previous one. Here, a dramatic amelioration is observed with *no* (or an unnoticeable) aggravation in the beginning. A careful review of all symptoms and their changes throughout the month confirms this report.

In such a case, the remedy was a perfect match to the resonant frequency of the patient, and moreover the chosen potency was as nearly perfect as can ever be expected. It may have been that the optimal potency for the patient was 195c, and a 200 was given. In such a perfect prescription, amelioration occurs without any significant aggravation. Again, the "second prescription" will then be to *wait* for a very long time (perhaps years)

before giving another remedy.

Another interpretation of this circumstance may be that the patient's condition was *already* aggravated to its maximum prior to the remedy. This means that the defense mechanism was at its highest pitch of activity before the medicine was administered. The correct remedy therefore simply produced an imperceptible aggravation followed by an amelioration. Such a circumstance is quite rare, but it can occur in chronic cases suffering very extremely at the outset of treatment. It is also commonly observed during acute ailments; this is the reason why it is usually said that aggravations are virtually never observed in acute illnesses.

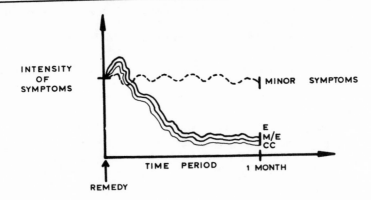

Figure 18:

CASE III:

Patient: "I feel better, but still have problems."

Case: Major symptoms ameliorated after an aggravation, while minor symptoms are unchanged.

Interpretation: Correct remedy. Good prognosis.

Prescription: Wait.

CASE III:

This situation is less clear in its interpretation. The patient reports an improvement in terms of the chief complaint, the mental/emotional state, and the energy, but some of the less important homeopathic symptoms (say, warmbloodedness, craving for sweets, sensitivity to noise, constipation, etc.) show no change. This situation is encountered in perhaps the majority of cured cases.

It is here that an overly perfectionistic homeopath can do a lot of harm. The prognosis in this circumstance is very good because all three of the major symptoms show a dramatic improvement following an aggravation. Treatment of the minor symptoms at this point must be avoided. If the pre-scriber is impatient, however, and gives another remedy based upon the remaining minor symptoms, the case may become disrupted.

The best course in such a case is to reassure the patient about the good response, and then to wait for a long time. Very likely, the minor homeopathic symptoms will gradually disappear over a period of three months or longer. They should not be prescribed upon at the moment. In case these minor symptoms remain with the patient after a long time, and if they are annoying, the homeopath should retake the case; most probably it will be found that one of the complementary remedies is then indicated.

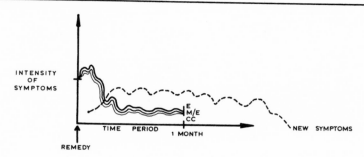

Figure 19:

CASE IV:

Patient: "I feel better, but I have a few new symptoms."

Case: Definite aggravation followed by amelioration, but some new symptoms develop which are characteristic of the remedy given.

Interpretation: Correct remedy, with "false proving." Good prognosis.

Prescription: Wait. New symptoms will disappear.

CASE IV:

This is another situation which is commonly encountered, and it represents another instance in which the homeopath is quite liable to make a serious mistake. The patient reports a dramatic improvement of all major symptoms, and further questioning reveals that there was an aggravation within the first few days. However, the patient reports new symptoms which are very characteristic of the remedy given.

For example, the patient may have initially complained of a lack of energy, recurrent aphthae, and herpetic skin eruptions. After taking the full case, Natrum muriaticum is prescribed. After one month, the patient says, "Boy, that is powerful stuff! Within a few days, I felt wiped out and all of my aphthae and herpes were much worse! However, since then they have disappeared. I have felt great, better than I have for twenty years! Now, though, I seem to get headaches at 10 A.M. several days of the week. Strange. I have never had headaches prior to taking this remedy." It is immediately realized that 10 A.M. headaches are very characteristic of Natrum muriaticum. The general state is improved, but a new symptom corresponding to the remedy is present.

This must not be misinterpreted as being a proving which should be antidoted. In fact, it confirms very nicely that the prescription was exact; the recommendation therefore must be, "Wait!" The new symptom is merely a manifestation of the remedy, and it will pass within a few weeks at the latest, leaving the patient feeling very well. This interpretation of the appearance of a new and characteristic symptom, however, is valid *only* when the general condition of the patient has been simultaneously ameliorated.

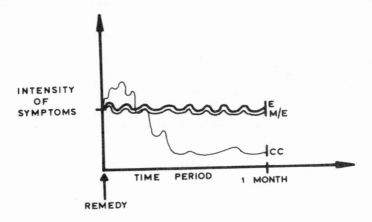

Figure 20:

CASE V:

Patient: "My main problem is better, but I am still not well."

Case: Chief complaint better after a brief aggravation, but other major symptoms unchanged.

Interpretation: 1) Very likely that deeper planes were relatively unaffected in the first place. 2) May be early phase of curative response.

Prescription: Wait.

CASE V:

Now we can begin to encounter cases in which the interpretation is less clear. The patient reports no change in energy or mental/emotional state, but the physical chief complaint shows a definite aggravation followed by dramatic amelioration.

Such an observation can occur in patients who have no problems with energy or mental/emotional states in the first place. There is little to expect on these levels simply because there were no problems to begin with. In the instance in which the patient did have some minor problems on mental/emotional levels, the change in the physical chief complaint may well be heralding an improvement on the other levels as well, but not enough time has yet elapsed to observe them. It is always a positive sign if even one of the major indicators—chief complaint, energy, or mental/emotional symptoms—changes favorably. It is furthermore encouraging that the chief complaint improved after an initial aggravation.

Even though the patient is not yet completely well, it is important to wait in cases such as this. A curative response is probably underway, and no chances should be taken which might interfere with it.

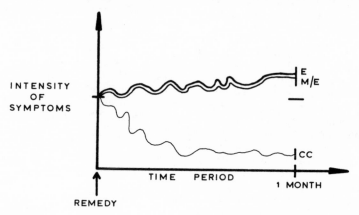

Figure 21:

CASE VI:

Patient: "I am better, but not really well."

Case: Chief complaint is better *without* aggravation, no change in energy or mental/emotional symptoms. No new symptoms.

Interpretation: Remedy close enough but not exact.

Prescription: Look again at original case to see if better remedy. 1) If cannot see a better original remedy, carefully retake the case. If remedy is clear, give it. 2) If no clear remedy upon re-taking the case, wait until new image becomes apparent.

301

CASE VI:

This case is similar to Case V, but with an important subtle difference. The patient reports some degree of worsening of symptoms on the energy and mental/emotional levels, but the chief complaint has definitely improved. After careful questioning, however, the homeopath discovers that the amelioration of the chief complaint was *not* preceded by an aggravation.

This amelioration without aggravation, coupled with a somewhat aggravated energy or mental/emotional state, represents an adverse circumstance. The remedy was close, but not exact. An improvement on physical levels combined with a decline on deeper levels means that the remedy has actually decreased the general health of the patient.

It is important to notice the drastically different interpretation in this case compared with Case V, even though the variations are quite subtle. This contrast underscores the importance of accurate reporting on the part of the patient, and the need for objective evaluation on the part of the prescriber. If a superficial impression were to be followed in such a case, an adverse influence would be allowed to continue unnecessarily. The mistake would become clear only after two or three months, during which time the patient's health may have deteriorated significantly.

The first step in managing such a circumstance is to look very carefully again at the original case. The initial remedy was close, but a better remedy is needed. If the original case was well-taken, a review may very well reveal the correct remedy. The homeopath, upon re-reading the original case, may say, "Oh my God! That's the true remedy. Why didn't I see it before?" This is a common event in the career of beginning homeopaths whose prescribing skills have yet to undergo further refinement.

If a more precise medicine is seen in the original case, then it should be given. This is so even though the current picture may have changed since the first prescription. Having been changed by an imprecise remedy, the current image is not to be relied upon for a new prescription.

If no remedy is clear upon review of the case, then the only alternative is to wait. Eventually (probably within a few weeks), the changes in the defense mechanism will stabilize into the original image. At that point, a completely re-taken case will most probably reveal a clear image, and then that remedy can be given.

The worse response would be to make a wild stab at the best possible remedy when the image is not yet clear. This would very likely result in further confusion of an already disordered case.

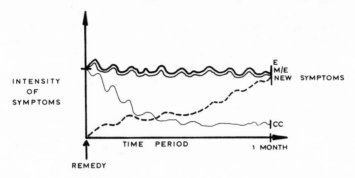

Figure 22:

CASE VII:

Patient: "My original problem is better, but now I have another one."

Case: Chief complaint better without aggravation, while new and deeper problem has emerged. No change in energy or mental-emotional state.

Interpretation: Suppressive and disruptive effect of medicine.

Prescription: 1) Study again the original case to discover the correct remedy in the first place. 2) If no remedy is apparent, antidote with allopathic drugs, coffee, or camphor, and then wait for new clear image to emerge.

CASE VII:

Here, we have a circumstance which is somewhat unusual, but by no means unheard of, especially in the first years of prescribing. The patient reports no significant change in energy or mental/emotional symptoms, and the chief complaint has diminished quite a bit, but some intense new symptoms have replaced it.

If the information is truly reliable, then we have suppressed one symptom and another has come up in its place. If, with this new symptom, there has not formed a new picture of another remedy and the case seems confused, then study again the original case to see if you can find a better remedy.

If no better medicine can be found from the original case, the best choice is to wait until the new symptoms subside and the image returns to its original state, provided the severity of the patient's condition allows it. If, however, the new state is causing a great deal of suffering, the best policy would be to try to antidote the action of the first remedy. This can best be done by giving ordinary allopathic drugs for palliation, or by having the patient drink significant amounts of coffee (or even by trying to rub large amounts of camphor into the skin). After a period of two or three weeks of allopathic treatment or coffee, stop the palliative or antidoting process and wait for one week to allow the system to settle into a new image. Then re-take the case and prescribe once again.

In such suppressed cases, it is very

303

important not to try to give a new remedy based upon the changed new image. This would likely lead to even further disordering of the case. It is also advisable not to try to antidote the remedy by another homeopathic medicine; any homeopathic remedy which can have an antidoting effect upon the system is likely to be close enough to the resonant frequency of the organism to cause further disturbance. It is much more desirable simply to simply allow time to produce a better image upon which to prescribe.

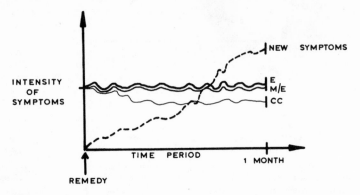

Figure 23:

CASE VIII:

Patient: "My original problem is a little better, but now there are some severe new changes."

Case: Chief complaint a *little* better, but new problems dominate the case. New remedy image is more full than originally.

Interpretation: One-sided case. Original remedy helped to bring out full picture.

Prescription: Give new remedy based on full current image.

CASE VIII:

This situation represents a somewhat unusual eventuality, but one which requires a good knowledge of homeopathy to interpret. The patient feels very little change in any realm, except that the chief complaint *might* be a little bit better. Meanwhile, however, a spectrum of new symptoms emerge which show even greater intensity than the original ailment and which now present a clear picture of a new remedy.

This is an example of what Hahnemann calls *one-sided cases* (described in Aphorisms 172-184). The initial disease image represented only a fragment of the totality. Hahnemann describes their cases as exhibiting only one or two symptoms upon which to prescribe, but in my experience there can be quite a few more. The primary principle involved here is that the full totality is not expressed in the initial image. This can occur for a variety of reasons: the case may have been severely suppressed by allopathic drugs, the patient may have become too withdrawn and "closed," or the energy

304

of the defense mechanism may have become excessively focused upon just a few symptoms.

In any case, the full image was not present initially, and the first prescription therefore was only partial to the full case. Nevertheless, it was close enough to create a beneficial effect, and the organism was then freed to express the full totality of symptoms. The patient may complain that harm has been created by the remedy because of all the new symptoms, but in reality the homeopath is now in a position to prescribe a truly curative remedy.

In this situation, the entire case must be carefully re-taken in order to elucidate the full totality. A new remedy should then be prescribed upon the full image. If a correct remedy is chosen, the ensuing response can be expected to be very favorable.

There are many homeopaths who talk about giving first prescriptions designed to "clear" a case. If many allopathic drugs have been given, or if other factors have produced confusion in a case, such homeopaths begin the case routinely (paying only scant attention to the full totality of symptoms) with Nux vomica, Pulsatilla, Carbo vegetabilis, or nosodes. The expectation is that the true constitutional prescription will later become clear. This is a confusion. Remedies can indeed "clear" a case if it is "one-sided," but only the most precisely chosen prescription will effect such a change. It takes considerable skill and thought to find such a remedy; it certainly cannot be done reliably by just a few minutes of routine prescribing. More likely, a routine prescription will further confuse the case, leading to even more difficulties later on.

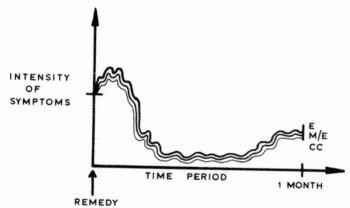

Figure 24:

CASE IX:

Patient: "I was much better, but now I'm worse again."

Case: Good amelioration following an aggravation, then a bit worse but still definitely better than before the remedy.

Interpretation: Patient became dis-

couraged after initial euphoria. Correct remedy. Good prognosis.

Prescription: Must wait. Another prescription at this point would probably cause a full relapse and disruption of the case.

CASE IX:

Now, let us return to a case in which true improvement has occurred. The patient reports a definite improvement for 20-25 days, but then a decline which the patient fears is the beginning of a relapse. In such cases, the homeopath must very carefully determine whether the patient is truly suffering as much as originally. It may be that even the suffering of the recent days is not nearly as bad as originally. It may also be discovered upon questioning that there was a definite aggravation preceding the amelioration.

In such a circumstance, it is quite likely that the patient has become overly elated from the dramatic relief, and now that he experiences some minor symptoms is afraid of a relapse. This psychology is analogous to that of a prisoner let out of prison, in whom there is an initial feeling of great liberation, a euphoria at being released from the burden of suffering; then, the realities of life faced by most of us are encountered. Some of the normal complaints due to everyday stresses begin to creep back, and the patient reacts in fear that the euphoric condition will not last. Discouragement sets in, and during the follow-up interview the patient is intent upon communicating the fear of relapse in order to convince the prescriber to give a "stronger" medicine.

In such a case, when the patient is still truly better, even though discouraged and fearful of relapse the homeopath must be very careful not to give another remedy. This is probably the most common mistake made by beginning prescribers. The interpretation is made that a higher potency is needed, or that another remedy must be given because of the "brevity" of the response. It is mistakenly concluded that the medicine has "worn off." This is a serious mistake because even a repetition of the same remedy in the same potency can disorder the action of the first remedy. Such disorder is later responded to by another remedy, and the process continues until the patient *truly* relapses back to the original state—but this time with symptomatology which perhaps no longer reveals a clear image.

This particular circumstance demonstrates most effectively of all the cases the need for caution and even suspicion on the part of the homeopath. The patient's descriptions must not be merely taken at face value. Otherwise, even a curative response may be missed because of the patient's desire to get the homeopath to respond. The pressures to prescribe another dose will be very great, but they must be resisted at all costs if the overall status of the patient is noticeably improved, even though the earlier amelioration was even more dramatic. Most likely, the seeming "relapse" will turn out to be merely a random fluctuation which, if left alone, will later show itself to be—*on the average*—progress toward cure.

306

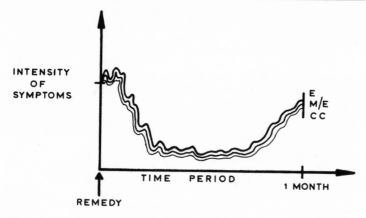

Figure 25:

CASE X:

Patient: "I was better, but now worse."

Case: Good amelioration following aggravation, then return to full relapse. Same remedy image.

Interpretation: Correct remedy but short effect. 1) May have been too low potency. 2) Remedy may have been antidoted.

Prescription: Re-take case to be *certain* the same remedy is indicated. If indeed it is the same remedy, give a higher potency, as long as there is no evidence of an antidote. If the remedy was definitely antidoted (by drugs, coffee, etc.), give the same potency.

CASE X:

Another patient may report an amelioration (following an initial aggravation) which is followed by relapse. In this instance, the homeopath discovers the relapse to be fully back to the original state in every respect. After careful questioning, the homeopath decides that the relapse is indeed complete, even though the initial response seemed highly curative.

There are two possible interpretations in such a situation. The obvious one is that the remedy was the precise *simillimum* but was somehow antidoted. The patient must be carefully questioned about all factors which

might have interfered with the medicine, even those factors which are relatively rare (discussed in Chapter 19). If the remedy *has* been antidoted, then a truly delicate decision must be made. In case the relapse presents exactly the same symptom picture, repeat the same remedy and the same potency. Sometimes you will find that during the relapse of the main complaint a different overall picture is emerging. In such case, a different remedy would be required. Therefore, the case must be carefully re-taken in order to determine which remedy to give.

Another possibility is that the original remedy was the *simillimum* but that the potency was too low. The remedy acted curatively, but it did not hold. In such a circumstance (which is quite unusual), the case must be carefully re-taken to be certain that the same remedy is still indicated; if so, a higher potency must be given.

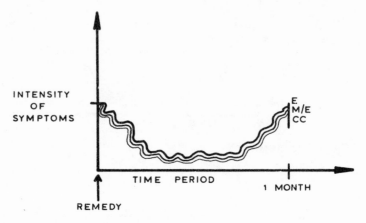

INTENSITY
OF
SYMPTOMS

TIME PERIOD

1 MONTH

REMEDY

Figure 26:

CASE XI:

Patient: "I was better, now the same as I was."

Case: Amelioration *without* aggravation, then return to full relapse.

Interpretation: Either 1) Partial remedy causing only a temporary, non-curative amelioration. Or 2) incurable case, especially if remedy image during relapse is changed.

Prescription: Interpretation 1) Look again at original case to find a better remedy. Interpretation 2) Find new remedy based on new image.

CASE XI:

As in Case X, the patient describes a definite amelioration, followed by a full relapse. However, this time careful questioning reveals that no aggravation occurred in the first few days. Of course, some patients may simply not clearly remember whether there was an aggravation, but this case applies primarily to those in whom there was definitely no aggravation, but an immediate amelioration, and finally a full relapse within one month.

Again, this example strongly underscores the importance of careful questioning during the follow-up visit. If the homeopath believes too readily the initial description of the patient, it is likely that the same remedy would be repeated. In this example, the seemingly unimportant inquiry into the presence or absence of an initial aggravation can make all the difference in proper interpretation.

Once it is definitely determined that there was no initial aggravation, there are two possible interpretations. On the one hand, the remedy may have been close, but only partial in its action. The response may have been merely temporary, noncurative, palliative—a "glancing" effect. (In such cases, however, an important clue is found in the fact that we never witness a *true* elevation of the energy level of the patient.) Considering this possibility, the homeopath must take a careful look at the original case to see if a more precise remedy might have been missed. If so, then the more precise remedy should be given at this point.

Another interpretation, however, is that this is an *incurable* case. This interpretation would apply most clearly to those cases with severe pathology. Another clue is elicited by re-taking the complete case. If the amelioration has occurred without an aggravation, is followed by a full relapse, and then the re-taken case reveals *a new image*, it is probable that the case is incurable. Let us take an example to make this clear. Suppose an elderly patient comes into the office complaining of cancer which involves several abdominal organs. The case is studied carefully, and Natrum sulphuricum 30 is given. On follow-up, the patient describes a dramatic "miraculous" amelioration of pains, but then after 10-15 days of amelioration returns fully to the original state. Careful inquiry is made into the first few days following the remedy, and the patient confirms that there was no aggravation. This is quite clear because the patient told all her friends about the "miracle" that seemed to have occurred immediately after taking the remedy. Next, the entire case is re-taken, and Natrum muriaticum is clearly indicated (less warmblooded, a strong craving for salt whereas before there was none, and a noticeable tendency toward claustrophobia has developed). This is an incurable case. The best that can be hoped for is palliation.

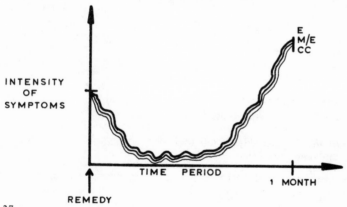

Figure 27:

CASE XII:

Patient: "I was better, but now even worse than I was before."

Case: Amelioration *without* aggravation, then worse than before remedy.

Interpretation: Incurable case. New image will be present.

Prescription: Give new remedy. Goal is palliation.

CASE XII:

This situation is identical to Case XI except that at the end of a month the patient feels *worse* than before taking the remedy. This definitely represents an "incurable" case, and it is very likely that a new image will be present. Incurable cases frequently experience responses after remedies, but the image continually shifts to new states.

It is fortunate that such cases do experience alleviation of symptoms for at least brief periods of time because palliation is thereby made possible. The prescriber must give a new remedy with each relapse. In this way, the patient can be successfully palliated without having to resort to allopathic drugs.

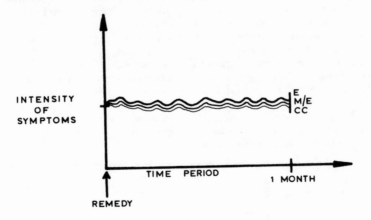

Figure 28:

CASE XIII:

Patient: "I am the same."

Case: "Open" patient. Indeed, no change.

Interpretation: 1) Remedy far off the mark. 2) Potency far from optimum potency. 3) Remedy has been spoiled prior to administration.

Prescription: Re-take the case and give the appropriate remedy.

CASE XIII:

Suppose a patient returns and reports absolutely no change. This impression is not accepted at face value, but further questioning nevertheless seems to bear it out. Further, suppose the patient is an "open" type person who would like very much to report some degree of change in order to please the prescriber.

There are three interpretations which might apply to this situation. First, and most likely, the remedy was far removed from the true *simillimum*. The procedure in this instance, of course, is to thoroughly re-take the case and study harder to find the true remedy.

Secondly, it may be that the correct

remedy was chosen, but the potency may have been far off the mark. Perhaps the case ideally required a 10M but was only given a 12×. This is a highly unlikely possibility, since a precise remedy will show some action at virtually *any* potency, but it is a consideration.

Finally, it must always be remembered that the remedy itself might have become inactivated in some manner. This consideration would be particularly likely if the homeopath were quite experienced and able to be very certain that the remedy image is clearly correct. In such a situation, it is reasonable to suspect the remedy itself; a repeat dose could then be given from the supply of a trusted homeopathic pharmacy. Of course, beginning prescribers in their relative ignorance consider this interpretation quite often. By far, however, the most likely interpretation is the first one listed—that the original remedy was far from the mark.

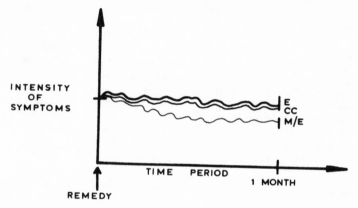

Figure 29:

CASE XIV:

Patient: "I am the same."

Case: "Closed" patient. Admits, "Well, I am less irritable with my husband, but then he has been nicer to me lately."

Interpretation: Remedy may be beginning to act, especially when a "closed" patient admits a change on an important level.

Prescription: Must wait.

CASE XIV:

Intellectualized, "closed" patients—people who tend to repress emotional expression—can present great difficulties for interpretation. Such people tend to intellectually "explain away" everything, so responses which are truly actions of the remedy are not reported because the patient attributes them to other influences. In addition, "closed" patients are generally unimpressed by any changes short of the dramatic. They are hard to convince, and therefore they tend to withhold some of the seemingly unimportant clues which signify movement toward cure.

The best way to illustrate this is by a case from my own experience. A

311

woman had been suffering severely from an extensive neurodermatitis for over 7 years. She was a "closed" patient, and the initial history was difficult to obtain. During the one-month follow-up visit, she reported no change at all. During careful questioning, she reluctantly admitted, "Well, I *am* less irritable with my husband, but then he has been nicer to me lately." This was the only change noted, but it was significant because it was an emotional symptom. In a "closed" patient, such symptoms are not easily given, so they carry more weight when they are expressed. For this reason, no further remedy was given. At the two-month follow-up visit, the patient still had noticed no change, but further questioning showed that the irritability continued to be even less. So, again no remedy was prescribed. Then, at about 2½ months after the first remedy, improvement in the skin began to occur, and by the three-month visit, the patient felt perfectly well in every respect, and the cure has lasted now for many years.

This case illustrates the extreme care required in evaluating the response to the remedy. The tendency to ignore the reduced irritability because it seemed easily explainable by other influences could have led to a disruptive second prescription in this patient. Especially after two months had passed with no "apparent improvement" according to the estimation of the patient, the temptation became very great to prescribe another dose. However, if the original remedy were to have been repeated, or a new remedy given, at either the one-month or two-month visits, it is very likely that ultimate cure would have been prevented. In such a serious case, any disruption can lead to enough disorder that it may become impossible to ever resume progress toward cure. This is why it is so very important to wait whenever there is improvement in any of the three major categories of symptoms—the mental/emotional symptoms, the energy, or the physical chief complaint.

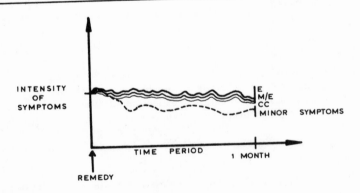

Figure 30:

CASE XV:

Patient: "I am the same."
Case: "Closed" patient. Finally admits improvement in a minor symptom only.

Interpretation: Uncertain effect. 1) May be early change from correct remedy. 2) May be only partial remedy. 3) May be merely random fluctuation after remedy far off the mark. Fluctuation may return to original state within a few weeks.

Prescription: Wait, for another month or so. Later, if there is no further improvement, seek a better remedy.

CASE XV:

A similar circumstance to Case XIV occurs when a "closed" patient reports no change whatsoever, and the only noticeable improvement found upon further questioning involves a minor symptom. For example, suppose there is no change in major symptoms, but a previously strong craving for salt has disappeared, or the patient no longer sticks feet out from under the covers at night.

Such a situation is difficult to interpret.

A) This minor change may be heralding the action of a precise remedy, and it should not be simply ignored in a "closed" patient who admits changes only reluctantly.

B) It may be that the change has occurred because the remedy is merely partial. It may be having only a "glancing" effect which is not reaching deeply enough into the organism and is not likely to last.

C) The third possibility is that the remedy was actually far from the mark, and the symptom change is merely an accidental fluctuation in the state of the patient.

If the remedy was precise, then more definite improvement will follow by the second month if nothing is done to disturb its action. If, however, the remedy was only partial or the symptom change is just a random fluctuation, then more time will reveal a return to the original state. The craving for salt will return, or the patient will again stick his feet out.

Therefore, the only course of action in such a case is to await further developments. Again, this case illustrates how important it is to go over every symptom in great detail. If the minor change is not noticed because of inadequate follow-up, the interpretation would be that the remedy was far from the *simillimum* and a new remedy should be given. This would be a mistake if the original medicine was in reality correct.

313

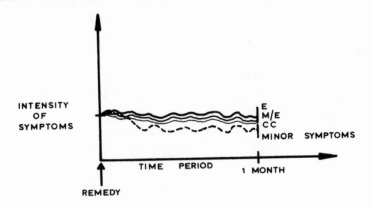

Figure 31:

CASE XVI:

Patient: "I am the same, but some symptoms have improved."

Case: "Open" patient. Wants to say he is better, but admits true improvement only in a few minor ways.

Interpretation: Remedy far from the *simillimum.*

Prescription: Re-take case and give another remedy.

CASE XVI:

This case is identical to Case XV except that here we are dealing with an "open" patient—a person who very much wants to offer some sign that he or she is better, or even to please the prescriber who has worked so hard on the case. In this instance, the seeming improvement is likely to be only apparent. An "open" patient would readily admit any improvement in *major* symptoms if actually present, so the fact that such a patient is able to report improvement of only a minor symptom is unimportant.

In this case, the minor improvement must be ignored. The case should be carefully re-taken and a new remedy prescribed.

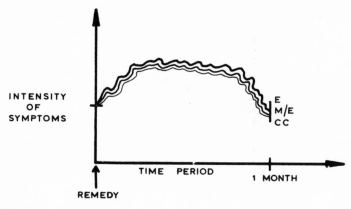

Figure 32:

CASE XVII:

Patient: "I have been worse."

Case: All symptoms worse, but better within past week.

Interpretation: Correct remedy.
Prescription: Wait.

CASE XVII:

Now we begin to evaluate prolonged aggravations. The first situation is one in which the patient reports having felt worse since taking the remedy. Upon questioning, however, it becomes clear that there has actually been improvement within the past 3-4 days to a week. At the moment of consultation, the patient is experiencing a definite improvement.

Generally, patients in this situation tend to ignore the recent improvement. They are patients with quite deep pathology who have been suffering a lot and are rather discouraged, and they want to convince the prescriber to do something more drastic to help them.

This pattern of change means that the remedy was the *simillimum* and that the patient can be expected to continue toward cure. The prognosis is quite good. Hence, the prescription must be to wait.

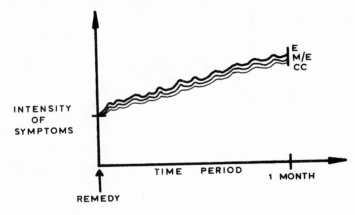

Figure 33:

CASE XVIII:

Patient: "I am much worse in every respect."

Case: Steady worsening of all symptoms.

Interpretation: 1) Allopathic drug discontinued, and remedy not close enough. 2) Remedy far off, had no effect, and disease getting out of control.

Prescription: Must find correct remedy. 1) If seems to be same remedy, must find even more confirmatory symptoms in order to safely repeat it, in which case a higher potency should be given. 2) If aggravation not serious, wait a few weeks for image to become more clear. 3) If becomes serious, *must be given the best possible remedy without delay.* 4) May have to find a remedy to merely palliate most serious symptoms.

CASE XVIII:

The least desirable circumstance for both patient and homeopath is a progressive worsening of symptoms after taking the remedy. All three major categories of symptoms become steadily worse, so that by the time of the follow-up visit, the situation is reaching a crisis point.

This situation occurs most commonly in patients who had been taking allopathic drugs and stopped them prior to taking the remedy; meanwhile, the homeopathic remedy was not correct. There is a natural aggravation which occurs upon discontinuation of many allopathic drugs anyway, but usually the administration of the correct remedy will alleviate this "rebound" aggravation. Thus the original prescription was not close enough to produce a curative effect.

If the patient had not been taking allopathic drugs prior to the remedy, then the only interpretation left is that the remedy was quite far removed from the exact *simillimum* and that the disease is following its natural course of deterioration.

The decision about the next course of action depends upon many factors:

316

the severity of the pathological condition, the type of case, the exact symptoms which are being aggravated, and how clear the image of the remedy seems to be. If the situation is becoming serious, then the best possible remedy must be immediately prescribed. In serious cases, it may even be necessary to enter with another remedy within a few days or a week, without waiting for the normal one-month follow-up visit. If by chance, the remedy image during the aggravation appears to be identical to the original prescription, then a higher potency must be given.

If the situation is clearly not serious and the remedy image is not yet clear, then the policy should be to wait until a clear image does emerge. (The reader will naturally understand the depth of knowledge a homeopath must have in order to be able to judge that a symptom-picture of a patient presents a clear, or as yet unclear, image of a remedy). It is not uncommon in such an aggravated case for a few symptoms to provide clues to what the next remedy will be, but one must wait as long as possible until the full image becomes clear. Of course, if the condition is deteriorating too rapidly, then one cannot wait, and must immediately give a remedy based upon the best possible image in the moment; but whenever possible it is better to allow the defense mechanism to provide a clear image. In such dramatic instances, in which the defense mechanism has been violently activated by the disease, it is probable that one will witness the emergence of a clear-cut picture of a remedy quite soon, in which case it will not be necessary to wait longer than perhaps two or three days before the clear image can be discerned.

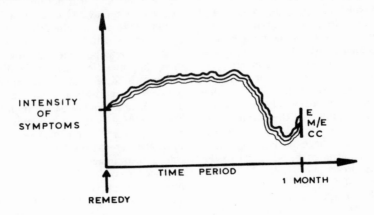

Figure 34:

CASE XIX:

Patient: "I have been worse, except for a brief time."

Case: Definite long aggravation, then better for 4 or 5 days, finally becoming worse again.

Interpretation: Nearly incurable case. Severe pathology. Poor prognosis. Pre-scriptions must be made very carefully.

Prescription: 1) Search for new remedy of the relapsed state. 2) If same image, repeat same remedy in higher potency. 3) If remedy image unclear, wait about 15 days for a new image.

CASE XIX:

Another adverse situation has occurred when the patient reports a strong, prolonged, and progressive aggravation followed by a distinct amelioration for only a short time (say, 4 or 5 days), and then becoming worse again.

The situation is *next to* incurable. There may be severe pathological changes such as cancer, deep psychosis, etc. The prognosis is poor, but some hope can be derived from the fact that even a brief amelioration has occurred. In other words, the defense mechanism is very weak, but not yet so weak that the case is incurable.

Prescribing in such cases is a very delicate matter. Virtually every prescription must be exactly correct if there is to be hope for a cure. Mistakes can very easily disorder such weakened defense mechanisms beyond hope of recovery.

The case must be taken in its relapsed state with great care. If a remedy is quite clear at that point, then it should certainly be given. More usually, however, the remedy will not yet be clear, and the homeopath must then wait for another 15 days or so in order to be sure about the next prescription. As mentioned before, these nearly incurable cases tend to change remedy images very frequently, so it is unlikely that the original remedy would again be indicated; if this does happen, however, then it should be given in a higher potency.

318

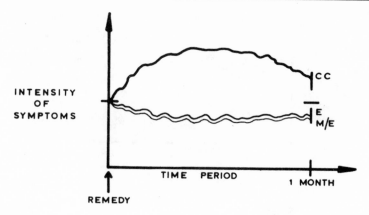

Figure 35:

CASE XX:

Patient: "I have been worse during the whole month."

Case: Chief complaint worse, but energy and mental/emotional states somewhat better.

Interpretation: 1) Probably local symptom previously suppressed by allopathic drugs. 2) Remedy is correct.

Prescription: Wait.

CASE XX:

It is not unusual to see a case in which the chief complaint has been aggravated during the whole of the month. Meanwhile, the energy level and mental/emotional states exhibit a slight degree of improvement. The patient, of course, reports feeling worse in general because, after all, how can the mental and emotional state be better when the physical suffering has been so intense? Nevertheless, careful questioning about every symptom will reveal no aggravation of the energy or mental/emotional states.

This situation is encountered most often in patients who have been using allopathic drugs to suppress a specific physical problem. Perhaps the patient has been using occasional applications of topical cortisone to control a skin eruption on the hands. The patient believes that the amount of cortisone being used is insignificant because it is "needed" only twice a week on an average; even so, the important point is not the dosage but the fact that the applications were enough to keep the symptom suppressed. Such cases frequently have a prolonged aggravation of the local symptom after discontinuing the cortisone and taking the correct remedy.

Therefore, the interpretation is that the remedy was the *simillimum*, and it is important to wait.

319

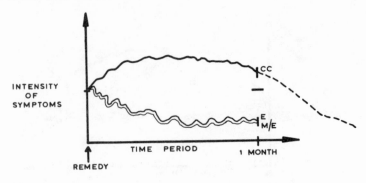

INTENSITY
OF
SYMPTOMS

TIME PERIOD

1 MONTH

REMEDY

Figure 36:

CASE XXI:

Patient: "I have been worse during the whole month."

Case: Chief complaint worse, the whole month. Others definitely better.

Interpretation: Correct remedy. Good prognosis.

Prescription: Wait.

CASE XXI:

This is very similar to Case XX, but here there is a very definite amelioration on the energy and mental/emotional levels. Even at the end of the month the patient reports that the physical chief complaint is also somewhat better than prior to taking the remedy.

This is a curative response, and the correct remedy was given. It is very desirable for an eruption to occur on the skin, or for a discharge to be produced from skin or mucous membranes, during a noticeable amelioration of symptoms from deeper levels of the organism. Such a response is definitely curative, and under no circumstances should the local symptom be allowed to be suppressed by any means. Such suppression would stop the cure and cause a further degeneration of the general health of the patient.

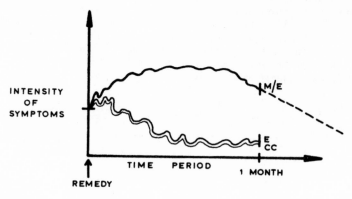

INTENSITY
OF
SYMPTOMS

M/E

E
CC

TIME   PERIOD   1 MONTH

REMEDY

Figure 37:

CASE XXII:

Patient: "I have been worse all month."

Case: Mental/emotional level worse, others better following aggravation.

Interpretation: Prolonged mental aggravation.

Prescription: Wait.

CASE XXII:

Some cases, especially those which originally are focused on the mental or emotional planes, will show a prolonged aggravation of mental or emotional symptoms while other minor symptoms are found to be improving and one or two symptoms, pathognomonic to the remedy prescribed, are showing up. At the end of a month, the mental/emotional state may still be worse than it was prior to taking the remedy, but the homeopath must not be misled into prescribing another remedy. From experience, it seems that deep mental or emotional cases tend to have aggravations which can last up to two months, but then a curative response follows if the action of the remedy is not interfered.

These cases, and others showing prolonged aggravations, can be very trying on both the patient and the ho-

meopath. The patient feels convinced that nothing beneficial is occurring, and indeed may believe that the disease is actually worse. The patient naturally, then, tries to convince the homeopath that "something *must* be done." This is an understandable feeling, but if the homeopath determines that the changes are following the laws of cure, he or she must have the courage to refuse to give a new remedy. Much support and reassurance must be given to the patient, but always the homeopath must appeal to the higher intelligence of the patient to continue to conform to the laws of healing. A curative response, especially when it necessitates a prolonged aggravation of symptoms, can be viewed as a kind of spiritual test which must be successfully passed for eventual cure to occur. The homeopath does not per-

321

form a service to the patient if a new remedy is administered out of false compassion at an incorrect moment.

Perhaps the most eloquent statement describing the pressures placed upon a homeopathic prescriber by a patient under aggravation is given by J.T. Kent: *"Sometimes the physician will be driven to his wit's end in dealing with these reactions. It.is sometimes a dreadful thing to look upon, and the physician may be turned out of doors. Let him meet it as a man; let him be patient with it, because the ignorance of the mother or the friends can be no excuse for his violation of principle, even once."*

Index

abdomen, 197-98.
  See also specific organs
absentmindedness. *See* Memory problems
accidents, 43
acne, 19.
  See also Skin ailments and eruptions
acquisitiveness, 28-29, 41, 42
acupuncture, 54, 67-68, 84, 90, 98, 265
acute illness, 187-89.
  See also specific illnesses
adrenal glands, 35
adrenocortex, 22
adrenocortical effect, 22
aerosol sprays, 12
Agaricus, 130
age, 43, 169
aggravation, 228, 230
ailments, 24-26.
  See also Disease
alcohol, 28, 102, 133, 163, 265
Allen, *Encyclopedia of Pure Materia Medica*, 155, 233, 244
allergies, 52, 186
  bronchial asthma, 6, 12, 18, 36-37, 52-53, 80, 129, 130, 135, 213
  eczema, 19, 36-37, 52-53, 124, 215
  hay fever, 116, 150, 185
  rhinitis, 18, 52, 53
allopathy, allopathic medicine, 6-7, 10, 12, 27
  damaging effect of, 10, 11, 81, 82, 110-11, 117
  fragmentation of, 19-20, 36-37, 38-39.
  See also Case-taking (homeopathic medicine); specific ailments and medicines
alternative therapies, 4, 38, 84, 270
  artificial, 37
  dynamic, 40, 78-79, 87
  electric, 76, 82
  herbal, 265
  insulin, 82
  natural, 37
  polarity massage, 265
  resonance, 114, 128, 146
  suppressive, 32, 109, 117, 130, 267-68.
  See also Case-taking (homeopathic medicine); specific ailments and medicines

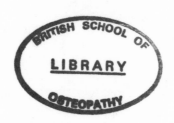

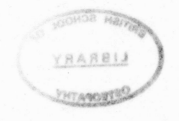

Selected Grove Press Paperbacks

62480-7   ACKER, KATHY / Great Expectations: A Novel / $6.95

17458-5   ALLEN, DONALD & BUTTERICK, GEORGE F., eds. / The Postmoderns: The New American Poetry Revised / $9.95

17397-X   ANONYMOUS / My Secret Life / $4.95

62433-5   BARASH, D. and LIPTON, J. / Stop Nuclear War! A Handbook / $7.95

17087-3   BARNES, JOHN / Evita—First Lady: A Biography of Eva Peron / $4.95

17208-6   BECKETT, SAMUEL / Endgame / $2.95

17299-X   BECKETT, SAMUEL / Three Novels: Molloy, Malone Dies and The Unnamable / $4.95

17204-3   BECKETT, SAMUEL / Waiting for Godot / $3.50

62064-X   BECKETT, SAMUEL / Worstward Ho / $5.95

17244-2   BORGES, JORGE LUIS / Ficciones / $6.95

17112-8   BRECHT, BERTOLT / Galileo / $2.95

17106-3   BRECHT, BERTOLT / Mother Courage and Her Children / $2.45

17393-7   BRETON, ANDRE / Nadja / $5.95

17439-9   BULGAKOV, MIKHAIL / The Master and Margarita / $4.95

17108-X   BURROUGHS, WILLIAM S. / Naked Lunch / $3.95

17749-5   BURROUGHS, WILLIAM S. / The Soft Machine, Nova Express, The Wild Boys: Three Novels / $5.95

62488-2   CLARK, AL, ed. / The Film Year Book 1984 / $12.95

17535-2   COWARD, NOEL / Three Plays (Private Lives, Hay Fever, Blithe Spirit) / $4.50

17219-1   CUMMINGS, E. E. / 100 Selected Poems / $2.95

17327-9   FANON, FRANZ / The Wretched of the Earth / $4.95

17483-6   FROMM, ERICH / The Forgotten Language / $6.95

17390-2   GENET, JEAN / The Maids and Deathwatch: Two Plays / $5.95

17838-6   GENET, JEAN / Querelle / $4.95

17662-6   GERVASI, TOM / Arsenal of Democracy II / $12.95

17956-0   GETTLEMAN, MARVIN, et. al. eds. / El Salvador: Central America in the New Cold War / $9.95

17648-0   GIRODIAS, MAURICE, ed. / The Olympia Reader / $5.95

62490-4   GUITAR PLAYER MAGAZINE / The Guitar Player Book (Revised and Updated Edition) / $11.95

62003-8   HITLER, ADOLF / Hitler's Secret Book / $7.95

17125-X   HOCHHUTH, ROLF / The Deputy / $4.95

62115-8   HOLMES, BURTON / The Olympian Games in Athens, 1896 / $6.95

17209-4 IONESCO, EUGENE / Four Plays (The Bald Soprano, The Lesson, The Chairs, and Jack or The Submission) / $4.95

17226-4 IONESCO, EUGENE / Rhinoceros / $4.95

62123-9 JOHNSON, CHARLES / Oxherding Tale / $6.95

17254-X KEENE, DONALD, ed. / Modern Japanese Literature / $12.50

17952-8 KEROUAC, JACK / The Subterraneans / $3.50

62424-6 LAWRENCE, D. H. / Lady Chatterley's Lover / $3.95

17016-4 MAMET, DAVID / American Buffalo / $4.95

17760-6 MILLER, HENRY / Tropic of Cancer / $4.95

17295-7 MILLER, HENRY / Tropic of Capricorn / $3.95

17869-6 NERUDA, PABLO / Five Decades: Poems 1925-1970. Bilingual ed. / $8.95

17092-X ODETS, CLIFFORD / Six Plays (Waiting for Lefty, Awake and Sing, Golden Boy, Rocket to the Moon, Till the Day I Die, Paradise Lost) / $7.95

17650-2 OE, KENZABURO / A Personal Matter / $6.95

17232-9 PINTER, HAROLD / The Birthday Party & The Room / $6.95

17251-5 PINTER, HAROLD / The Homecoming / $4.95

17539-5 POMERANCE, BERNARD / The Elephant Man / $4.25

17827-0 RAHULA, WALPOLA / What the Buddha Taught / $6.95

17658-8 REAGE, PAULINE / Story of O, Part II; Return to the Chateau / $3.95

62169-7 RECHY, JOHN / City of Night / $5.95

62001-1 ROSSET, BARNEY and JORDAN, FRED, eds. / Evergreen Review No. 98 / $5.95

62498-X ROSSET, PETER and VANDERMEER, JOHN / The Nicaragua Reader / $8.95

17119-5 SADE, MARQUIS DE / The 120 Days of Sodom and Other Writings / $12.50

62009-7 SEGALL, J. PETER / Deduct This Book: How Not to Pay Taxes While Ronald Reagan is President / $6.95

17467-4 SELBY, HUBERT / Last Exit to Brooklyn / $2.95

17948-X SHAWN, WALLACE, and GREGORY, ANDRÉ / My Dinner with André / $5.95

17797-5 SNOW, EDGAR / Red Star Over China / $8.95

17260-4 STOPPARD, TOM / Rosencrantz and Guildenstern Are Dead / $3.95

17474-7 SUZUKI, D. T. / Introduction to Zen Buddhism / $2.95

17599-9 THELWELL, MICHAEL / The Harder They Come: A Novel about Jamaica / $7.95

17969-2 TOOLE, JOHN KENNEDY / A Confederacy of Dunces / $3.95

17418-6 WATTS, ALAN W. / The Spirit of Zen / $3.95

GROVE PRESS, INC., 196 West Houston St., New York, N.Y. 10014